A Diagnostic Guide to Clinical Gastroenterology

CW01507074

Edited by

D. Kumar, Consultant General and Colorectal Surgeon, St George s Hospital Medical School, London, UK

J. Christensen, Professor, Division of Gastroenterology and Hepatology, Department of Internal Medicine, University of Iowa College of Medicine, Iowa City, Iowa, USA

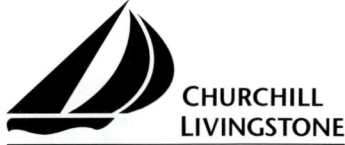

CHURCHILL
LIVINGSTONE

NEW YORK EDINBURGH LONDON MADRID MELBOURNE SAN FRANCISCO AND TOKYO 1996

CHURCHILL LIVINGSTONE
Medical Division of Pearson Professional Limited

Distributed in the United States of America by Churchill Livingstone Inc., 650 Avenue of the Americas, New York, N.Y. 10011, and by associated companies, branches and representatives throughout the world.

© Pearson Professional Limited 1996

First published 1996, reprinted 1997

British Library Cataloguing in Publication Data
A catalogue record for this book is available from the British Library.

Library of Congress Cataloging in Publication Data
A catalog record for this book is available from the Library of Congress.

Medical knowledge is constantly changing. As new information becomes available, changes in treatment, procedures, equipment and the use of drugs become necessary. The editors/authors/contributors and the publishers have, as far as it is possible, taken care to ensure that the information given in this text is accurate and up to date. However, readers are strongly advised to confirm that the information, especially with regard to drug usage, complies with latest legislation and standards of practice.

The
publisher's
policy is to use
**paper manufactured
from sustainable forests**

Printed in Hong Kong

A Diagnostic Guide to Clinical Gastroenterology

For Churchill Livingstone

Commissioning Editor: Sheila Khullar
Project Editor: Antonia Seymour
Project Controller: Sarah Lowe
Cover Design: Andrew Jones
Indexer: Nina Boyd

Contents

SECTION 2   Objective assessment of common clinical symptoms

Contributors

M. J. Benson Senior Registrar in Gastroenterology, St George's Hospital, London, UK

C. K. Burnett Functional Gastrointestinal Disorders Center, University of North Carolina, Chapel Hill, North Carolina, USA

J. Christensen Professor, Division of Gastroenterology and Hepatology, Department of Internal Medicine, University of Iowa College of Medicine, Iowa City, Iowa, USA

J. L. Conklin Associate Professor, Division of Gastroenterology and Hepatology, Department of Internal Medicine, University of Iowa College of Medicine, Iowa City, Iowa, USA

E. Elias Consultant Gastroenterologist, Liver Unit, Queen Elizabeth Hospital, Edgbaston, Birmingham, UK

D. F. Evans Gastrointestinal Science Research Unit, St Bartholomew's & The Royal London School of Medicine and Dentistry, Queen Mary and Westfield College, London, UK

A. M. Gudgeon Derbyshire Royal Infirmary, London Road, Derby, UK

R. Hutchinson Queen Elizabeth Hospital, Edgbaston, Birmingham, UK

D. B. Jones Washington University of Medicine, Saint Louis, Missouri, USA

D. Kumar Consultant Surgeon/ Senior Lecturer, Department of Surgery, Colorectal Surgery Unit, St George's Hospital Medical School, London, UK

R. J. Leicester Consultant Colorectal Surgeon, St George's Hospital, Blackshaw Road, London, UK

A. Mendoza Research Fellow, Liver Unit, Queen Elizabeth Hospital, Birmingham, UK

F. A. Mitros Professor, Department of Pathology, University of Iowa, University Hospital, Iowa, USA

S. Morgan Associate Professor of Nutrition Sciences and Medicine, University of Alabama at Birmingham, Birmingham, Alabama, USA

J. A. Murray Assistant Professor, Division of Gastroenterology and Hepatology, Department of Internal Medicine, University of Iowa College of Medicine, Iowa City, Iowa, USA

J. F. C. Olliff Consultant Radiologist, Queen Elizabeth Hospital, Edgbaston, Birmingham, UK

S. S. C. Rao Assistant Professor, Division of Gastroenterology and Hepatology, Department of Internal Medicine, University of Iowa College of Medicine, Iowa City, Iowa, USA

N. Soper MD Associate Professor of Surgery, Washington University of Medicine, Saint Louis, Missouri, USA

R. W. Summers Professor, Division of Gastroenterology and Hepatology, Department of Internal Medicine, University of Iowa College of Medicine, Iowa City, Iowa, USA

W. E. Whitehead Division of Digestive Diseases, University of North Carolina, Chapel Hill, North Carolina, USA

D. L. Wingate Gastrointestinal Science Research Unit, St Bartholomew's & the Royal London School of Medicine and Dentistry, Queen Mary and Westfield College, London, UK

Preface

The sub-speciality of gastroenterology has made significant advances over the last few decades. Our understanding of the pathophysiology of various disorders of the gastrointestinal tract has also improved. New approaches have been added to the already existing diagnostic tests. These developments have widened the diagnostic workup of common gastrointestinal complaints. This book aims to bring together the current knowledge to provide a clinically useful text. Its aproach emphasises the practicality and the useful application of all types of test now used in diagnosis in gastroenterology. The tests to be discussed include classical history-taking and physical examination in addition to modern laboratory procedures. The book is intended as a practical guide to the diagnostic approach in gastroenterology in the modern era.

The first section is devoted to the test procedures themselves. The usefulness, the indications for and the shortcomings of the tests in addition to brief summaries of the methods have been provided.

The second section deals with the application of the tests. The common presenting complaints are treated here as problems susceptible to analysis via the various tests discussed in the first section. The emphasis is on differential diagnosis and a rational analysis of the symptom-complex to lead the reader through various steps to a final diagnosis.

It is hoped that this book will provide a practical and clinical guide to medical and surgical gastroenterologists, trainees and medical practitioners in allied specialities.

Devinder Kumar   **James Christensen**
London   Iowa City

Available tests

Clinical history and examination
J. Christensen

INTRODUCTION

The information gained from interviewing and examining patients guides all subsequent aspects of the physician–patient interaction. The completeness and accuracy of the clinical history and examination determine both the efficiency of diagnosis and the success of treatment. The interview is the beginning of diagnosis and the end as well, for the diagnosis reached must explain fully all the features of the illness discovered in the clinical interview.

The assessment of complaints and physical abnormalities, sometimes called the 'art of medicine', is not an art but, like a science, a body of knowledge susceptible to organization, analysis and evaluation. This knowledge comes to us more through oral tradition than from archives or texts. Its importance varies among the various specialties of medicine but gastroenterologists especially rely upon this science.

This chapter organizes the elements of the clinical history and examination in gastroenterology – the 'bedside logic' of gastroenterology. The assertions made reflect the general experience, but almost nothing said here has been subjected to systematic testing. Our modern interpretations of symptoms and physical abnormalities rest on the observations of generations of perceptive gastroenterologists and surgeons.

GENERAL APPROACH TO THE HISTORY

The clinical interview is simply a conversation. As such, it works best when the discourse is friendly, when it has a focus or direction and when the participants respect and trust one another. But a clinical interview rarely starts out easily. The physician wants information but haste and distractions may impede him. The patient wants help and understanding but fear and guilt may get in his way.

Some simple arrangements can facilitate the beginning of the interview. The physician and the patient must seat themselves in the positions that are usual for persons who are conversing seriously. This means that both must be seated with their heads at about the same level. When one conversant's head is much higher than the other's, the difference implies a dominance which can prevent easy discourse. The two conversants should face each other obliquely, not directly, face-to-face. The latter position is usual in confrontational and intimate conversations. A slight obliquity in position encourages the relaxed exchange of information. Conversations rarely go easily over barriers like tables or desks but work better when the conversants are separated only by empty space, about 3 to 6 feet.

The physician must lead the clinical interview, acting as the host and directing the conversation, if it is to accomplish its purpose. Several simple maneuvers taken at the outset establish this relationship. First, a neutral person (a nurse, clerk or receptionist) should bring the patient to the examining room so that the physician enters after the patient is seated. Second, a formal introduction and shaking of hands establishes the seriousness of the interview. Third, the question of the presence of third parties should be settled at once.

The clinical conversation is essentially one-to-one and it involves private matters. Thus, third parties should be excluded unless the patient, directly or indirectly, indicates that another person can be present. Relatives, spouses or close friends may help in adding or confirming elements of the history but they can also interfere. They are essential in cases where the subject is impaired or unreliable. The presence of strangers, even medical personnel such as nurses or medical students, sometimes seriously interferes with the clinical conversation. The physician who senses that the presence of others is impairing the interview should either exclude those persons immediately or arrange for a subsequent interview alone.

Some physicians avoid taking notes during the conversation, for it can interfere with the natural flow of the conversation to do so. Sometimes, however, especially in respect to remote events such as the past medical history or the history of family illnesses, one must take notes. At the end of the interview the account of the current symptoms can be written from memory and the notes can be used to reconstruct the rest of the account.

ELEMENTS OF THE CLINICAL INTERVIEW

A clinical interview falls quite naturally into three elements. The patient expounds the facts in the first stage, the physician explores them in the second and the two participants together review them in the third. It is useful to think of these as the opening, middle and end conversations.

The opening conversation normally starts with an open-ended question from the physician: 'How can I help you?' or 'What can I do for you?' or 'Tell me all about your problem'. In the case of a specific referral the physician should know the reason for the referral and the patient will know this. A wholly neutral and open-ended question in such a situation may make the patient believe that the physician is forgetful or distracted, so the opening question should make it clear that the physician knows the reason for the referral when he does.

Once the physician has indicated that the patient should begin to speak, most patients will launch into an account of the illness. This may be long and detailed or brief and incomplete. Patients often ramble. If this happens, the physician should interrupt, pick up the thread of the story and get the patient back on course, but then let the story proceed to the end.

The patient's account in the opening conversation almost never tells the physician all he needs to know. Usually, it only sketches the nature of the complaint with an incomplete chronology. The physician requires far more information than the opening conversation usually provides if he is to make a useful analysis of the story. Patients, however, cannot be expected to know all that the physician needs to know. They reveal only what seems important to them. The physician must find out what he needs to know in the subsequent middle conversation.

In the middle conversation, the physician explores the story of illness in such a way as to discover features of the illness that he must know about. This part takes the form of questions and answers. It is an interrogation. For that reason, the physician must emphasize his seriousness of purpose by maintaining good eye contact, by avoiding note taking and by not tolerating interruptions to the interview.

Here the physician begins to test hypotheses about the origin of the complaints. He asks specific questions designed to allow inferences as to the organ of origin of the symptoms or the nature of the pathologic process. He generates questions to test hypotheses as they develop.

Some patients, being eager to help, tend to respond to questions with the answers they infer the physician wants to hear. To avoid this source of error, the physician must not ask leading questions, questions formulated in such a way as to suggest a desired answer.

In the end conversation, the physician, having exhausted the questions that have occurred to him in the explorations of the middle conversation, undertakes a brief summary. In this, the physician repeats the account of the illness in detail as he has come to understand it. He gives the patient a chance to clarify, asking 'Have I missed anything?' or 'Is that correct?'. In the end conversation, the positions of the conversants are reversed. The physician speaks and the patient listens. For this reason, the patient is beginning to find out what the physician thinks. At this point, therefore, the perceptive physician may discover areas in which the patient has been less than forthcoming – fear of cancer, peculiar dietary practices, drug abuses, peculiar sexual practices and the like. Such sensitive areas may be explored quite naturally by the physician in the end conversation as he summarizes his understanding of the illness, when direct questions about them earlier might have seemed confrontational or threatening. At this point, also, the observant physician can look especially carefully for well-known signs of anger, embarrassment, fear or depression as he observes the patient responding to his revelation of his own thinking (Boxes 1.1–1.4).

Box 1.1 Some signs that mainly indicate anger or resentment

Clenching the jaws
Clenching the fists
Uncrossing the legs and sitting upright
Gripping the table or chair
Smoking or asking to smoke
Glancing angrily at a relative

Box 1.2 Some signs that mainly indicate embarrassment

Leaning back and crossing the legs and/or arms
Rubbing the palms of the hands together
Partially covering the jaw or mouth with the hand
Smoothing the hair
Breaking eye contact with you
Glancing fearfully at a relative

Box 1.3 Some signs that mainly indicate fear

Constant and intense eye contact
Sweating and/or pallor
Clutching or rubbing a piece of clothing, a handkerchief, a piece of tissue or a purse
Shifting the chair away from you
Inappropriate laughter, giggling or smiling
Abnormally rapid or deep breathing

Box 1.4 Some signs that mainly indicate depression

An expressionless face
Paucity of body movements
Avoidance of eye contact
A slumping posture
Difficulty in following the line of conversation
Poor grooming

SPECIFIC FEATURES OF GASTROINTESTINAL COMPLAINTS

Later chapters of this book deal with the assessment of specific common gastrointestinal complaints, including dysphagia, pyrosis, chest pain, dyspepsia, nausea, abdominal pain, bloating, gas, diarrhea, constipation, incontinence, anorectal pain and bleeding per rectum. The full analysis of these complaints requires the consideration of six general features, as follows: *character, location, chronology, aggravating factors, relieving factors* and *related symptoms*. Not all these factors are useful in the analysis of all complaints, but they are useful in all sensory complaints.

Patients rarely provide a full description of a pain or a sensation. The *character* of a sensation always proves most useful in the analysis. The physician must ask for specific descriptions in sensory complaints, asking 'What does it feel like?' or 'What words can you use to describe it?' or offering lay terms to allow patients to choose those that describe the sensation. Severity, a part of character, is an especially subjective matter. It can be judged by discovering the extent to which the complaint interferes with normal activities or it can be graded on a scale of 1 to 10.

When a patient indicates the *location* of a pain or sensation, he usually puts his whole hand to the area. If he is asked to use one finger to show the sites of origin and radiation of a pain, the information is usually useful.

A precise *chronology* always facilitates the interpretation of symptoms. Patients rarely volunteer this but the physician wants details: time of onset, nature of onset, rate of progression, duration, intervals of attacks and remissions and so on. Patients are usually fairly confident about the chronology of events of recent and sudden onset, but vague about the timing of complaints of remote or insidious onset. The physician can fruitfully use special events to explore chronology, such as seasonal changes in weather, holidays, historical or political events and birthdays.

Aggravating factors need exploration. Many of the principal complaints in gastroenterology are made worse by normal gastrointestinal events, such as eating and defecation. Others may be affected by such non-gastrointestinal functions as deep breathing, coughing, certain postures and physical activities. Knowledge of specific aggravating factors often goes far to explain the origin of complaints.

Relieving factors, like aggravating factors, require exploration. Many gastrointestinal complaints abate with normal gastrointestinal functions and with various self-treatments. Such information is not often volunteered. The physician must ask about all treatments that have been tried, both successfully and unsuccessfully.

The principal symptoms of gastrointestinal disease uncommonly occur alone, but patients may fail to notice or to describe *related symptoms*. Since they are valuable in the analysis of an illness, they must be asked about. One must be alert to both gastrointestinal and non-gastrointestinal symptoms. Also, gastrointestinal symptoms may reflect primary disease in other systems. For example, nausea and vomiting can reflect intra-cranial disease. The absence of related symptoms may be as important as their presence.

CLARITY IN COMMUNICATION

The two most common reasons patients give for their dissatisfaction with medical care relate to verbal communication. Patients often complain both that 'the doctor doesn't listen to me' and that 'I don't understand what the doctor says'.

Although insufficient time may account in part for the first of these complaints, linguistic problems account for both. The vocabularies of physicians and patients can differ greatly. Highly educated people may use different words from poorly educated people. Persons whose native language is not English may use terms different from those used by native English speakers. Even in the native English-speaking world, different terms or pronunciations can be used for the same thing. The physician must be aware of all this if he wishes truly to understand his patients. Conversely, when physicians use their own technical vocabulary in addressing patients, uncomprehending patients often fear to interrupt to ask for definitions.

Only the physician can rectify the pervasive problem of poor communication. First, he must be aware of the idiosyncratic usages of the population he cares for. When he hears terms he does not understand, he must ask for clarification. Second, he must explain things to patients in terms that he knows they understand. Sometimes, effective communication requires the plainest possible language. The physician must not refrain from using it.

THE SUMMARY CONVERSATION

At the end of the clinical examination, the physician prepares to proceed to objective testing in his search to establish a diagnosis. The tests chosen will have been established by the elements of the history and the abnormalities detected on physical examination. At this point, the physician should have in mind a list of diagnostic possibilities. He should explain them to the patient at this point both as a matter of courtesy and as a means to allay fear. The physician must not make a firm statement about diagnosis at this point. Premature decision making can be disastrous. He should explain the tests he proposes to do, why he wants to do them, what he expects to learn from them and in what order he will do them. Patients deserve to know what is going to happen next. Time spent at this point by the physician summarizing his thoughts and his plans can do much to allay anxiety and reduce delay when the tests are done.

THE ABDOMINAL EXAMINATION

The examiner of the abdomen uses the four techniques of physical examination in a particular order: inspection, auscultation, palpation and

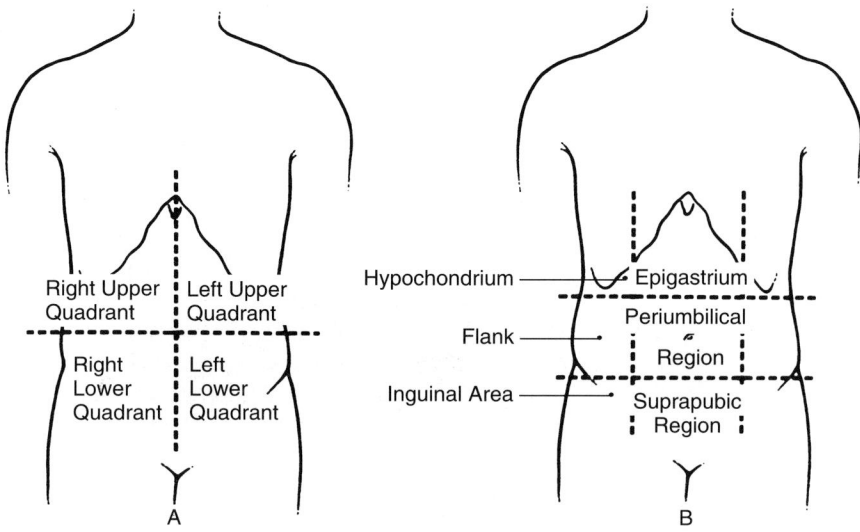

Figure 1.1   Two systems for mapping the abdomen.

percussion. Auscultation precedes palpation because palpation may excite peristalsis to create sounds which can obscure vascular sounds.

The best *position of the abdomen* for inspection is the full supine position with the legs fully extended. After auscultation the abdomen should be slightly flexed because a relaxed abdomen facilitates palpation. This can be done by slightly raising the head and chest and slightly flexing the hips and knees. In the absence of an adjustable examination table, the examiner can use pillows.

A *surface map* of the abdomen facilitates the description of the location of abnormal findings (Fig. 1.1). The simpler system (Fig. 1.1A) involves drawing two imaginary lines through the umbilicus, one craniocaudad and the other transverse. The four regions so delineated are the *right* and *left, upper* and *lower quadrants.* The more complex map (Fig. 1.1B) involves four lines: two craniocaudad lines drawn through the nipples and two transverse lines, one connecting the most caudal points of the costal margins and the other connecting the two superior iliac crests. The nine regions so delineated are the *right* and *left hypochondria* and the *epigastrium,* the *right* and *left flanks* and the *periumbilical region,* the *right* and *left inguinal regions* and the *suprapubic region.*

Inspection of the abdomen

Lighting. Inspection should include inspection with an oblique light. An oblique light can sometimes make an enlarged organ or a mass cast a shadow. Sometimes such a structure can be seen better than it can be felt. If no fixed source of oblique light is available, one can use a flashlight with the overhead light dimmed or extinguished.

The configuration of the abdomen (Fig. 1.2). In most people without

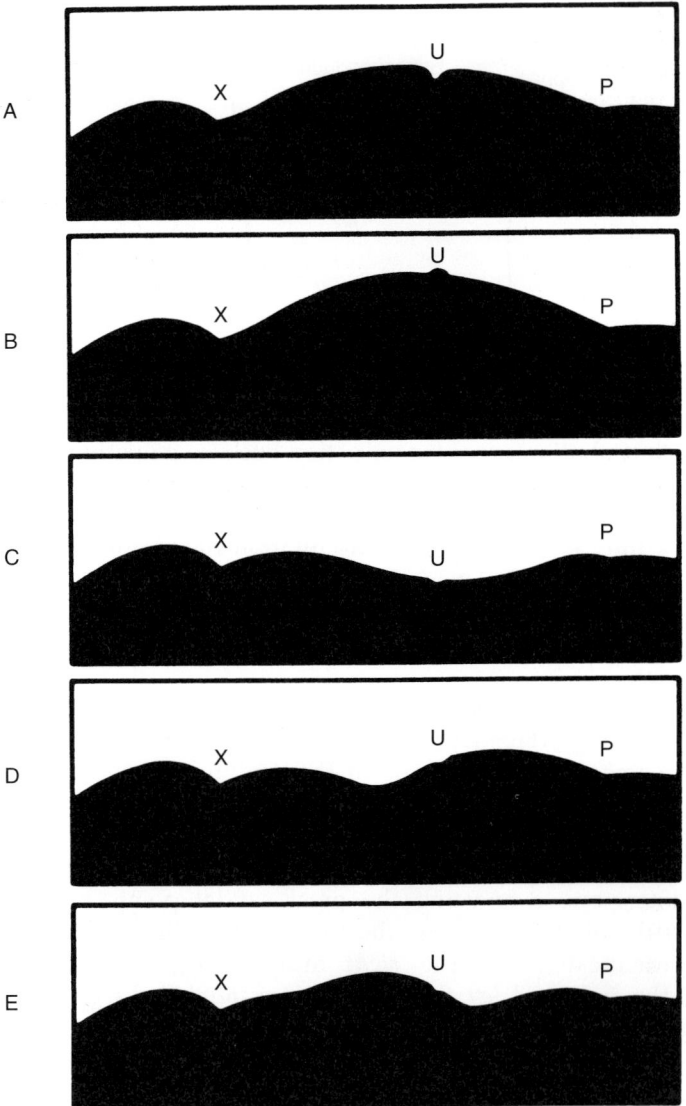

Figure 1.2 Several abdominal configurations as shown in silhouette. X: xiphoid process, U: umbilicus, P: pubis. A: obesity or distension by gas. B: ascites. C: the scaphoid abdomen. D: a distended bladder. E: massive hepatomegaly.

excess adiposity and normal musculature, the relaxed abdominal wall sinks slightly within the bony margins of the abdomen to produce a scaphoid ('boatlike') configuration.

In very muscular persons, the abdominal wall does not sink and the margins of the two rectus muscles (the most superficial abdominal muscles) are visible along with the rectus inscriptions, fibrous transverse bands that indent the surfaces of these two muscles. The margins and inscriptions of the rectus muscles can, in very muscular persons, be mistaken easily for the edges of viscera, so their positions should be discovered at inspection before palpation (Fig. 1.3).

The medial edges of the rectus muscles normally touch at the midline but some separation can occur, especially between the xiphoid and the umbilicus, as a congenital or acquired defect. In such a *diastasis recti*, the palpable medial edges of the rectus muscles also can be mistaken for palpable viscera. If the patient raises his head for a moment, the fascia between the separated rectus muscles bulges forward to make clear the positions of the medial borders of the muscles.

In people with some adiposity and normal musculature, the abdomen often presents a slightly rounded contour. When this is extreme, the abdomen is said to be *bulging* or *protuberant*. Such prominence may only represent fat, but it can also represent gas, ascites, intraabdominal tumor or a feces-packed colon. Fat can sometimes be distinguished from gaseous

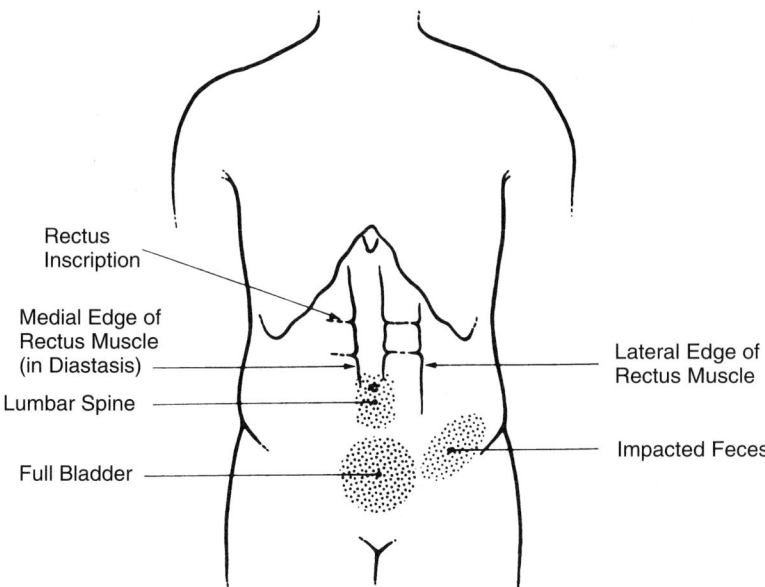

Figure 1.3 Some features of the normal abdomen that can be mistaken for abnormalities.

or fluid distension by inspection of the flanks. When generalized abdominal enlargement represents fat, the flank has a more rolled appearance in cross-section while ascites and gas produce a smoother curvature, often called *bulging flanks* (Fig. 1.4).

The surface of the supine abdomen is normally *symmetrical* right to left. Distension from an enlarged organ or other mass may produce asymmetric abdominal protuberance. Masses in the abdominal wall and the retraction of surgical scars can also lead to abdominal asymmetry. The physician can assess symmetry by viewing the abdomen from a position taken at the head or the feet of the patient.

Inspection with oblique light can reveal a greatly enlarged organ or a mass when its border casts a shadow. The location and shape of the shadow suggests the organ that is enlarged. When such shadows lie in the upper abdomen, the shadow moves with respiration if the mass lies next to the diaphragm and is not fixed. This is commonly the case with an enlarged liver or spleen. A distended stomach does not move with breathing because it is deformed rather than shifted by the moving diaphragm. A greatly distended gallbladder can sometimes be seen better than it can

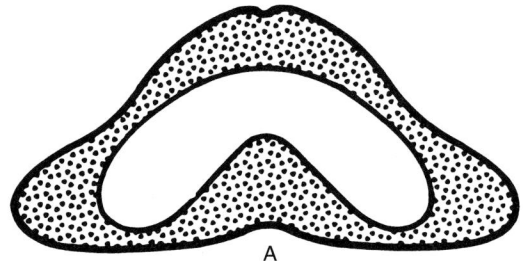

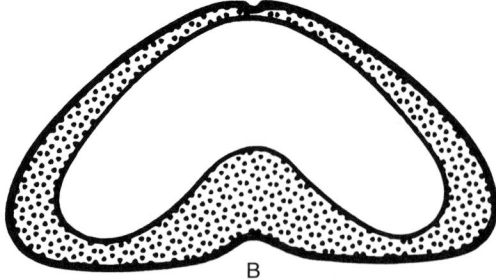

Figure 1.4 The configuration of the flanks. A: obesity. B: ascites and gas.

be felt, appearing as a smooth globular mass that moves with respiration. Visible midline masses in the lower abdomen most commonly constitute a distended bladder or an enlarged uterus. Lateral lower abdominal masses, rarely seen except in very thin people, are either greatly enlarged kidneys or masses arising from the colon.

The umbilicus. The normal umbilicus is a symmetrical indentation in most people though it may be nearly flat in very slender persons. A protruding or everted umbilicus may reflect only a herniation, a widening of the normal umbilical ring (a fascial defect in the linea alba) to admit a little fat or intestine. Such a widening may be congenital or acquired as a consequence of prolonged abdominal distension from, often, ascites. The umbilicus may rarely drain fluid, clear yellow ascitic fluid when ascites is extreme or feculant fluid when an enteric fistula has formed in inflammatory or malignant disease. Umbilical nodules are usually lipomas, but malignant nodules can form if intraabdominal tumors extend along the umbilical ligament. Umbilical stones, concretions of desquamated epidermal cells and dirt, sometimes form in those who do not clean the umbilicus.

The abdominal skin. The lower abdomen is rarely tanned by the sun except in the very vain, so that disorders characterized by abnormal pigmentation may be most evident there. One should look there for jaundice. Bruising may also appear in the lower abdomen in people who have bleeding disorders or in people who inject things there. Periumbilical bruising can signify massive retroperitoneal hemorrhage, as occurs in hemorrhagic pancreatitis. The blood dissects between the fascial layers of the abdominal wall to come to the surface at the umbilicus (and occasionally in the flanks). The bruise is 'black and blue' at first, fading to a yellow pigmentation which persists for many days.

Abdominal striae, commonly called 'stretch marks', appear as parallel discontinuous rows of marks where the skin appears to be thin, shiny and either very pale or violaceous. Striae arise from rapid abdominal distension, commonly in pregnancy or in those who take large doses of corticosteroids. The violaceous hue signifies a recent origin. The striae turn white after about 6 months.

Abdominal scars, like striae, remain violaceous for about 6 months before fading. Abdominal scars present a record of abdominal traumas (including operations) so the physician should note their number, locations and configurations, asking the patient about the circumstances surrounding each one (Fig. 1.5). This often clarifies a complex surgical history.

Abdominal abrasions may be the only evidence of generalized pruritus. Patients may scratch more intensely there because the abdomen is easy to reach and because abrasions there do not show. Rapid abdominal distension can make the abdomen itch.

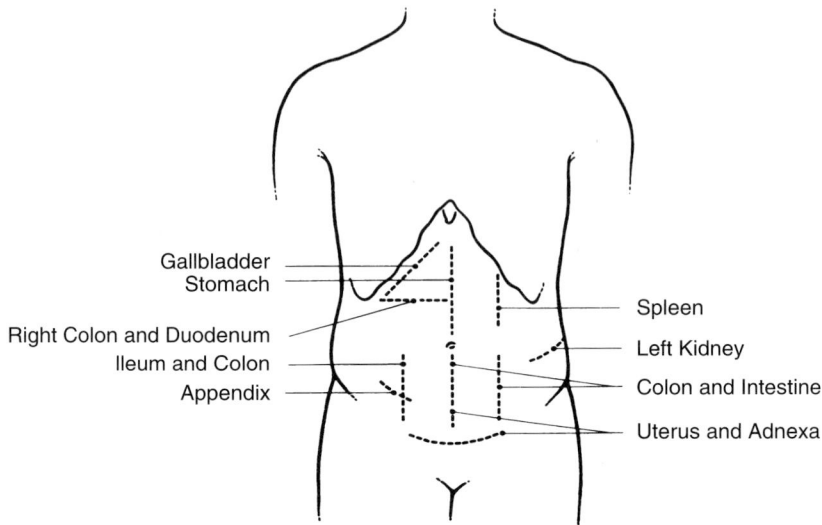

Figure 1.5   The positions of abdominal scars can suggest the organ that was operated on.

The veins of the anterior abdomen. The abdominal veins, normally obscure, can sometimes be seen in the very thin or the very old when the skin and subcutaneous fat are thinned. Generalized abdominal distension can also make them visible. Visibility of these veins alone is not useful information but the direction of their blood flow is because, connecting through the umbilicus to the portal venous system, they constitute a portal–systemic venous shunt pathway. Blood in these veins normally flows away from the umbilicus, cephalad above it and caudad below it (Fig. 1.6). Obstruction of the inferior vena cava below the hepatic veins can reverse the flow in the veins over the lower abdomen and obstruction of the superior vena cava can reverse flow in those over the upper abdomen. In portal venous obstruction the direction of flow is normal but the increased volume of flow distends the veins, making them very prominent and even varicose.

Visible peristalsis. Recurring rippling movements across the abdomen, best seen with oblique lighting, are instantly recognizable as visible peristalsis. Their appearance can be normal in very thin or emaciated persons but they are an important sign of disease in those of more normal adiposity or nutrition. They usually reflect contractions of the small intestine since that organ contacts most of the anterior abdominal wall, but they may also arise from the stomach. If they occur in a setting of symptoms that suggest obstruction in the gastrointestinal tract, they strongly support that diagnosis. Neonates with hypertrophic pyloric stenosis often exhibit visible gastric peristalsis but adults with gastric outlet obstruction rarely do.

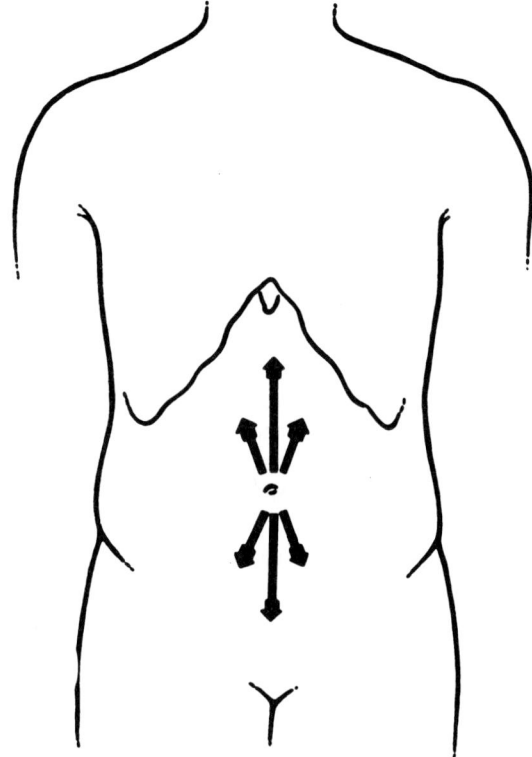

Figure 1.6 Flow in the superficial abdominal veins is normally away from the umbilicus.

Visible pulsations. A pulsating aorta is commonly visualized in very thin people and in aged persons with arteriosclerosis, aortic tortuosity or a widened pulse pressure. Visible aortic pulsation is thus not in itself abnormal but it may signify aneurysmal dilatation of the aorta.

Auscultation of the abdomen

Technique. Auscultation is often neglected or cursory in the routine abdominal examination because it is so often unproductive. On the other hand it can give a major clue in vascular disease or suggest certain visceral disorders.

To listen properly takes time. The physician should sit down and rest the diaphragm of the stethoscope on the abdomen without pressure. He should warm the stethoscope first, coat it with lubricating gel if the abdomen is hairy (to minimize friction-induced sounds) and leave it in one place for a long time, listening carefully. Bowel sounds are usually loud while vascular sounds are faint. Bowel sounds generally spread widely so that a single listening site, usually adjacent to the umbilicus, provides an adequate evaluation. Vascular sounds spread less so the listener must listen over the vessels more directly (Fig. 1.7).

Arterial sounds. Arterial sounds (*bruits*), harsh high-pitched sounds in tempo with the arterial pulse, can be normal events in the abdomen, especially in the elderly. The turbulent arterial flows that produce them can arise from acute angulations at arterial branch points, from vascular tortuosity, from arteriosclerotic plaques, from compression, from aneurysmal dilatation or from increased blood flow to a vascular tumor (such as hemangioma or hepatoma). Bruits most commonly occur over the liver and spleen, the aorta and the splenic and renal arteries.

Bruits over the liver or spleen must be considered abnormal. Those over the aorta and splenic arteries may not be abnormal because tortuosity alone can produce them. Rarely, the murmur of aortic stenosis may be heard over the aorta in the upper abdomen. Bruits over the renal arteries can suggest renal artery stenosis but many cases of renal artery stenosis lack bruits.

Venous sounds. A low-pitched continuous *venous hum* is abnormal in the abdomen, nearly always signifying increased flow through a portal–systemic venous shunt. It is best heard where such shunts are most common, in the region of the liver and spleen and in the periumbilical area.

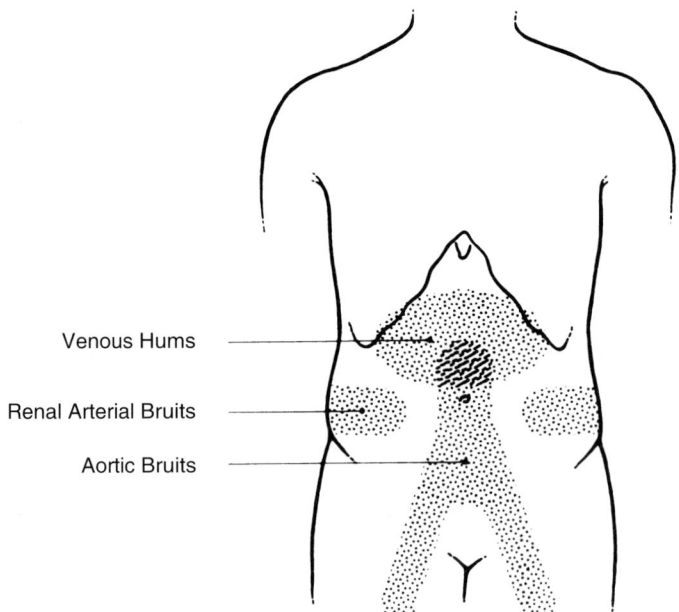

Venous Hums

Renal Arterial Bruits

Aortic Bruits

Figure 1.7 The locations of vascular sounds heard in the abdomen.

Intestinal sounds. Contractions of the muscular intestinal walls propel the liquid–gas mixture contained in the lumen, vibrating the gut wall to produce the gurgling bowel sounds. The sounds persist in fasting because of the presence of swallowed air and secreted fluid. Thus, they are heard (intermittently) at all times except when contractions are absent. The sounds can vary in intensity, so that the absence of bowel sounds, the main point to be established in listening, can only be concluded after listening for a full 5 minutes or so. The absence of bowel sounds identifies ileus. In intestinal obstruction, without accompanying ileus, the listener may hear intermittent runs of high-pitched 'tinkling' bowel sounds. These musical notes, like the sound of a damped high-pitched bell occurring in short bursts, are not always heard in bowel obstruction but their presence favors obstruction over ileus. Their exact origin is not clear.

Succussion splash. After a meal and after drinking, a large volume of fluid and swallowed air accumulates in the stomach. If the examiner shakes the patient's abdomen while listening, he can hear the splash at the gas–liquid interface. When this succussion splash is heard many hours after a period of eating or drinking, it signifies gastric retention, either from obstruction or ileus.

Peritoneal friction rub. Respiration normally moves the upper abdominal viscera, rubbing peritoneal surfaces together. In peritonitis, before exudate has separated the inflamed surfaces, this movement produces a dry, soft scraping sound, a friction rub. It can often be heard after a needle biopsy of the liver where it signifies bleeding at the liver surface. It can also accompany splenic infarction or abscess and neoplastic disease at the surface of the liver.

Palpation of the abdomen

Technique. Palpation, the major technique in the abdominal examination, can reveal the sizes and shapes of masses and organs and the location and degree of tenderness. Accuracy in palpation requires a relaxed abdominal wall, achieved when necessary by slight flexion of the thoracic spine and of the hips and knees produced with appropriately placed pillows. Convention dictates palpation from the patient's right side. The examiner who learns to use the right side cannot easily shift to the left. The examiner does a better job if he is comfortable, relaxed and patient, qualities which are better achieved if he can sit rather than stand at the bedside.

Most patients expect palpation to be uncomfortable and tense the abdominal muscles in anticipation. A gentle touch, a steady, deliberate approach and warm hands can all do much to alleviate protective responses. Occasional patients are so ticklish that good palpation is impossible. In this case, the examiner should ask the patient to rest his fingertips on the back of the examiner's hand and follow it about. This works because one cannot tickle oneself, as all children know.

Survey palpation. A good examination begins with a quick and light palpatory survey of the whole abdomen. This helps, first, to allay the patient's fear and, second, to discover areas of great tenderness before deep palpation begins. If the history has suggested that one area is very tender, the examiner should begin elsewhere and reserve the tender area until last.

The examiner explains his intentions continuously as he lightly palpates in all quadrants, seeking to find any tenderness or resistance. In doing this, he notes the consistency or 'feel' of all areas palpated, searching for the rigidity that may signify peritonitis, the firmness overlying a mass and the spongy feel of an abdomen filled with ascitic fluid.

Specific palpation for tenderness. The initial survey palpation will have suggested matters requiring more careful exploration and should have allayed some of the patient's anxiety. Then the examiner can proceed to a deeper and more detailed search for palpable abnormalities.

The examiner must be especially alert to *tenderness*. When he finds it he must assess its degree, location and depth. The degree of tenderness, a subjective matter, can be assessed only relative to the degree of pressure. Some patients are stoic, so the careful examiner watches the patient's face as he palpates tenderness. The examiner should map the location of tenderness first by discovering the margins of the tender area and then by seeking the point of maximum tenderness with one finger. Sometimes the patient, again using one finger, can find this point much more accurately and quickly than the examiner can. The location of this point strongly suggests the organ of origin.

It is easy to confuse superficial tenderness or abdominal wall tenderness with visceral tenderness. The former comes with light pressure, the latter with deeper pressure, but this distinction may be fuzzy. A clearer distinction is achieved by the *abdominal tension test* (or *Carnett's test*). Here the examiner uses light palpation to find a point of maximal tenderness. Then, holding his finger on the spot with a steadily maintained pressure just sufficient to produce a stable low level of pain, he asks the patient to tense the abdominal muscles. The patient can do this by raising the head, by raising the heels with legs extended or by 'bearing down'. The examiner can feel the abdominal muscles tighten under his finger. Pain of intraabdominal or visceral origin lessens as the contracted muscle pushes the finger out and away, but pain arising at that point in the abdominal wall itself is increased or, at least, unchanged. The test can fail when the abdominal muscles are very weak and when the examiner is feeling through a diastasis recti. Abdominal wall pain can arise from inflammation and trauma in the abdominal wall, but it more commonly seems to be neuropathic, a part of a generalized sensory neuropathy or, more often, a local neuropathy producing a 'trigger point'. The finding of cutaneous hyperesthesia by the use of standard neurological techniques helps to confirm neuropathic abdominal wall pain.

Sometimes, much is made of *rebound tenderness* as a sign of peritonitis. In this sign, greater pain occurs a moment after the deeply applied finger is withdrawn than occurred with the deep palpation itself. *Percussion tenderness* is just as reliable and a much less painful sign of peritoneal irritation.

Specific palpation of the right hypochondrium. Palpation to discover the size, consistency, surface contour and tenderness of the liver begins with the finding of the caudal border of the right lobe. In most normal people the border either cannot be felt at all or appears only in deep inspiration. Its discovery can be made with several different positions of the examining fingers (Fig. 1.8). The fingers are put into position and, as the patient inspires deeply, the liver edge moves across the examiner's fingers. Once the position of any point on the caudal border of the right lobe is discovered, the same technique can be used to trace that border to the left lobe and to discover the firmness and tenderness of the organ and

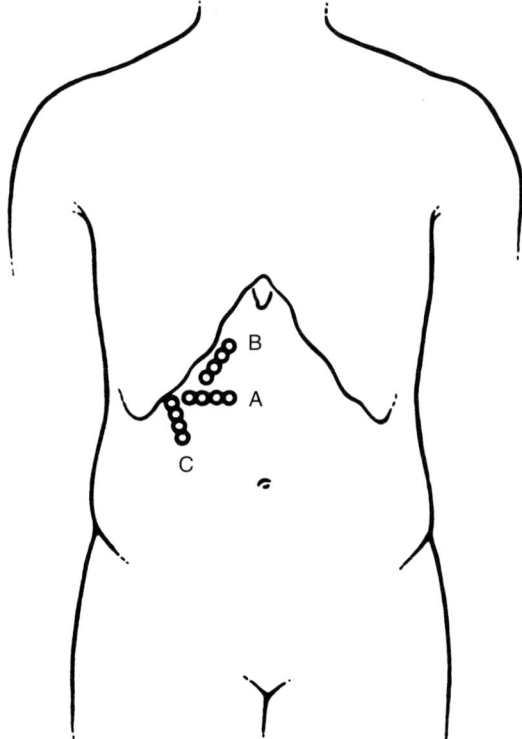

Figure 1.8 Three ways to position the fingers in feeling for the liver.

the smoothness or regularity of the border. Similarly, the distance between the palpated border of the right lobe and the percussed level of the hepatic dome can be measured (Fig. 1.9). The liver edge is normally smooth, soft and non-tender, but estimates of abnormality are necessarily subjective. Size is less subjective, the normal liver being less than 12 cm wide in the measurement from the percussed hepatic dome to the palpated border of the right lobe in the anterior axillary line.

Specific palpation of the epigastrium. In the epigastrium, where the relevant organs are the stomach, duodenum, pancreas and left hepatic lobe, the examiner uncommonly detects masses but commonly must explore tenderness. The left lobe of the liver is the commonest site of epigastric masses. Gastric and pancreatic tumors are rarely palpable, but inflammation in these organs regularly induces epigastric tenderness. When the physician anticipates epigastric tenderness, he first should define the margins of the tender area by approaching it from the sides and below. Then, with graded degrees of pressure he should find the point of maximal tenderness. It is useful to use one finger, systematically exploring the tender zone in a grid pattern and repeating the process for confirmation. The location of the point of maximal tenderness can strongly suggest the organ of origin. A sharply localized point at the midline or just to the right of the midline suggests the duodenal bulb as the source.

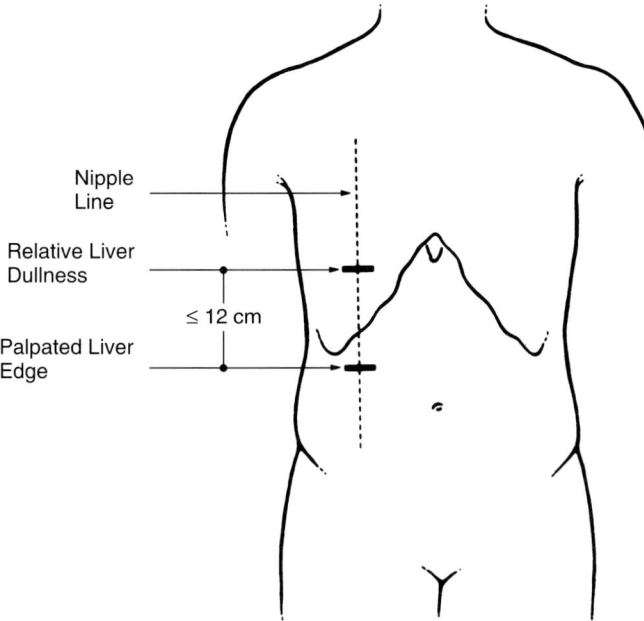

Nipple Line

Relative Liver Dullness

≤ 12 cm

Palpated Liver Edge

Figure 1.9 'Liver span'.

Gastric tenderness produces a more diffuse zone extending to the left of the midline. Pancreatic tenderness is usually broad and diffuse, not a point. Epigastric pressure producing a pain that radiates broadly suggests a diffuse inflammatory process, such as occurs in pancreatic inflammation or subhepatic abscess.

Location of the point of maximal tenderness near the xiphoid process should prompt the examiner to manipulate that process or to probe the xiphosternal joint to establish that the pain arises from *xiphalgia* rather than the viscera. Xiphoid pain, arising from traumatic or idiopathic costo-chondritis, often radiates into the epigastrium to be confused with visceral pain. In such a case, the rib margins themselves are often tender as well. A related source of epigastric tenderness is the *slipping rib*, in which the motion of an unusually mobile 10th or 11th rib against the adjacent ribs or costal cartilages sets up an inflammation with pain radiating into the epigastrium. This problem can best be identified by demonstrating pain on direct manipulation of that rib.

Specific palpation of the left hypochondrium. The left hypochondrium is relatively difficult to examine because it is far away when the examiner is at the patient's right side and because the examiner particularly needs to feel far up under the rib cage where the spleen lies. Almost all masses in this area arise from the spleen, the splenic flexure of the colon or the pancreas. Much less commonly, they represent the left hepatic lobe or the left kidney.

Examination of the area with the patient in the normal body position can miss masses if they lie deep or far to the left. A better technique involves placement of a pillow under the patient's lumbar area to exag-gerate lumbar lordosis and thus make accessible the deep recess of the hypochondrium. It helps as well for the examiner to use his subordinate hand to elevate the left flank as he probes. Another useful technique is to roll the patient to the right side with the knees drawn up. This makes the viscera fall forward against the abdominal wall, giving the examiner better access to them.

While a mass in this area is usually splenic, the examiner can establish this conclusion more securely if he looks for the motion of the mass with respiration. The spleen, being both mobile and contiguous with the diaphragm, moves with breathing while most other sources of masses do not. Because the spleen touches the diaphragm so far to the left, its motion follows an arc toward the umbilicus rather than following the cephalo-caudad axis (Fig. 1.10). When the spleen is very large, its movement is reduced, but the greatly enlarged spleen is identifiable from the finding of the *splenic notch*, a palpable indentation on the medial border representing the splenic hilum (Fig. 1.11).

The examiner should look for the tenderness and the firmness of a palpable spleen. A spleen that has enlarged rapidly, either from inflammation or passive congestion, is soft and tender. Slow enlargement, in contrast, tends to produce a harder and less tender spleen.

Specific palpation of the periumbilical area. The main structures to think of in the periumbilical area are the aorta and the pancreas. Since the aortic bifurcation lies at about the level of the umbilicus the examiner should feel for the aorta mainly just above the umbilicus (the position of the umbilicus is highly variable). The pancreas, too, usually lies just above the umbilicus.

It is easy to feel the aorta in thin people, less so in fat people and it is more prominent in the old than in the young. A palpable aorta, especially in the presence of a bruit, always suggests an aortic aneurysm. Masses that overlie the aorta can transmit systolic aortic pulsation and so be mistaken for aneurysm. One must detect systolic lateral expansion to distinguish an aortic aneurysm. The examiner can assess lateral expansion of a pulsating midline periumbilical mass by pressing with one hand on each side of the mass and feeling for the systolic expansion. This is not a highly discriminatory technique. Masses that transmit the aortic pulse can

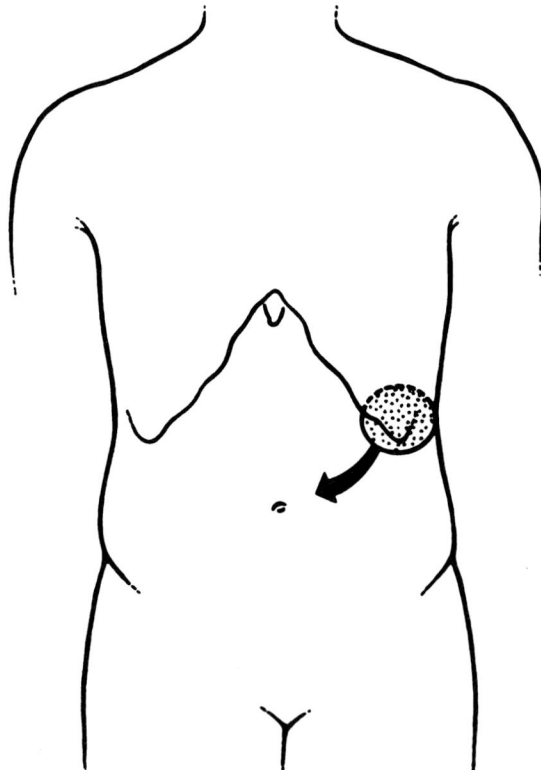

Figure 1.10 In respiration the spleen moves along an arc toward the umbilicus because of its position on the diaphragm.

sometimes be detected as such by their nodularity, irregularity or lack of a smooth tubular or fusiform shape.

Both the normal and the abnormal pancreas are rarely palpable as masses, but pancreatic disease often manifests itself to the examiner as tenderness. Some slight tenderness over the pancreas is normal so that the degree of tenderness becomes critical. When periumbilical or epigastric tenderness is present and the history suggests pancreatic disease, the *jar test* can be a useful maneuver. This test takes advantage of the fact that an inflamed organ hurts if it is shaken and that the pancreas is firmly fixed to the spine. A jarring force applied to the spine shakes the pancreas more than it does those viscera which are less tightly adherent to the spine or suspended on mesenteries. The examiner asks the patient to extend one leg and then he strikes the heel sharply, looking for a momentary pain in the midabdomen in response. A graded series of blows, beginning with a very gentle tap, prevents the induction of a severe pain and provides a rough measure of the magnitude of the inflammation. Furthermore, if the

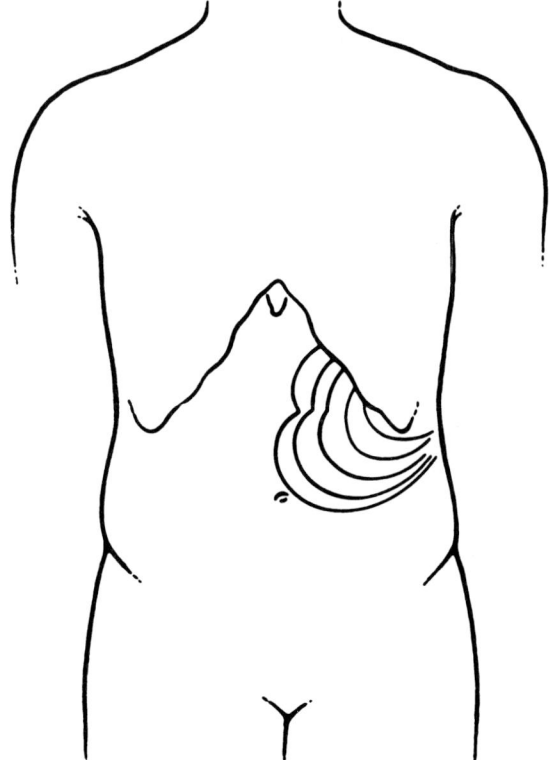

Figure 1.11 The greatly enlarged spleen can be recognized as such by the palpable notch on its medial border, representing the splenic hilum.

patient is not told what the examiner is looking for, the test can be quite objective, at least the first time it is done. It can provide a useful bedside assessment of the resolution of pancreatitis. Since other structures are attached tightly to the spine, the test is not specific for pancreatic inflammation. It is positive in peritonitis, in retroperitoneal or subhepatic abscess and in inflammatory disease involving the spine itself.

Specific palpation of the flanks. Since the viscera in the flanks lie deep, the examiner must pull them forward with the subordinate hand while he feels with the dominant hand. Since motion often facilitates the perception of masses at palpation, he should move his subordinate hand in and out. The organs to feel for are the kidneys and the colon.

The normal kidney is rarely palpable except in the very slender. The kidney shows little or no movement with respiration and its margins are rarely distinct. It is soft and its surface usually feels smooth even when it is greatly enlarged by tumors or cysts. The normal kidney can be quite tender, but the tenderness of an infected kidney or a perinephric abscess is extreme.

Apart from kidneys, masses in the flank usually represent colonic tumors. They are often quite mobile, but they do not move with respiration. They are commonly nodular, hard and moderately tender.

Percussion of the abdomen

Done after palpation, percussion is useful only for a few specific purposes: to find ascites, to measure organs and to explore tenderness when it is too severe to explore by palpation. One taps the abdomen with one or two fingers of the dominant hand, using a finger of the subordinate hand as a plessimeter. Gas in the intestine makes most of the abdomen resonant. Dullness only occurs at points where a solid organ or mass encounters the abdominal wall. In mapping such areas of dullness, the examiner delivers taps along a series of straight lines, moving from resonance to dullness, noting the points where the sound changes.

Generalized abdominal percussion. Normal abdominal resonance extends only as far in the flanks as the intestine extends. The presence of an increased amount of gas in the gut produces hyperresonance in which the resonant note is higher in pitch and more 'musical' than normal. This is hard to judge and useful only with really major abdominal distension from gas. Among the organs, only the stomach can be identified as such when the gaseous distension is localized.

Generalized abdominal percussion finds its major use in the detection of ascites, in the search for shifting dullness and for a fluid wave. *Shifting dullness* takes advantage of the flotation of the gas-filled intestine in the pool of ascitic fluid. The examiner percusses the level of dullness in one flank, then rolls the patient toward that side and, after a minute or so,

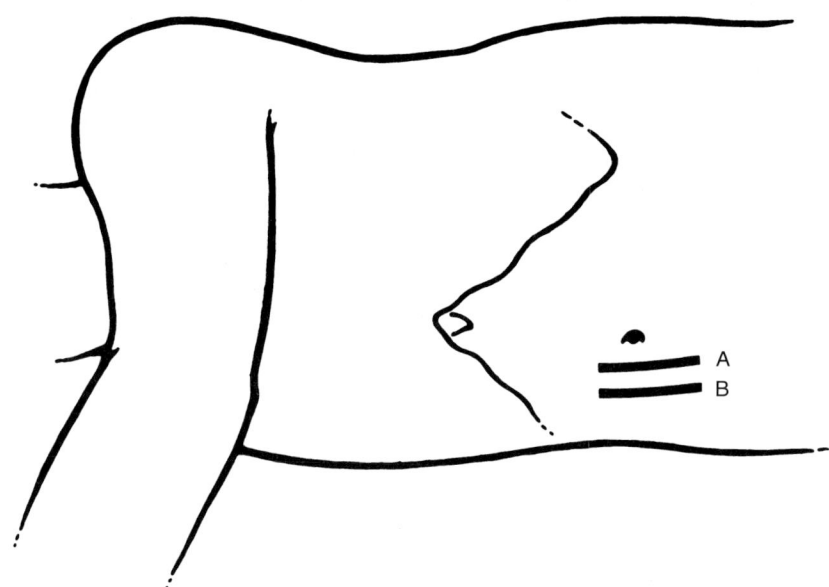

Figure 1.12 In shifting dullness, the percussed level of flank dullness moves from B to A as the patient is rolled to his side.

percusses for the level of dullness again in the same flank. The presence of ascites moves the level of dullness toward the midline as the ascitic pool shifts (Figs 1.12 and 1.13). The search for a *fluid wave* takes advantage of the incompressibility of liquid as compared to gas. A wave motion passes through a fluid mass with little damping or dissipation. The examiner simply taps sharply in one flank, below the estimated fluid level, and feels for the transmission of the pulse below the estimated fluid level in the other flank. The ulnar margin of another person's hand is pressed in the abdominal midline to dampen transmission of the pulse through the abdominal wall. Both these tests for ascites lack sensitivity so a negative test means nothing, but a positive test can be convincing. Both tests should be repeated several times to ensure reproducibility.

Specific organ percussion. In hepatomegaly or splenomegaly, the edges of the organs may be obscure on palpation because of fat, ascites, the abdominal configuration or the softness of the organ. In such a case percussion can reveal the organ when palpation cannot. The examiner percusses along a series of straight lines, moving from resonance to dullness, perpendicular to the anticipated edge of the organ, noting the points where resonance diminishes. When massive ascites obscures palpation, an enlarged and suspended organ or mass, usually the liver or spleen, can be detected by *ballottement*. The examiner taps forcefully and directly over the suspected organ and leaves his fingers indenting the

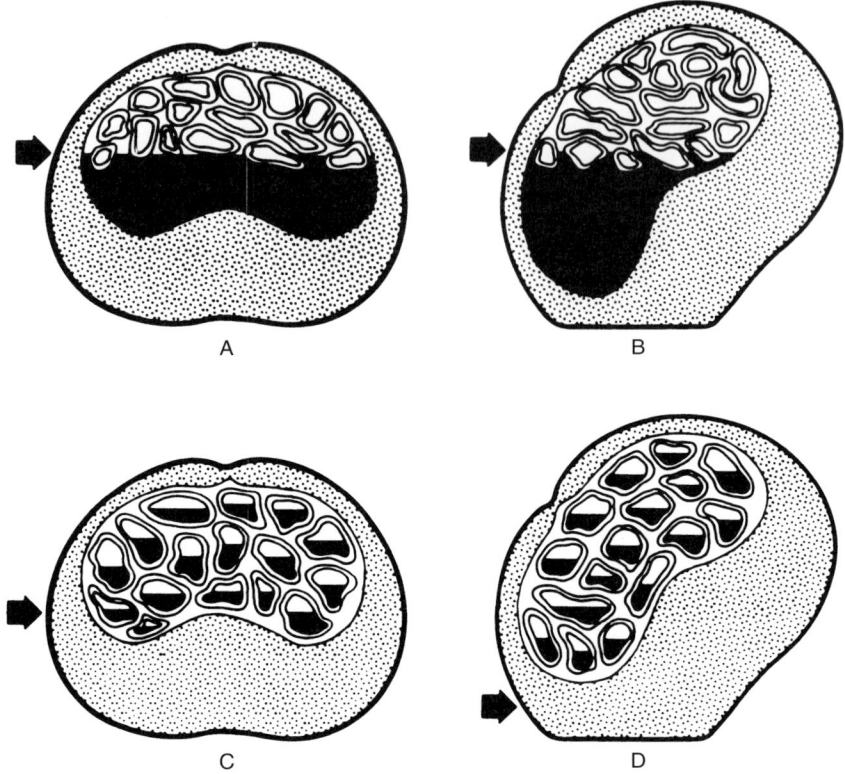

A   B

C   D

Figure 1.13 How the presence of much ascites causes shifting dullness. A and B: the gas-filled bowel floats so that the dullness level (arrows) moves in rotation. C and D: the fluid-filled bowel retains its position in rotation so that the level of dullness remains the same.

abdominal wall. The floating organ, displaced away from the abdominal wall, bounces back toward it with enough force that the examiner can feel it a second or so after he taps. This works well only when the organ is quite firm. The method allows assessment of both the firmness and size of the organ.

Percussion can be used to map tenderness when it is too great to be assessed easily by palpation. Light taps, both direct and through a plessimeter finger, are effective, tolerable and reliable in mapping tenderness.

Fist percussion is used more widely than it should be to assess tenderness deep in the splenic and hepatic fossae. It can produce much pain if done too forcefully, as it usually is. One first taps very gently with a clenched fist over the lower ribs, using the subordinate hand as a plessimeter. The force can be increased as necessary in a series of taps to estimate the degree of tenderness.

THE ANORECTAL EXAMINATION

Osler offered the definition of a consultant as a physician who does rectal examinations! Anorectal examination, long advocated as a necessary part of any routine examination, still seems to be neglected even in patients whose complaints are gastrointestinal. Patients resent them because of the indignity and discomfort, both of which can be minimized by the physician.

Perianal inspection and palpation

The examination is best done with the patient in the knee–chest position and with a very strong light.

The *perianal skin* is normally hyperpigmented for a variable distance around the orifice. Chronic inflammation tends to enhance this pigmentation. Abrasions in the area signify pruritus ani.

Perianal openings may appear as pits or, more commonly, as small firm nodules, heaps of inflamed skin, which obscure the pits. The relatively large opening of a *pilonidal sinus*, in the posterior midline near the coccyx, commonly lies in a field of inflamed skin and may exude foul matter and hair. The much smaller openings of *perianal fistulae*, fistulous tracts from the crypts of the anorectum to the skin around the anal canal, may lie in any perianal quadrant and at a variable distance from the anal orifice. Those seen posteriorly usually connect to posterior crypts and those anteriorly connect to anterior crypts. Those very near the anus usually communicate to anterior crypts. Those with active inflammation may seep feculent fluid and lie in an obviously inflamed area. Those with less active infection (often as a consequence of treatment) may be buried in a skinfold. The examiner must spread the skin to find them.

Perianal masses are common. *Pilonidal cysts* lie over the coccyx in the posterior midline. *Genital warts* are usually multiple, firm, pigmented nodules surrounding the anal orifice. The soft, smooth and pliable *skin tag*, having the color of normal perianal skin, is usually a solitary small structure at the end of a radiating perianal skinfold. There can be several. *External hemorrhoids* may resemble skin tags except that they can be recognized from their color as blood-filled. An enlarged *anal papilla*, a dense, firm, smooth, somewhat triangular white-pink mass, may emerge from the anal canal on straining. Carcinoma of the anal canal is usually visible as a multinodular and/or ulcerated firm mass.

A *fissure* in the anal canal often extends externally far enough that the examiner can see one end of it if he spreads the perianal skin to flatten the radiating folds.

During the examination, the examiner should ask the patient to bear down or strain for a moment. This can reveal or exaggerate hemorrhoids, enlarged anal papillae or rectal prolapse.

Digital examination of the anal canal. The 'rectal examination' is best done with the patient in the knee–chest position along with perianal inspection, because the examiner can reach so far up the anterior and lateral walls in this position. The gloved finger, coated with lubricant (an anesthetic lubricant in patients with much inflammation), is passed slowly and gently, the examiner sliding it in an arc curving over the perineal body.

With the finger just seated in the canal, the examiner presses gently in all quadrants of the canal. A fissure will usually express itself as a sharp, stabbing and focused pain with this maneuver and so the examiner will learn exactly where to look for a fissure when he uses the sigmoidoscope.

The examiner then seeks palpable abnormalities in the anal canal. Hemorrhoids can be felt only if they are large and thrombosed. Enlarged papillae are not palpable. A stricture can be felt as a fixed narrowing which does not yield to force or does so only with great pain. Malignant tumors are usually readily detected as large, nodular firm masses. The examiner then asks the patient to squeeze, allowing him to judge the competence of sphincter function.

Then, passing the fingertip into the rectum, the examiner first palpates the prostate or cervix anteriorly and the coccyx posteriorly. With these as landmarks, the examiner can describe the locations of palpable pararectal masses, cysts or abscesses. In appropriate cases, he should feel carefully for the hard nodular *rectal shelf*, representing an intraabdominal malignant tumor implanted in the *pouch of Douglas* anteriorly.

FURTHER READING

Christensen J 1987 Bedside logic in diagnostic gastroenterology. Churchill Livingstone, New York

Davenport H 1982 Physiology of the digestive tract, 5th edn. Year Book Medical Publishers, Chicago

DeGowin E L, DeGowin R L 1994 Bedside diagnostic examination, 6th edn. Macmillan, New York

Engle G L, Morgan W L (eds) 1993 Interviewing the patient. W B Saunders, Philadelphia

Gelin L–E, Nyhus L M, Condon R E (eds) 1969 Abdominal pain: a guide to rapid diagnosis. J B Lippincott, Philadelphia

Granger D N, Barrowman J A, Kvietys P R 1985 Clinical gastrointestinal physiology. W B Saunders, Philadelphia

Greenberger N J (ed) 1986 Gastrointestinal disorders: a pathophysiologic approach, 3rd edn. Year Book Medical Publishers, Chicago

Johnson L 1985 Gastrointestinal physiology, 3rd edn. C V Mosby, St Louis

Judge R D, Zuidema G D (eds) 1982 Clinical diagnosis: a physiological approach, 4th edn. Little, Brown & Co, Boston

Silen W 1983 Cope's early diagnosis of the acute abdomen, 16th edn. Oxford University Press, New York

2

Imaging in gastroenterology
J. Olliff

There are now many ways to image the gastrointestinal tract and related structures. This chapter lists the methods currently used widely in practice, with indications, contraindications and notes about technique and interpretation.

Many of the imaging investigations listed below involve the use of ionizing radiation. This should be remembered when requesting such investigations, especially in patients who have repeated follow-ups or women of childbearing age. Examinations involving ionizing radiation of the lower abdomen and pelvis are not advised in patients who may be pregnant.

PLAIN RADIOGRAPHY
Lateral soft tissue neck

Indications

1. Suspected foreign body.
2. Suspected perforation.

Chest X-ray

Indications (in gastroenterology)

1. Suspected perforation (Fig. 2.1).
2. Suspected aspiration.
3. Suspected foreign body.

The erect chest X-ray centered at the diaphragm is the investigation of choice for detecting extraluminal air. If the patient is not well enough to have an erect film, a left decubitus film of the abdomen can be performed. These films can demonstrate as little as 1–2 mL of free air (Miller & Nelson 1971).

The plain film requires maintenance of position for 10 minutes or more so that small amounts of gas can collect either just below the diaphragm or lateral to the liver.

Mediastinal air and/or pleural fluid should be looked for in patients suspected of esophageal perforation following instrumentation or ingestion of a foreign body.

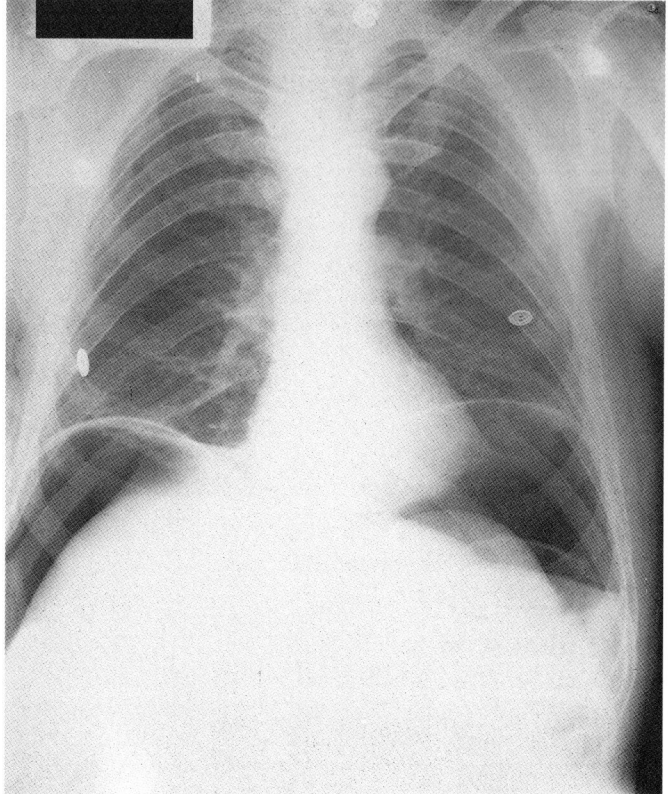

Figure 2.1   X-ray showing gas under both hemidiaphragms.

Plain abdominal film

Indications

1. Intestinal obstruction (Fig. 2.2).
2. Calcification.
3. Suspected ischemia.
4. Intestinal transit studies.
5. Inflammatory bowel disease (Fig. 2.3).

Contraindications

1. Pregnancy

The plain abdominal film is most helpful for detecting intestinal obstruction. The exact site of obstruction can be difficult to judge on plain film since there may be many loops of fluid-filled bowel interposed between

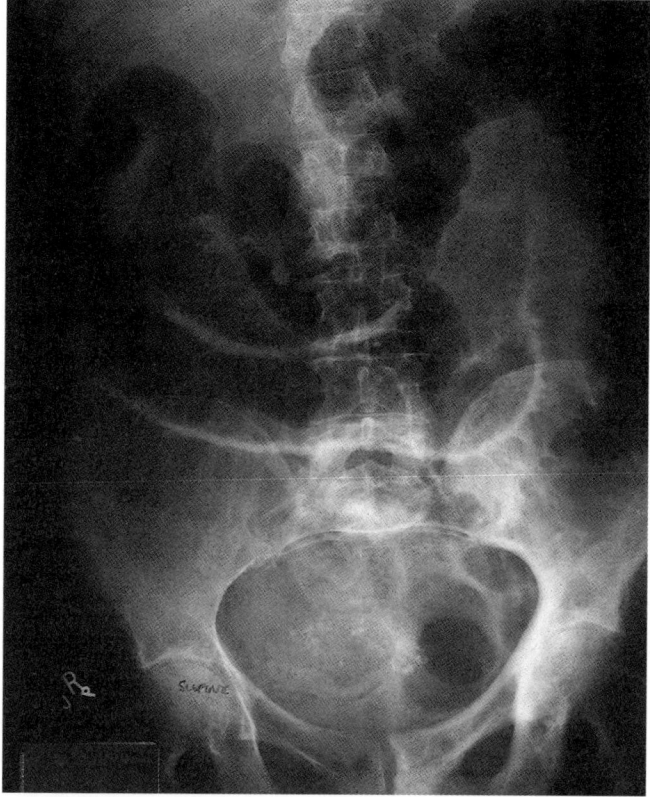

Figure 2.2   Plain abdominal X-ray showing intestinal obstruction.

the actual obstruction and distal air-filled loops (Love 1973). Cecal and sigmoid volvulus, however, do give a distinctive pattern on plain film allowing the diagnosis to be made and often indicating the approximate point of obstruction. The normal caliber of the proximal jejunum should be less than 3.5 cm, of the mid small bowel less than 3 cm and of the ileum less than 2.5 cm.

The presence of extraluminal air should also be assessed on a supine abdomen. If large amounts are present, both sides of the bowel wall may be seen and air may be seen in Morrison's pouch and outlining the fissure of the ligamentum teres. Retroperitoneal free gas may also be assessed and in this situation the renal outlines will appear unusually sharp.

Focal collections of air within abscesses may also be seen on a supine abdominal film. Bowel wall thickening may be seen in conditions such as ischemia, inflammatory bowel disease, etc.

An erect abdominal film is not needed either to assess the presence of

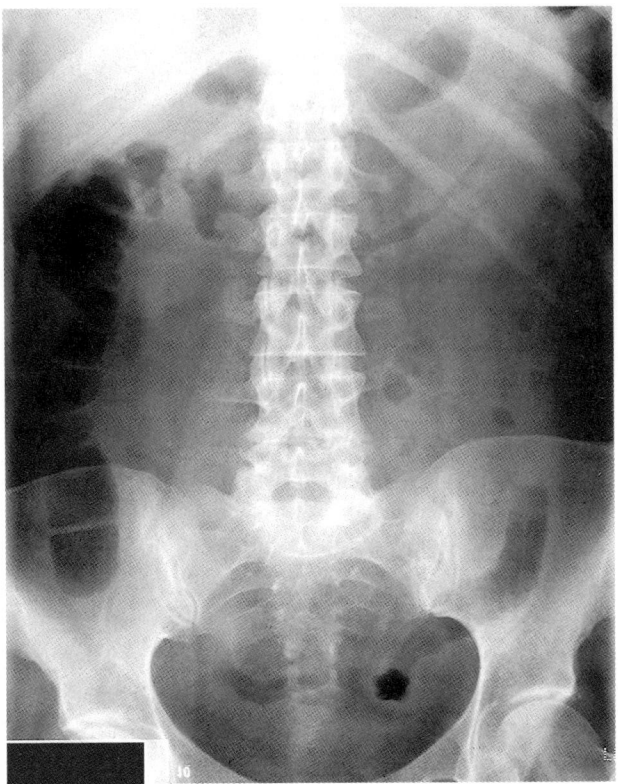

Figure 2.3 Plain abdominal film showing narrowing of the distal transverse colon and mucosal thickening.

extraluminal gas, since this is better seen on an erect chest X-ray, or to diagnose intestinal obstruction.

Gas may also be seen within the biliary tree in patients who have had a sphincterotomy, have a biliary enteric anastomosis or who have recently passed a gallstone. Gas in the portal veins appears as gas shadows which extend to the periphery of the liver because of portal vein blood flow. Gas may also be seen in splenic or mesenteric veins and within the bowel wall. This is seen in necrotizing enterocolitis, following umbilical vein catheterization and in erythroblastosis fetalis. In adults it is a grave prognostic sign in patients with mesenteric infarction and can be seen following embolus of air during double contrast barium enema in patients with severely ulcerated large bowel. It has been described in hemorrhagic pancreatitis.

Calcification may be looked for on a plain film within the gallbladder, pancreas and renal tract.

Free intraabdominal fluid results in medial displacement of the colonic gas shadows from the properitoneal fat line. It also leads to a ground glass appearance.

Intestinal transit

Colorectal function and constipation can be investigated by the assessment of the passage of ingested radioopaque markers (Fig. 2.4). On day 0 the patient ingests one capsule containing 20 radioopaque markers. Plain films of the abdomen are taken each day for the next 5 days. If more than 50% of the markers have been eliminated by day 5 the study is considered normal (Mezwa et al 1993).

If more than ten markers are retained the distribution of these can be documented and localization made of the abnormal segment of the gut. A film only on day 5 will give a gross evaluation of the degree of constipa-

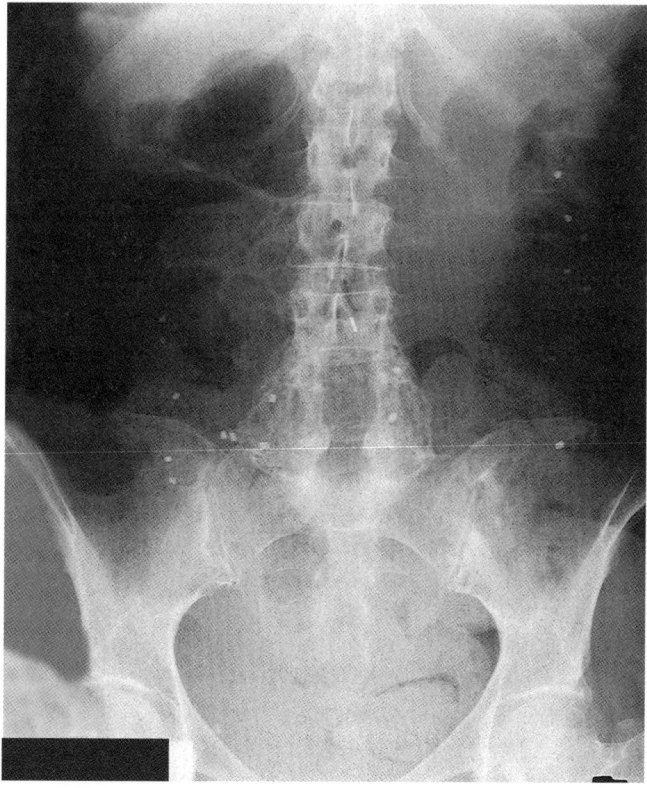

Figure 2.4 Plain abdominal X-ray showing retention of radioopaque markers in a patient with chronic constipation.

tion but will not assess any retrograde propulsion of colonic contents. Cathartics and laxatives should not be taken for 48 hours before and during the study.

CONTRAST RADIOGRAPHY
Oral cholecystography

Indications

1. Suspected cholelithiasis.
2. Suspected gallbladder mass.

This method has largely been replaced by ultrasound but it may be needed in patients in whom ultrasound has failed, usually due to obesity. It may also be used if ultrasound is doubtful in the diagnosis of a small, chronically contracted gallbladder. It is sometimes used to assess gallbladder function although this also may be done by ultrasound.

Barium swallow

Indications

1. Dysphagia.
2. Pain.
3. Assessment of tracheoesophageal fistula in children.

Barium swallow should not be used to assess anastomoses postoperatively because barium aspiration can be fatal. Water-soluble contrast media should be used in its place in this instance and also if the patient is suspected of aspirating for any other cause.

Barium swallow provides a dynamic evaluation of motility and double contrast films demonstrate morphology. Water-soluble contrast media should be used if perforation is suspected.

Swallowing dynamics are best examined using cineradiography or videofluoroscopy. The following features may be analyzed: tongue movement; soft palate elevation; epiglottic tilt; laryngeal closure; pharyngoesophageal segment (cricopharyngeal) opening and pharyngeal peristalsis (Lowe & Rubesin 1993).

Double contrast spot films may then be taken. The presence of gastroesophageal reflux may be assessed by tipping the patient head down or by asking him to cough.

A double contrast study has a sensitivity of 75–90% in diagnosing reflux esophagitis, depending on the severity (Creteus et al 1983, Graziani et al 1983, Koehler et al 1980). The barium swallow may also be used to diagnose infectious and drug-induced esophagitis.

Aspiration occurs when contrast medium enters the laryngeal vestibule between swallows during normal respiration. If this is suspected, a water-soluble contrast medium should be used rather than barium. It is associated with stasis in the pharynx. This may be due to neuromuscular disorders, tumor, pharyngeal pouch or diverticulum. Aspiration can also occur during gastroesophageal reflux or may be due to an obstruction in the lower esophagus. A prominent cricopharyngeus is also seen often in patients with gastroesophageal reflux or esophageal obstruction. It may also be due to abnormal pharyngeal peristalsis. Pharyngeal diverticula and pouches may be demonstrated by barium swallow, a Zenker's diverticulum often being associated with gastroesophageal reflux and hiatus hernia (Lowe & Rubesin 1993).

Malignant pharyngeal and esophageal tumors may be diagnosed by their irregular narrowing of the lumen associated with mucosal destruction ulceration and shouldering. Narrowing of the esophagus by mediastinal tumors causes an extrinsic mass effect unless the tumor directly invades the esophagus. Smooth esophageal narrowing may be due to previous radiotherapy, caustic ingestion and dermatological disorders. An esophageal web appears as a narrow shelflike band usually in the cervical esophagus. Esophageal varices may be missed if the esophagus is distended.

Barium swallow may also be used to evaluate various motility disorders including achalasia, diffuse esophageal spasm, etc.

Barium meal (Fig. 2.5)

Indications

1. Dyspepsia.
2. Weight loss.
3. Upper abdominal mass.
4. Gastrointestinal hemorrhage.
5. Partial obstruction.

Contraindications

1. Complete large bowel obstruction.
2. Suspected site of perforation (unless a water-soluble contrast medium is used rather than barium sulfate).

A gas-producing agent is swallowed. The patient then drinks the barium. The patient is turned to achieve adequate coating of the stomach and double contrast views are obtained. An IV injection of a smooth muscle relaxant (buscopan or glucagon) is given and views of the duodenum are taken.

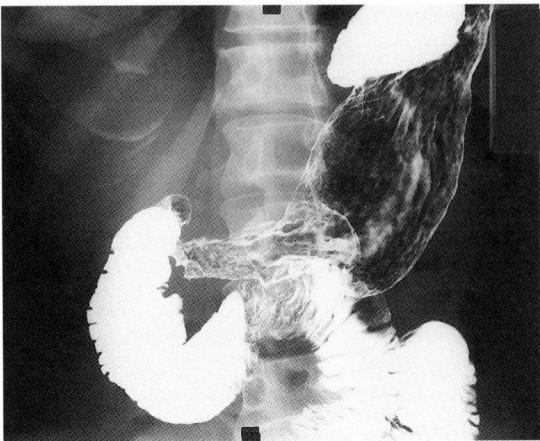

Figure 2.5 Barium meal showing carcinoma of the gastric antrum.

Barium meal may be used to diagnose gastritis and peptic ulceration. Ulcers greater than 5 mm in size are more likely to be detected on barium study than smaller ones. The size of the ulcer has no relationship to the presence of carcinoma (Levine 1994). There is debate whether barium studies can distinguish benign ulcers from malignant ones. Earlier single contrast barium studies suggested that 6–16% of gastric ulcers that appeared to be benign were malignant but more recent double contrast studies have suggested that virtually all gastric ulcers with an unequivocally benign appearance on double contrast studies are, in fact, benign lesions (Thompson et al 1983, Levine et al 1987). Ulcers that have an equivocal suspicious appearance should be evaluated endoscopically. Erosive gastritis is fairly frequently seen on double contrast studies but rarely on single contrast studies. Atrophic gastritis, eosinophilic gastritis and involvement of the stomach by Crohn's disease may also be shown. Benign tumors such as hyperplastic polyps and adenomatous polyps may be demonstrated. Congenital conditions such as ectopic pancreatic rests and duplication cysts can also be seen.

Barium follow-through/small bowel meal

Indications

1. Pain.
2. Diarrhea.
3. Bleeding.
4. Partial obstruction (Fig. 2.6).

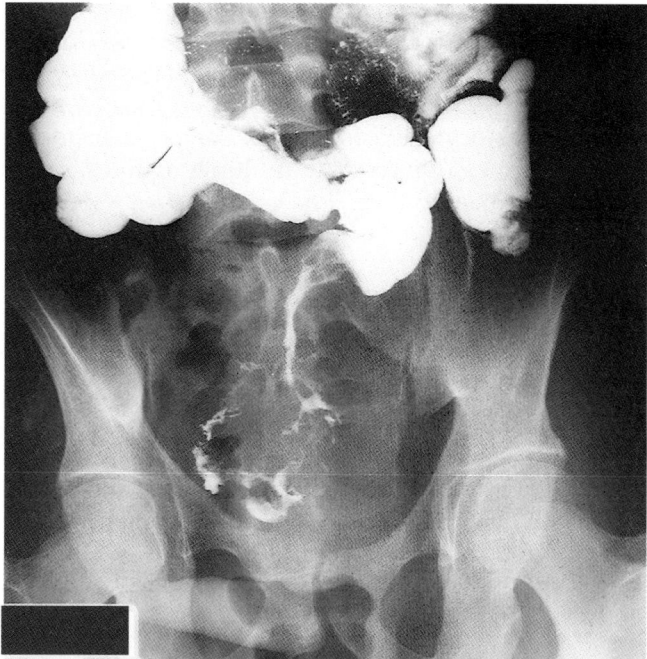

Figure 2.6   Barium contrast radiograph showing a long stricture in the ileum due to Crohn's disease.

Contraindications

1. Complete obstruction.
2. Suspected perforation unless a water-soluble contrast medium is used rather than barium sulfate.

This is generally better performed as a dedicated study rather than a study following a barium meal. The relaxant given for a barium meal will hinder the passage of barium through the small bowel.

The conditions demonstrated by a small bowel meal and small bowel enema may be divided into those that give dilatation of small bowel loops (mechanical obstruction, celiac disease, tropical sprue, dermatitis herpetiformis, scleroderma, postvagotomy) and those that give dilatation with thickened folds (ischemia, Crohn's disease, radiotherapy, lymphoma, Zollinger–Ellison syndrome) (Chapman & Nakielny 1995). Other conditions may give rise to strictures, e.g. Crohn's disease, ischemia, radiotherapy, tumors, tuberculosis and actinomycosis.

Some conditions give rise to thickened folds in non-dilated small bowel which are irregular and distorted, e.g. Crohn's disease, Zollinger–Ellison syndrome, lymphoma, metastases, carcinoid and tuberculosis, which all give localized involvement. Other conditions, such as amyloidosis, eosinophilic enteritis, mastocytosis, Whipple's disease, Crohn's disease, giardiasis and strongyloides, give rise to widespread changes. Some conditions, such as nodular lymphoid hyperplasia, Crohn's disease, Whipple's disease, mastocytosis, lymphoma, polyposis, metastases, typhoid and yersinia infection, can give rise to multiple nodules within the small bowel (Chapman & Nakielny 1995).

Small bowel enema

Indications

1. As for small bowel meal.

It is more time-consuming for the radiologist and more unpleasant for the patient but it allows better visualization of the small bowel.

A Bilboa-Dotter tube or similar with a guidewire is introduced into the duodenum and advanced to the level of the ligament of Treitz. Dilute barium is then run in quickly or dilute barium followed by methyl cellulose. Spot films are taken of the barium column and its leading edge at regions of interest until the colon is reached.

Complications

1. Aspiration.
2. Perforation of the bowel by the guidewire.

For discussion, see under small bowel meal, above.

Barium enema

Indications

1. Change in bowel habit.
2. Pain.
3. Mass.
4. Melena.
5. Large bowel obstruction.

Contraindications

1. Toxic megacolon.
2. Pseudomembranous colitis.
3. Rectal biopsy within the previous 7 days.

Patient preparation is important to obtain a clear colon. A disposable enema catheter is inserted into the rectum; it is then connected to the barium reservoir and handpump. IV injection of muscle relaxant (buscopan or glucagon) is given. Barium is infused to the region of the splenic flexure. Air is then gently pumped into the bowel which forces the column of barium round to the cecum. This produces a double contrast effect.

Complications

1. Perforation of the bowel.
2. Venous extravasation.
3. Water intoxication.
4. Intramural barium.
5. Cardiac arrhythmia due to rectal distension.
6. Transient bacteremia (patients with prosthetic heart valves should receive prophylactic antibiotic cover).
7. Side-effects of muscle relaxant.

Barium enema may be difficult for a frail or elderly patient to tolerate and in those patients who have tortuous long colons it may be difficult to reach and adequately coat the cecum. Barium enema will outline diverticula and show the muscle hypertrophy. A diagnosis of perforated diverticulitis can only be made when there is extravasation of contrast material from a diverticulum. Computed tomography (CT) is more sensitive for the diagnosis of diverticulitis with inflammatory changes in the pericolic fat being seen in 98% of patients (Balthazar 1994). Barium enema may be used to document the distribution of active disease in patients with ulcerative colitis or Crohn's disease. Again, mesenteric involvement and abscess formation are better demonstrated by CT.

Colonic polyps and colonic cancer may be diagnosed by barium enema (Fig. 2.7). There is debate whether colonoscopy is superior to contrast enema for the detection of polypoid lesions but there may be failure to reach the cecum in up to 25% of cases in colonoscopy. Thoeni and Laufer (1994) claim that colonoscopy and double contrast enema examinations have comparable overall accuracy with the detection of approximately 90% of lesions.

Benign strictures secondary to ischemia or long-standing inflammatory bowel disease are also demonstrated by barium enema.

The instant barium enema

This is performed without bowel preparation because a colon involved by inflammatory bowel disease does not contain fecal residue.

Indications

1. Extent and severity of disease in active ulcerative colitis.

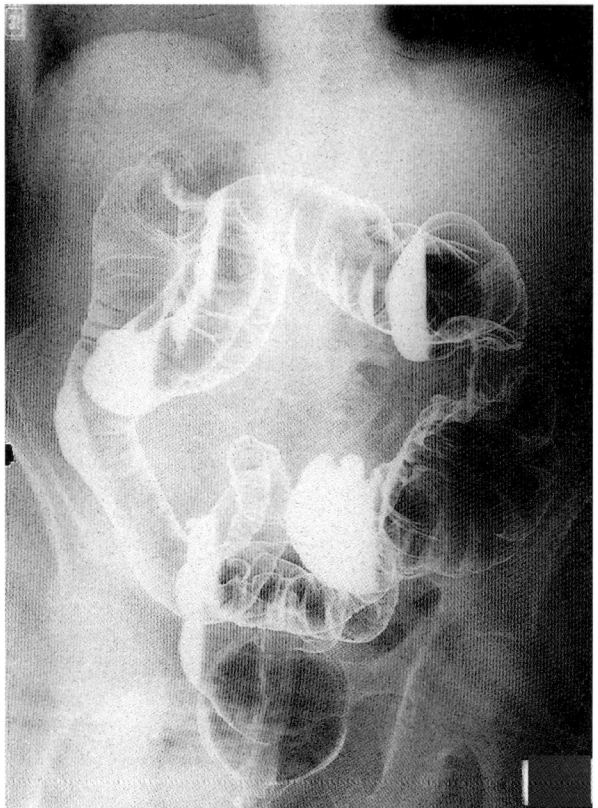

Figure 2.7 Double contrast barium enema showing an 'apple core' lesion in the descending colon suggesting a carcinoma.

Contraindications

1. Toxic megacolon.
2. Rectal biopsy within the previous 7 days.
3. Long-standing ulcerative colitis – this is not the examination to exclude a carcinoma.
4. Crohn's colitis unless there is severe anal disease making bowel preparation intolerable.

Barium enema reduction of an intussusception

Contraindications

1. Evidence of peritonitis or perforation.
2. Advanced intestinal obstruction.

Defecating proctography (Mezwa et al 1993)

Indications

1. Abnormal intestinal transit study markers accumulating in rectum and sigmoid.
2. Difficulty in emptying rectum.
3. Sensation of rectal obstruction.
4. Unexplained rectal bleeding.
5. Mucous discharge.
6. Incontinence.
7. Urge to defecate.
8. Incomplete evacuation.
9. Perineal pain.
10. Suspected prolapse.
11. Aided evacuation.

The vagina is marked with gel and water-soluble contrast medium (Mezwa et al 1993). Barium paste is then introduced into the rectum and the patient placed on a commode. Films are taken in natural position while the patient is at rest, straining and with maximum squeezing. Features that should be assessed are (Mathieu et al 1984):

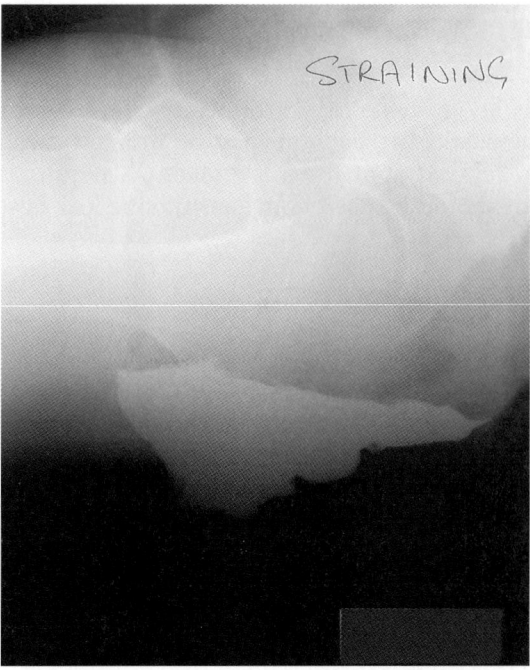

Figure 2.8   Barium proctogram from a patient with a large anterior rectocele.

1. the anorectal angle (85–130°);
2. obliteration of the posterior impression by puborectalis sling;
3. the aperture of the anal canal;
4. evacuation of rectal contents;
5. pelvic floor descent (should be less than 2–3 cm);
6. presence of rectocele or enterocele (Fig. 2.8);
7. internal intussusception;
8. rectal prolapse.

Sinogram

Indications

1. Investigation of a sinus/fistula.

Water-soluble contrast medium is used. A fine catheter is inserted into the orifice of the sinus and contrast medium injected with screening. Films are taken as required.

Loopogram and retrograde ileogram

Indications

1. To investigate the bowel proximal to a colostomy or ileostomy (Fig. 2.9).

The tip of a Foley catheter is introduced a few centimeters into the appropriate stoma and the balloon may be inflated carefully. Barium is run into the bowel and spot films are taken as required. Water-soluble contrast medium should be used if an anastomotic leak is suspected.

Intravenous cholangiography

Indications

These are subject to debate at present. Forty five percent of examinations may not provide adequate visualization of the biliary tree and there may be a significant diagnostic error even in adequate studies (Goodman et al 1980). Many of the indications can be resolved by other imaging modalities, e.g. ultrasound, CT and ERCP.

1. Further assessment of non-functioning gallbladder.
2. Postcholecystectomy patients with recurrent symptoms.
3. Preoperatively to exclude common bile duct calculi (the biliary tract is only likely to be visualized when the serum bilirubin is less than 50 micromoles per liter).

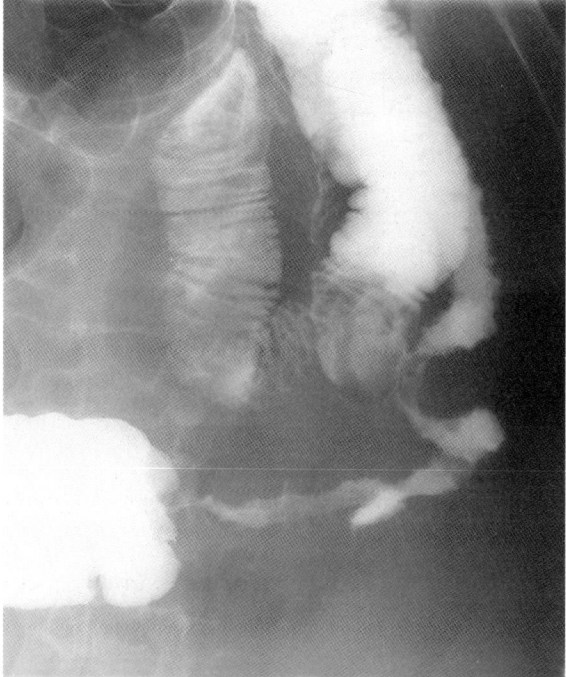

Figure 2.9   Retrograde barium contrast study showing recurrent Crohn's disease at the ileocolonic anastomosis (courtesy of Dr A. Grundy).

Contraindications

1. Severe hepatorenal disease;
2. Oral cholecystography within the previous week; because the incidence of toxic effects is increased, the ducts are less likely to be visualized.

A slow infusion of 100 mL of biligram (meglumine ioglycamate) for infusion over 45–60 minutes, endobil (meglumine iodoxamate) for infusion over 15–30 minutes or biliscopin (meglumine iotroxate) for infusion over 15–30 minutes. Films are taken at the end of the infusion and every 15 minutes until contrast medium reaches the duodenum. Tomography may be helpful. Glucagon 1 mg IV after the first infusion film may improve visualization of the common bile duct (Evans & Whitehouse 1980).

Complications

1. Mortality rate of one in 5000.
2. Impaired liver function – dose related.
3. Uricosuric action.

4. Precipitation of Bence-Jones protein and IgM macroglobulin.
5. Renal impairment, less common with oral cholecystographic agents.

Postoperative (T-tube) cholangiography

Indications

1. To exclude biliary tract calculi following surgery of the common duct.
2. After liver transplantation to assess the biliary anastomosis.

Examination is performed in non-transplant patients on or about the tenth postoperative day prior to pulling out the T-tube. The drainage tube is clamped off near the patient and cleaned. A 23 gauge butterfly needle, extension tubing and syringe are assembled and filled with contrast medium, all air bubbles being expelled. The needle is then inserted into the tubing and contrast injected into the T-tube.

Complications

1. Injection of contrast medium under high pressure into an obstructed tract can rarely produce septicemia.

Percutaneous transhepatic cholangiography

Indications

1. Undiagnosed jaundice, particularly when it is believed to be due to extrahepatic obstruction.

Contraindications

1. Bleeding propensity.
2. Platelet count less than 100 000.
3. Prothrombin time 2 seconds greater than control.
4. Biliary tract sepsis.
5. Hydatid disease.

Surgical facilities should be available. Prophylactic antibiotics are necessary 24 hours before and for 3 days after the examination. A fine flexible 22 gauge needle is inserted into the liver during suspended respiration using local anesthesia. Contrast medium is then injected under fluoroscopic control while the needle is slowly withdrawn until a duct is entered. If no ducts are entered on the first attempt, further attempts are made. The procedure is abandoned after ten attempts if a duct has not been entered. Contrast medium is injected to fill the duct system and to define the lower end of an obstruction.

Complications

1. Bacteremia, septicemia and endotoxic shock.
2. Bile leakage may lead to biliary peritonitis. This is more likely with ducts under pressure and if there are multiple puncture attempts but less likely if a drainage catheter is left in situ.
3. Cholangitis.
4. Subphrenic abscess.
5. Hemorrhage.
6. Puncture of extrahepatic structures (usually no serious sequelae).
7. Intrathoracic injection.
8. Shock, owing to injection into the region of the celiac plexus.

Angiography

Indications

1. Gastrointestinal bleeding (Fig. 2.10).
2. Detection of vascular tumors.
3. Further assessment of focal liver lesions following ultrasound, CT or magnetic resonance imaging (MRI).

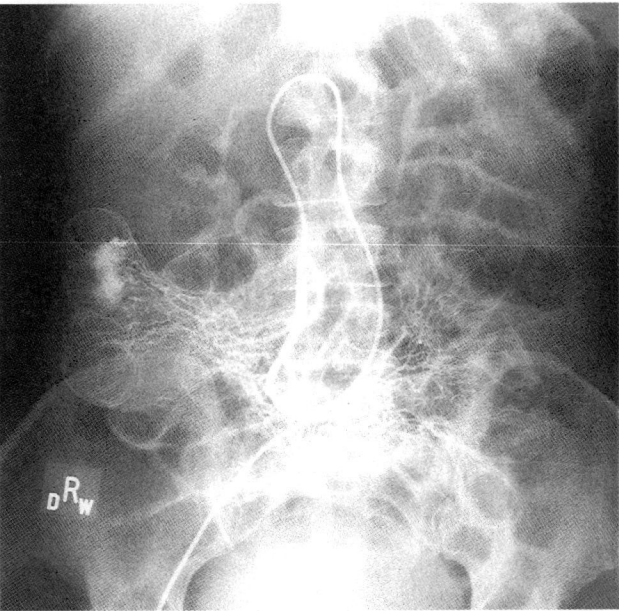

Figure 2.10   Angiogram showing the bleeding site in the ileum (courtesy of Dr A. Grundy).

Contraindications (relative)

1. Recent barium may obscure the examination.
2. Bleeding tendency.

Generally puncture is made into a femoral artery using the Seldinger technique. A guidewire is passed into the artery with a catheter following. Selective catheterization of the vessels of interest is performed and contrast medium is generally injected via a pump. Films may be obtained to show the arterial and/or venous phase. Catheterization and injection of the celiac axis and SMA will allow assessment of the portal venous system.

Complications

1. Hematoma.
2. Pseudoaneurysm formation at the puncture site.
3. Allergy to contrast medium.

ULTRASOUND

Ultrasound does not use ionizing radiation and so does not have its attendant risks. Ultrasound machines are relatively inexpensive and are generally portable, allowing the patient to be examined at the bedside or in clinics. Doppler ultrasound allows assessment of flow within vessels and the addition of color flow Doppler greatly enhances its usefulness.

Ultrasound of liver

Indications

1. Suspected focal or diffuse liver disease.
2. Staging of known extrahepatic malignancy.
3. Right upper quadrant pain or mass.
4. Hepatomegaly.
5. Jaundice.
6. Abnormal liver function tests.
7. Pyrexia of unknown origin.
8. Ultrasound guided biopsy.

Ultrasound allows assessment of the liver texture with recognition of generalized disorders, e.g. fatty liver (Taylor et al 1986, Saverymuttu et al 1986) and cirrhosis (Joseph et al 1991, Di Lelio et al 1989, Newbury & Clarke 1979). Focal lesions can be identified although ultrasound is not as sensitive as CT and MRI (Wernecke et al 1991). It will allow differentiation between fluid and solid lesions and can be used to guide percutaneous biopsy.

Flow and direction of flow may be assessed within the portal vein, hepatic veins and hepatic arteries. The intrahepatic and extrahepatic biliary tree may also be assessed. The internal diameter of the common hepatic duct is 4 mm or less in a normal adult; 5 mm is borderline, 6 mm is considered dilated. The lower common duct (common bile duct) is normally 6 mm or less but distinction of the common hepatic duct from the common bile duct depends on identification of the insertion of the cystic duct which is often not possible with ultrasound.

Ultrasound of the gallbladder and biliary system

Indications

1. Suspected gallstones.
2. Right upper quadrant pain.
3. Jaundice.
4. PUO and acute pancreatitis.
5. To assess gallbladder function.
6. Guided percutaneous procedure.

It is imperative that the gallbladder is scanned in a fasted patient. Stones can be recognized within the fluid-filled gallbladder because of their echogenic appearance and posterior acoustic shadowing (Fig. 2.11). Fasting gallbladder volume may be assessed by measuring longitudinal transverse and AP diameters. The normal gallbladder contracts, reducing the volume by more than 25% 30 minutes after a standard fatty meal. There is disagreement as to whether the normal common bile duct dilates after cholecystectomy. The common bile duct may measure more than 6 mm in these patients but if the patient is symptomatic further investigation by ERCP is required. The common bile duct should never measure more than 1 cm in these patients.

Ultrasound of the pancreas

Indications

1. Suspected pancreatic tumor.
2. Pancreatitis with complications.
3. Epigastric mass.
4. Epigastric pain.
5. Jaundice.
6. Ultrasound guided biopsy.

Again the patient should be scanned fasted. In a young adult the texture of the pancreas is very similar to that of the liver but increasing age causes

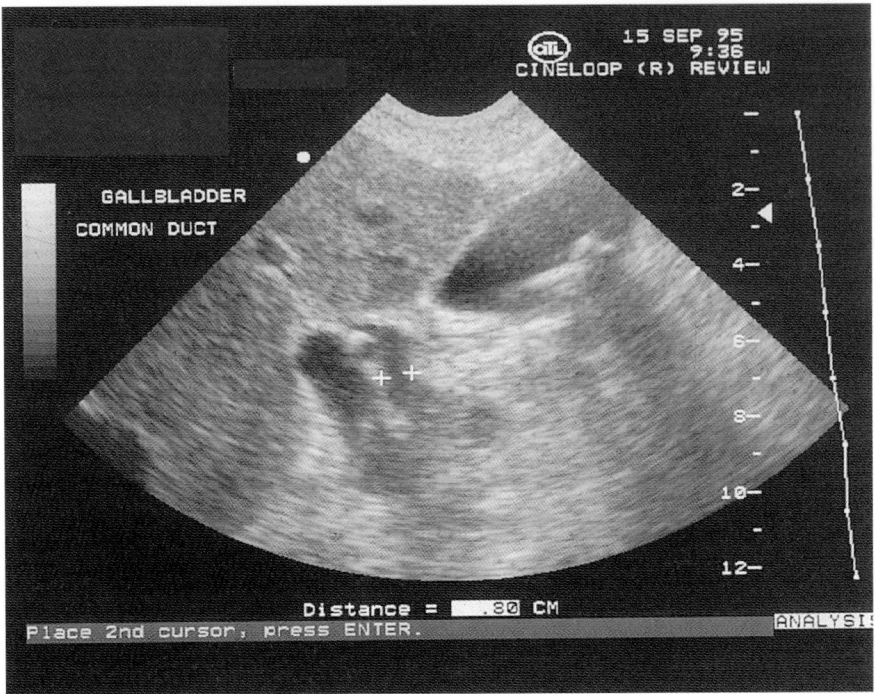

Figure 2.11 Ultrasound scans showing gallbladder with multiple stones and dilatation of the common bile duct.

increasing fatty infiltration of the pancreas which results in the pancreas becoming more echogenic.

The normal pancreatic duct should not measure more than 3 mm in the head or 2 mm in the body. The normal AP diameter of the pancreatic head is 2.7 ± 0.7 cm and the craniocaudal measurement is 3.6 ± 1.2 cm (Haber et al 1976). Coarsening of the echotexture is recognized in patients with chronic pancreatitis; the presence of duct dilatation and pancreatic stones may also be seen. Ultrasound will readily detect peripancreatic fluid collections if these are not obscured by bowel gas.

Ultrasound of the spleen

Indications

1. Portal hypertension.
2. Left upper quadrant pain.
3. Left upper quadrant mass.

The normal spleen is homogeneous in echotexture and measures less than 13 cm in length. The vessels at the splenic hilum may be assessed using ultrasound and Doppler and this allows recognition of lienorenal shunting and other collateral vessels.

Ultrasound of gut and peritoneum

Indications

1. Mass.
2. Abdominal distension.
3. Suspected appendicitis.
4. Inflammatory bowel disease.

Ultrasound has established a role in the investigation of suspected acute appendicitis. The diameter of the normal appendix is usually 5 mm or less, of an inflamed one 6 mm or more (Puylaert 1994). The ultrasonographer may diagnose an abscess which can then be drained percutaneously and recognize an inflammatory mass but not be able to differentiate between inflamed bowel wall and adjacent fat and an established abscess. CT will be necessary in this situation. Ultrasound can show thickening of bowel wall but may not be able to differentiate between inflammation and tumor. It has been suggested that ultrasound can be used to follow up patients with Crohn's disease to assess response to treatment (Dubbins 1984).

COMPUTED TOMOGRAPHY (CT)

CT of the abdomen

Indications

1. Staging known gastrointestinal malignancy (Fig. 2.12) and assessment of response to treatment (Fig. 2.13).
2. Investigation of mass.
3. Investigation of suspected gastrointestinal malignancy especially in patients unable to tolerate barium examination (Fig. 2.14).
4. Abnormal LFTs – after ultrasound.
5. Inflammatory bowel disease.
6. Pancreatitis.
7. PUO.
8. Diagnosis of recurrent rectal cancer.

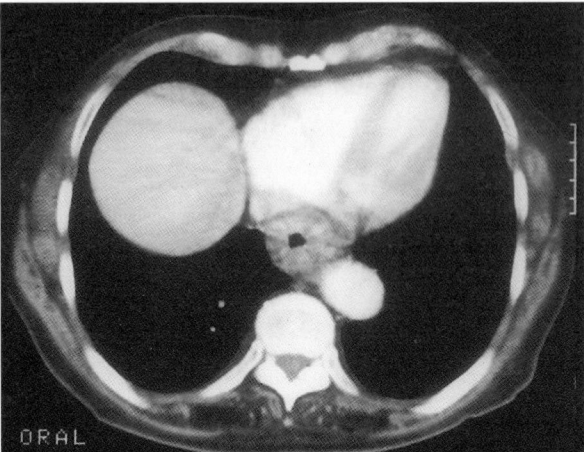

Figure 2.12 CT scan showing the lower esophageal wall with tumor abutting the aorta.

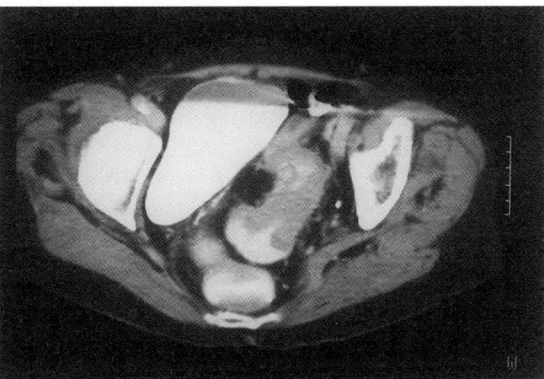

Figure 2.13 CT scan showing typical 'apple core' appearance of a carcinoma of the sigmoid colon.

9. Trauma – suspected organ rupture or laceration.
10. CT guided interventional procedures.

Contraindications

1. Pregnancy.
2. Allergy to IV iodinated contrast medium (relative: CT scan could be performed without contrast).

Computed tomography uses a finely collimated X-ray beam and detectors which rotate around the patient producing generally an axial image after

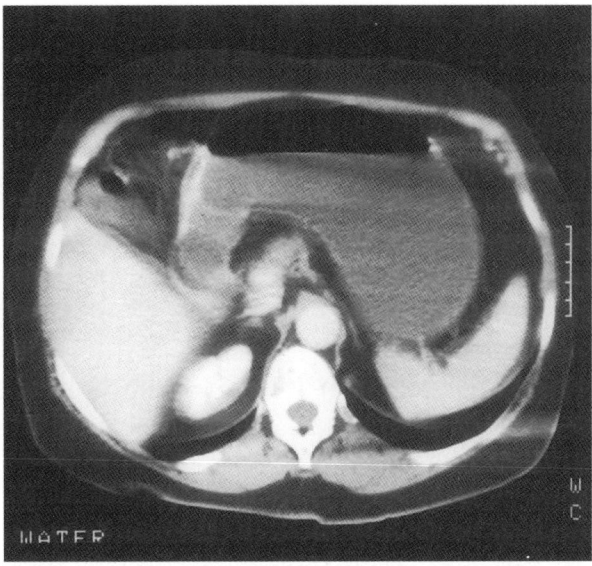

Figure 2.14 CT scan following intravenous contrast medium with the stomach distended with water showing a focal area of thickening in the antrum.

computerized processing of the digital information. Its use has increased since its introduction in the early 1970's and it now contributes heavily to the total national radiation dose. The average effective dose from a CT of the abdomen is equivalent to 4 years of natural background irradiation (Chapman & Nakielny 1993).

CT of the liver

Indications

See above. CT is more sensitive than ultrasound for detection of focal hepatic lesions, but dynamic IV contrast enhanced CT scans should be obtained (Fig. 2.15).

CT of the pancreas

Indications

See above. Again dynamic IV contrast enhanced scans should be obtained. Precontrast scans may be useful to detect pancreatic calcification. Post-contrast CT scans are useful in patients with acute pancreatitis to assess the degree of pancreatic necrosis and to detect abscess or pseudocyst formation.

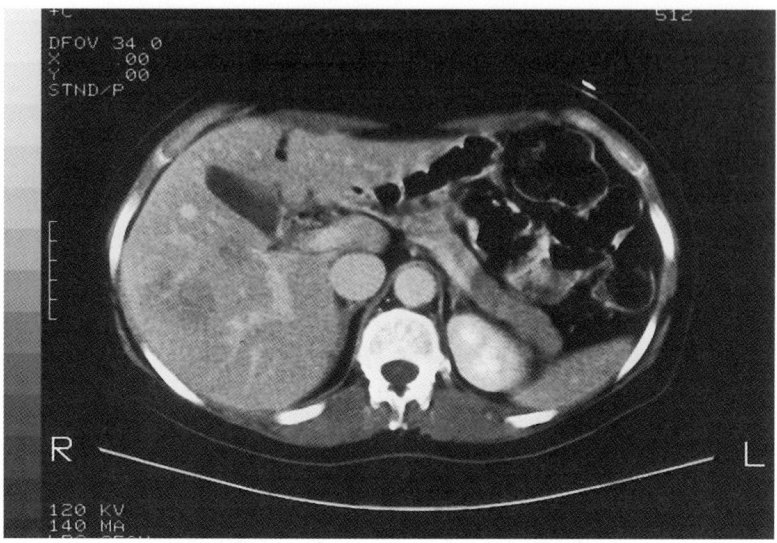

Figure 2.15 Enhanced CT showing metastatic deposits in the liver (courtesy of Dr A. Grundy).

CT of the spleen

Indications

See above. Focal splenic defects following IV contrast enhancement may be due to cyst, tumor, abscess or infarction.

CT of the gut (Fig. 2.16)

Indications

See above. CT is commonly used to investigate patients with carcinoma of the esophagus and stomach to assess resectability of the local tumor and to detect distant metastases. Abnormal lymph nodes are recognized on CT by an increase in size from normal. CT cannot distinguish between reactive and involved lymph nodes or detect micrometastases in normal sized nodes. This lowers the accuracy of CT in staging nodal disease. CT is more accurate in staging advanced tumors than in finding early ones. The accuracy of CT for staging esophageal cancer (combined data from six series reported by Halvorsen & Thompson 1989) ranges from 98% for the detection of liver metastases to 70% for the detection of mediastinal adenopathy.

CT is reasonably accurate at determining the presence of local invasion with accuracies of 97% for tracheobronchial invasion, 94% for aortic

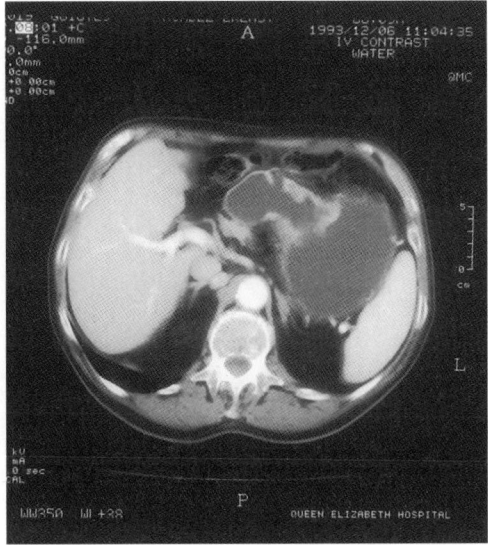

Figure 2.16 CT scan showing recurrent gastric cancer following previous gastroenterostomy.

invasion and 94% for pericardial invasion. For gastric cancer, CT has an overall accuracy of 72% when compared to surgery (Kleinhaus & Militianu 1988). Another study comparing preoperative CT and operative staging in 75 patients demonstrated that 31% of patients were under-staged and 16% overstaged by CT (Sussman et al 1988).

CT is used less often to stage colorectal cancer, resectability being judged on clinical examination. CT has recently been shown to have an accuracy of 52% for the local staging of rectal cancer compared with an accuracy of 81% for transrectal ultrasound (Goldman et al 1991). It may be used to investigate more advanced tumors and to assess response to radiotherapy or chemotherapy.

Separation of bowel loops on barium studies in patients with Crohn's disease may be due to lymphadenopathy, fibrofatty proliferation, phleg-mon or abscess (Gore 1989). CT can be used to differentiate between these in a patient with an unexplained fever. It can also be used to exclude an abscess elsewhere in the abdomen or pelvis. The large bowel will be opacified if oral contrast is given 24–48 hours before the CT examination is performed and CT can then be used to exclude a lesion of significant size in a patient too infirm to undergo barium enema (Day et al 1993). This technique may not show small polyps, but these are unlikely to be significant in a patient who is this unwell.

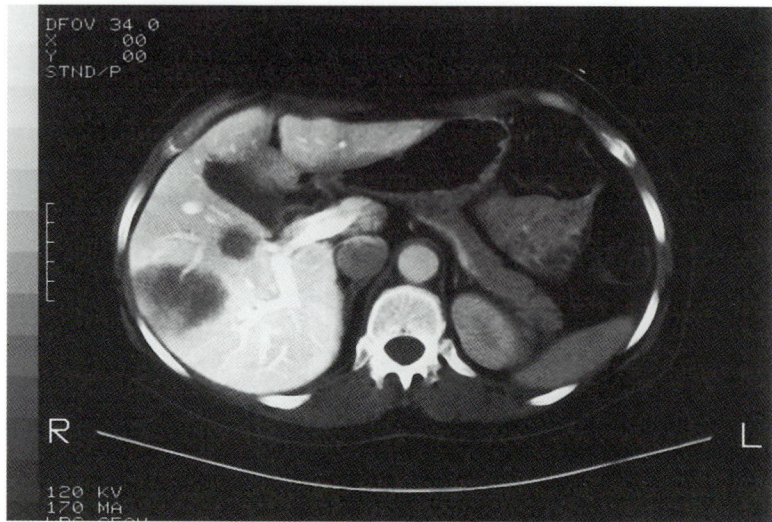

Figure 2.17 CT portogram showing metastatic deposits in the liver (courtesy of Dr A. Grundy).

CT arterioportography

Indications

1. Suspected focal hepatic lesions usually prior to surgical resection (Fig. 2.17).

Contraindications

1. Allergy to IV iodinated contrast medium.

This is currently the most sensitive imaging technique for the detection of focal liver metastases but it is invasive. It is used as part of the assessment of patients who are to undergo hepatic resection for liver metastatic disease (Soyer et al 1992, McGrath et al 1993).

MAGNETIC RESONANCE IMAGING (MRI)

This is a relatively new addition to diagnostic imaging. This technique requires a homogeneous magnetic field, most commercial units operating at 0.5–1.5 Tessa (T) field strength, and radiowaves. Its main advantages are the ability to image in any plane, a soft tissue contrast superior to that of CT and the absence of ionizing radiation. Its uses are still evolving but currently it has been proved to be similar to CT for the detection of focal hepatic lesions (Wernecke et al 1991) and staging rectal cancer (Thoeni 1991). At present it lacks a good bowel contrast agent which also allows assessment of bowel wall. Intravenous gadolinium is used in much the same way as IV iodinated contrast agents in CT. Flowing blood will give rise to a flow void on spin echo sequences and MR angiography can be performed to assess major vessels. Gadolinium-enhanced images can be obtained to assess portal vein patency. It is contraindicated in the first trimester of pregnancy.

MRI of the liver

Indications

1. Right upper quadrant mass.
2. Detection of focal hepatic disease.
3. Staging of hepatic tumors.

Specific liver MR contrast agents are being developed which will increase sensitivity to focal disease (Mitchell 1993, Rofsky et al 1993, Ni et al 1993). At present gradient echo T1 weighted breathhold and T2 spin echo sequences are standard. T2 weighted spin echo sequences with a long echo time may allow differentiation of cavernous hemangioma and cysts from other solid liver lesions. A turbo T2 weighted spin echo sequence with a long echo time can be used to examine the biliary tree.

MRI of the pancreas

Indications

1. Suspected islet cell tumor.
2. Investigation of suspected pancreatic mass.
3. Chronic pancreatitis.

MRI is proving to be the investigation of choice in patients with suspected islet cell tumors (Semelka et al 1993a). It can be used to detect and stage pancreatic cancer (Vellet et al 1992, Semelka et al 1993a) and some authors claim that the development of fibrosis can be detected at an early stage in patients with chronic pancreatitis (Semelka et al 1993b). Calcification is not as easily recognized on MRI as CT. It has little place in the diagnosis of acute pancreatitis but can detect fluid collections.

MRI of the pelvis

Indications

1. Staging rectal cancer.
2. Assessment of perianal disease in inflammatory bowel disease.
3. Detection of recurrent disease.

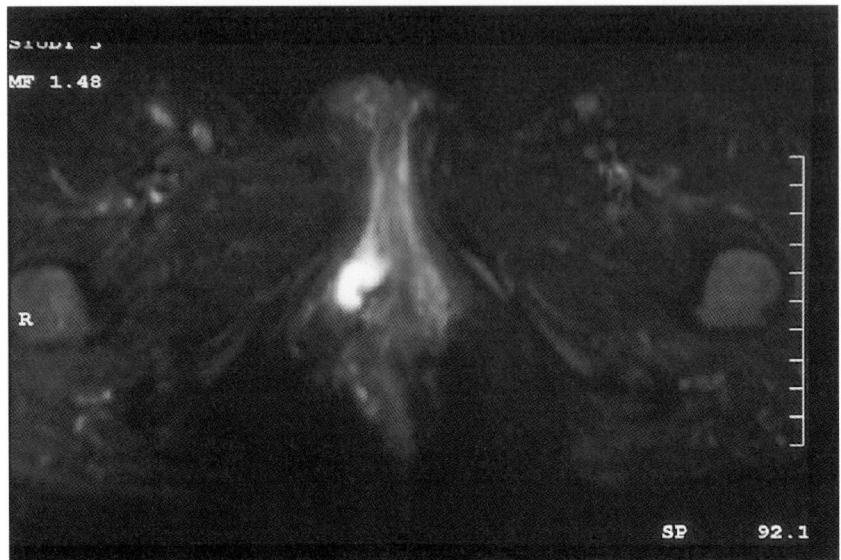

Figure 2.18 MRI scan showing right perianal fistulae and a focus of sepsis in relation to the right labium.

Comparisons of CT, MRI and transrectal ultrasound (TRUS) to determine the most effective imaging technique for preoperative staging and follow-up for recurrence have shown MRI to be similar to CT for the preoperative staging but that MRI and TRUS are superior to CT for the detection of recurrent disease (Krestin et al 1988, Gonberg et al 1986, Waizer et al 1991, Thoeni 1991).

The use of an endorectal coil will improve accuracy of the staging of rectal cancer (Chan et al 1991). Dynamic MRI imaging has been suggested for the diagnosis of recurrent rectal cancer (Muller–Schimpfle et al 1993).

MRI has recently been shown to be extremely useful in the assessment of perianal disease in patients with Crohn's disease and in patients with complex perianal fistulae (Koebel et al 1989, Barker et al 1994) (Fig. 2.18). The use of coronal and axial scans using T1 weighted spin echo and STIR sequences allows the recognition of tracks and abscesses and their relationship to the sphincters and levator ani muscles.

NUCLEAR MEDICINE

These techniques use radioisotope-labeled substances which therefore result in the patient receiving ionizing radiation.

Radionuclide gastroesophageal reflux study

Indications

1. Diagnosis and quantification of gastroesophageal reflux.
2. Assessment of response to treatment.

Radiopharmaceuticals

^{99m}Tc colloid or ^{99m}Tc DTPA mixed with acidified orange juice/normal milk feed (babies).

Radionuclide gastric emptying

Indications

1. Gastric stasis and dumping.
2. Diabetic gastropathy.
3. Gastric positioning.
4. Assessment of side-effects of drugs altering gastric motility.

Contraindications

1. Vomiting.

Radiopharmaceuticals

No standard has yet been developed and emptying rate is influenced by the content of the 'meal'. For further information see Chapman & Nakielny 1993 and Harding & Robinson 1990.

Radionuclide bile reflux study

Indications

1. Persistent symptoms postgastrectomy.
2. Persistent symptoms postcholecystectomy.

Radiopharmaceuticals

^{99m}Tc labeled derivatives of iminodiacetic acid (HIDA) 75–150 MBq

Radionuclide Meckel's diverticulum scan

Indications

1. Suspected Meckel's diverticulum.

Radiopharmaceuticals

^{99m}Tc pertechnetate 200–400 MBq max.

Radionuclide investigation of gastrointestinal (GI) bleeding

Indications

1. Active GI bleeding.

Contraindications

1. No active bleeding.
2. Slow bleeding less than 0.1 mL/min.
3. Recent barium study (may obscure bleeding site).

Radiopharmaceuticals

1. ^{99m}Tc in vivo labeled red blood cells 400 MBq max.
2. ^{99m}Tc colloid 400 MBq max. shown to be less sensitive (Harding & Robinson 1990).

Radiolabeled colloid liver scan

Indications

1. Hepatic space-occupying lesions – not as sensitive as ultrasound, CT or MRI.
2. Diffuse liver disease.

Radiopharmaceuticals

^{99m}Tc colloid 80 MBq max. Hemangiomas will show an area of increased blood volume on blood pool images using ^{99m}Tc labeled blood cells (Front et al 1981, Moinuddin et al 1985).

Dynamic radionuclide hepatobiliary imaging

Indications

1. Suspected acute cholecystitis – after normal US.
2. Suspected biliary obstruction – after normal US.
3. Assessment of neonatal jaundice.
4. Suspected bile leak – after normal US.

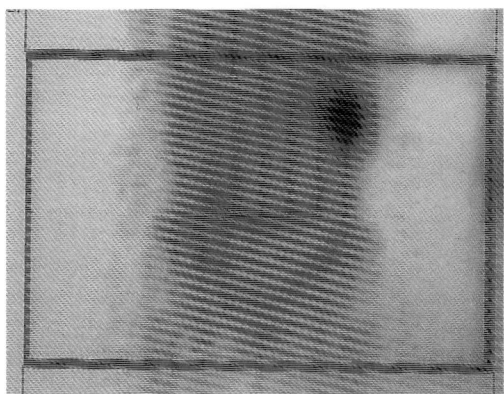

Figure 2.19   Radio labeled white cell scan showing uptake in the whole colon and rectum.

Radiopharmaceuticals

99mTc-diethyl-iminoacetic acid (HIDA).

111Indium labeled leukocytes scan (Fig. 2.19)

Indications

1. Suspected inflammatory bowel disease.
2. Suspected abscess.

Radiopharmaceuticals

111Indium 20 MBq max. (67Gallium citrate may be superior for chronic infection).

Imaging

111Indium labeled leukocytes at 3, 24 and possibly 48 hours postinjection; 67Gallium citrate 48 and 72 hours postinjection.

FURTHER READING

Balthazar E J 1994 Diverticular disease. In: Textbook of gastrointestinal radiology. W B Saunders, Philadelphia, pp 1092–1097

Barker P G, Lunniss P J, Armstrong P, Reznek R H, Cotton K, Phillips R K 1994 Magnetic resonance imaging of fistula in ano: technique, interpretation and accuracy. Clinical Radiology 49: 7–13

Chan T W, Kresser H Y, Milestone B et al 1991 Rectal carcinoma: staging of MR imaging with endorectal surface coil. Radiology 181: 461–467

Chapman S, Nakielny R 1995 Aids to radiological differential diagnosis, 3rd edn. Baillière Tindall, Eastbourne, pp 164–170

Chapman S, Nakielny R 1993 A guide to radiological procedures, 3rd edn. Baillière Tindall, London

Creteur V, Thoeni R F, Federle M P et al 1983 The role of single- and double-contrast radiography in the diagnosis of reflux oesophagitis. Radiology 147: 71–75

Day J J, Freeman A H, Coni N K, Dixon A K 1993 Barium enema or computed tomography for the frail elderly patient. Clinical Radiology 48: 48–51

Di Lelio A, Cestari C, Lomazzi A, Beretta L 1989 Cirrhosis: diagnosis with sonography study of the liver surface. Radiology 172: 389

Dubbins P A 1984 Ultrasound demonstration of bowel wall thickness in inflammatory bowel disease. Clinical Radiology 35: 227

Evans A F, Whitehouse G H 1980 Further with glucagon enhanced cholangiography. Clinical Radiology 31: 663–665

Front D, Royal H D, Israel O, Parker J A, Kolodney G M 1981 Scintigraphy of hepatic haemangioma; the value of ^{99m}Tc-labelled red blood cells. Journal of Nuclear Medicine 22: 684–687

Goldman S, Arvidsson H, Norming G, Lagersteadt U, Magnusson I, Friseu J 1991 Transrectal ultrasound and computed tomography in pre-operative staging of lower rectal adenocarcinoma. Gastrointestinal Radiology 16: 259–263

Gonberg J S, Friedman A C, Radecki P D, Grumbach K, Caroline D S 1986 MRI differentiation of recurrent colorectal carcinoma from post-operative fibrosis. Gastrointestinal Radiology 11: 361–363

Goodman M W, Ansel H J, Vemnes J A, Lasser R B, Silvis S E 1980 Is intravenous cholangiography still useful? Gastroenterology 79: 642–645

Gore R M 1989 CT of inflammatory bowel disease. Radiologic Clinics of North America 27: 717–729

Graziani L, De Nigris E, Pesares A et al 1983 Reflux oesophagitis: radiologic endoscopic correlation in 39 symptomatic cases. Gastrointestinal Radiology 8: 1–6

Haber K et al 1976 American Journal of Roentgenology 126: 624

Halvorsen R A, Thompson W M 1989 CT of oesophageal neoplasms. Radiologic Clinics of North America 27: 667–685

Harding L K, Robinson P J A 1990 Hepatobiliary studies: localization of gastrointestinal bleeding. In Ell P J (ed) Clinician's guide to nuclear medicine: gastroenterology. Churchill Livingstone, Edinburgh, pp 116–128

Harding L K, Robinson P J A 1991 Gastric emptying. In: Ell P J (ed) Clinician's guide to nuclear medicine: gastroenterology. Churchill Livingstone, Edinburgh, pp 22–30

Joseph A E A, Saverymuttu S H, Al-Sams et al 1991 Comparison of liver histology with ultrasonography in assessing diffuse parenchymal liver disease. Clinical Radiology 43: 26

Kleinhaus U, Militianu D 1988 Computed tomography in the pre-operative evaluation of gastric carcinoma. Gastrointestinal Radiology 13: 97–101

Koebel G, Schmiedl U, Majer M C, Weber P, Jenss H, Kueper K, Hess C F 1989 Diagnosis of fistulae and sinus tract in patients with Crohn's disease: value of MR imaging. American Journal of Roentgenology 152: 999–1002

Koehler R E, Weyman P J, Oakley H F 1980 Single- and double-contrast technique in oesophagitis. American Journal of Roentgenology 135: 15–19

Krestin G P, Stiebrich W, Friedmann G 1988 Recurrent rectal cancer: diagnosis with MR versus CT. Radiology 168: 307–311

Levine M S, Creteur V, Kressel H Y et al 1987 Benign gastric ulcers: diagnosis and follow-up with double contrast radiography. Radiology 164: 9–13

Levine M S 1994 Peptic ulcers. In: Textbook of gastrointestinal radiology. W B Saunders, Philadelphia

Love L 1973 Large bowel obstructions. Seminars in Roentgenology 8: 299–322

Lowe G H S, Rubesin S E 1993 Contrast evaluation of the pharynx and oesophagus. Radiologic Clinics of North America 31: 1265–1291

Mathieu P, Pringet J, Bodar P 1984 Defaecography: description of a new procedure and results in normal patients. Gastrointestinal Radiology 9: 247

McGrath F P, Malone D E, Dobranowski J, Stevenson G W 1993 Editorial. CT portography and delayed high dose iodine CT. Clinical Radiology 47: 1–6

Mezwa D G, Seczko P J, Besanco C 1993 Radiology evaluation of constipation and anorectal disorders. Radiologic Clinics of North America 31: 1375–1393

Miller R E, Nelson F W 1971 Roentgenographic demonstration of tiny amounts of free intraperitoneal gas: experimental and clinical studies. American Journal of Roentgenology 112: 574–585

Mindelsen R, Le Court J J 1980 Hepatic and perihepatic radiolucencies. Radiologic Clinics of North America 18: 221–238

Mitchell D G 1993 Hepatobiliary contrast material: a magic bullet for sensitivity and specificity? Radiology 188: 21–22

Moinuddin M, Allison J R, Montgomery J H, Rockett J F, McMurray J M 1985 Scintigraphic diagnosis of hepatic haemangioma. American Journal of Roentgenology 145: 223–228

Muller–Schimpfle, Brix G, Layer G et al 1993 Recurrent rectal cancer: diagnosis with dynamic MR imaging. Radiology 189: 881–889

Newbury K, Clarke M 1979 The accuracy of ultrasound in the detection of cirrhosis of the liver. British Journal of Radiology 52: 945

Ni Y, Marchal G, Yu J et al 1993 Experimental liver cancers: Mn-DPDP-enhanced rims in MR – microangiopathic-histologic correlation study. Radiology 188: 45–51

Puylaert J B C M 1986 Acute appendicitis – ultrasound evaluation using graded compression. Radiology 158: 355

Puylaert J B C M 1994 Acute appendicitis. In: Dubbins P A, Joseph A E A (eds). Ultrasound in gastroenterology. Churchill Livingstone, New York

Rofsky N M, Weinreb J C, Bernadino M E et al 1993 Hepatocellular tumors: characterisation with Mn DPDP-enhanced MR imaging. Radiology 188: 53–59

Saverymuttu S H, Joseph A E A, Maxwell J L 1986 Ultrasound scanning in the detection of hepatic fibrosis and steotosis. British Medical Journal 292: 13

Semelka R C, Cummins M, Shoemet J P, Yasse C S, Kroeker M A, Greenburg H M 1993a Islet cell tumours: a comparison of detection by dynamic contrast enhanced CT and MRI with dynamic gadolinium enhanced imaging and fat suppression. Radiology 190: 799–802

Semelka R C, Shoemet J P, Kroeker M A, Micflikier A B 1993b Chronic pancreatitis: MRI features using pre and post intravenous gadolinium DPTA, breathhold, FLASH and fat suppressed spin echo. Journal of Magnetic Resonance Imaging 3: 79–82

Soyer P, Levesque M, Elias D, Zeitoun G, Roche A 1992 Detection of liver metastases from colo-rectal cancer: comparison of intraoperative ultrasound and arterial portography. Radiology 183: 541–544

Sussman S K, Halvorsen R A, Illescas F F et al 1988 Gastric adenocarcinoma: CT versus surgical staging. Radiology 167: 335–340

Taylor K J W, Riely T A, Lax S et al 1986 Ultrasound attenuation in normal liver and in patients with diffuse liver disease: importance for that. Radiology 160: 65

Thoeni R F 1991 Colorectal cancer: cross-sectional imaging for staging of primary tumour and detection of local recurrence. American Journal of Roentgenology 156: 909–915

Thoeni R F, Laufer I 1994 Polyps in cancer. In: Textbook of gastrointestinal radiology. W B Saunders, Philadelphia

Thompson G, Somers S, Stevenson G W 1983 Benign gastric ulcer: a reliable radiologic diagnosis? American Journal of Roentgenology 141: 331–333

Vellet A D, Romano W, Bach D B et al 1992 Adenocarcinoma of the pancreatic ducts: comparative evaluation with CT and MR imaging at 1.5T. Radiology 183: 87–95

Waizer A, Powsner E, Russo I et al 1991 Prospective comparison study of magnetic resonance imaging versus transrectal ultrasound with pre-operative staging of follow-up of rectal cancer. Diseases of the Colon and Rectum 34: 1068–1072

Weott J F, Selsen B 1961 Gas in the portal venous system. American Journal of Roentgenology 86: 920–929

Wernecke K, Rummeny E, Bongart Z G et al 1991 Detection of hepatic masses in patients with carcinoma: comparative sensitivity of tomography CT and MR imaging. American Journal of Roentgenology 157: 731–739

3

Nutritional assessment of patients

S. L. Morgan

INTRODUCTION

The patient with gastrointestinal disease presents an interesting challenge for nutritional assessment and nutritional support (Floch 1981). The major causes of nutrient deficiency are decreased intake, decreased absorption, decreased utilization, increased losses and increased requirements. Specific examples of these nutrient deficiencies in patients with gastrointestinal disease are presented in Table 3.1. Not only are patients predisposed to nutrient deficiencies because of their underlying disease(s), but malnutrition alters small bowel structure and function. It has been demonstrated that the DNA, RNA, protein and water content of the small bowel fall during starvation, thereby possibly further contributing to malnutrition (Steiner et al 1986, Gleeson et al 1972, Levine et al 1974, McMahon & Bistrian 1990).

The rationale for doing a nutritional assessment is to estimate body composition, evaluate nutrient deficiencies and excesses and determine how states of deficiency and excess affect the physiologic functioning of the patient. This evaluation then serves as a basis for plans for nutrient repletion and support. The human body can be visualized as a variety of tissue compartments (Lusaki 1987, McMahon & Bistrian 1990, Heymsfield & Waki 1991, Roubenoff & Kehayias 1991). The body may be divided into skeletal tissue, lean body mass (LBM) and fat mass compartments. The skeleton represents on average 10% of body weight. An average male is 13–17% body fat and an average female is 20–24% body fat. Lean body

Table 3.1 Mechanisms of nutrient deficiencies in patients with gastrointestinal disease

Mechanisms of nutrient deficiency	Examples in patients with gastrointestinal disease
Decreased intake	Anorexia from underlying disease, inability to buy and prepare food
Decreased absorption	Short bowel syndrome, pancreatitis with fat malabsorption, loss of disaccharidases with n.p.o. status
Decreased utilization	Drug–nutrient interactions, such as use of the antifolate, methotrexate
Increased losses	Fat malabsorption, glucosuria
Increased requirements	Sepsis, exacerbations in inflammatory bowel disease

mass comprises approximately 75% of body weight with water occupying 73.2% of the LBM. Body muscle mass then can be grossly divided into skeletal muscle and visceral (circulating) proteins. The physical examination, anthropometrics, biochemical tests and specialized tests are used to further evaluate the size of these compartments.

The nutritional assessment and care of patients with gastrointestinal disease are best handled by a team of healthcare professionals. Physicians should be actively involved in all phases of nutrition support. Registered/licensed dietitians are uniquely qualified to translate the science of nutrition into practical food choices. Pharmacists, nurses and social workers are also important parts of the nutrition team. The nutritional assessment should be recorded as a part of the physical examination. Daily progress reports should reflect nutritional and metabolic progress. Such an assessment can best be done by historical, clinical, biochemical and anthropometric methods. A reasonable approach is using the traditional SOAP format where S = SUBJECTIVE, O = OBJECTIVE, A = ASSESSMENT and P = PLAN.

SUBJECTIVE

History

The nutrition history is a part of the subjective assessment. Information to be solicited includes:
- usual body weight;
- recent weight loss or weight gain;
- presence of diseases affecting digestion or absorption and other coexisting medical conditions;
- dentition and chewing difficulties;
- nausea and vomiting;
- diarrhea and/or constipation;
- ability to buy and prepare foods;
- medications and their dosages;
- supplemental vitamin and mineral use.

The mnemonic INTAKES can be used to remember key factors which may alter nutritional status.

A dietary history is a key part of the nutritional assessment and is taken to outline the usual eating habits of the individual so that the adequacy of dietary intake can be evaluated. A dietary history may be taken in several ways. The question 'What did you have to eat yesterday?' can be used. Particular attention should be paid to methods of food preparation, portion sizes and added condiments. The use of food models can make the dietary history more exact. In the absence of food models, measuring cups and spoons can help to more accurately estimate portion sizes. A 3-day

I = Involuntary weight loss or weight gain. The actual body weight should be compared with the usual and ideal body weights. The presence of edema may make it difficult to assess actual body weight.

N = Nurturing. Many psychological and psychosocial factors affect nutritional status. The ability to perform activities of daily living such as shopping, food preparation and self-feeding is important for nutritional status. Psychiatric diseases such as depression can contribute to impaired intake.

T = Tooth loss. Chewing difficulties, dry mouth and swallowing difficulties can adversely affect nutritional status.

A = Additional medical and surgical diseases affect nutrient intake, absorption, metabolism, losses and requirements. Sepsis is an example of a state which greatly increases nutrient requirements.

K = K(c)ash. The inability to buy food and medications can cause nutrient deficiencies.

E = Eating poorly. This involves an assessment of the quantity and quality of foods selected. Selection of foods with empty calories (fat and sugar) fall in this category.

S = Substances. Drug–nutrient interactions are important in the pharmacology of many commonly prescribed drugs (Roe 1985, 1989).

dietary recall gives a better indication of dietary patterns than a 1-day recall of intake, but it is logistically more difficult to perform (Stuff et al 1983, Sorenson et al 1985). If multiple days of intake are requested, patients may be asked to keep food diaries.

The food frequency questionnaire is another approach to taking a dietary history (Sampson 1985). Such a questionnaire estimates how often, on average, an individual consumes food in the categories of fruits, vegetables, dairy, meat, breads and cereals and alcohol. The food frequency questionnaire can complement the 1-day dietary recall and better define usual intake patterns. Table 3.2 shows a form that incorporates questions in the nutritional history and a space for a dietary history as well as a food frequency assessment.

The food guide pyramid (Fig. 3.1) from the United States Department of Agriculture can be used as a benchmark to assess the adequacy of dietary intake. Information obtained from the food frequency questionnaire and the 1-day dietary recall can be compared with the food guide pyramid guidelines for an assessment of adequacy. It is suggested that healthy Americans consume 6–11 servings of bread, cereal, rice and pasta, 3–5 of vegetables, 2–4 of fruits, 2–3 servings of milk, yoghurt and cheese and 2–3 servings of meat, poultry, fish, dry beans, eggs and nuts per day. One serving is defined as:

- **Bread:** one slice of bread, 1 ounce of ready-to-eat cereal, 1/2 cup cooked rice or pasta;
- **Vegetables:** one cup raw or 1/2 cup cooked vegetable, 3/4 cup vegetable juice;
- **Fruit:** one medium piece of fruit, 1/2 cup of chopped, cooked or canned fruit, 3/4 cup of fruit juice;

Table 3.2   Nutrition history assessment form

FORM FOR NUTRITIONAL ASSESSMENT

Name: _____ Medical record number: _____
Age: _____ Date of Birth: _____
Diagnoses: _____
Height: _____Weight: _____
Usual body weight: _____% Ideal body weight: _____
Recent weight loss or gain: _____
Anthropometrics: triceps skinfold: _____ Midarm muscle circumference: _____
Chewing, swallowing, nausea, vomiting, diarrhea, constipation: _____
Social factors: _____
Nutritional diagnosis: Marasmus _____ Kwashiorkor _____ Mixed _____
Other deficiencies: _____
Estimated caloric needs: _____

Women: BEE = 655.10 + 9.56 (W) + 1.85 (H) − 4.68 (A) _____
Men: BEE = 66.47 + 13.75(W) + 5(H) − 6.76(A), _____
where: W = weight in kg, H = height in cm, A = age in years
Activity and stress factors (1.2 − 1.5 × BEE for maintenance, 2 × BEE for weight gain,
for marasmus begin feeding at 0.8 × BEE) _____
Caloric goals: _____

One Day Dietary Recall

1st Meal	Snack	2nd Meal	Snack	3rd Meal	Snack

Food frequency

Food	How often consumed in a week	Parenteral or Enteral feeding	Medications:
		TPN	
Meat, fish, poultry		Dextrose: Protein: Fat:	
Milk		Electrolytes:	
			Nutritional supplements:
Fruits		Enteral feeding	
Vegetables		Formula:	
Breads and starches		Rate:	
Alcohol			
Sweets			
Salt			

Comments:

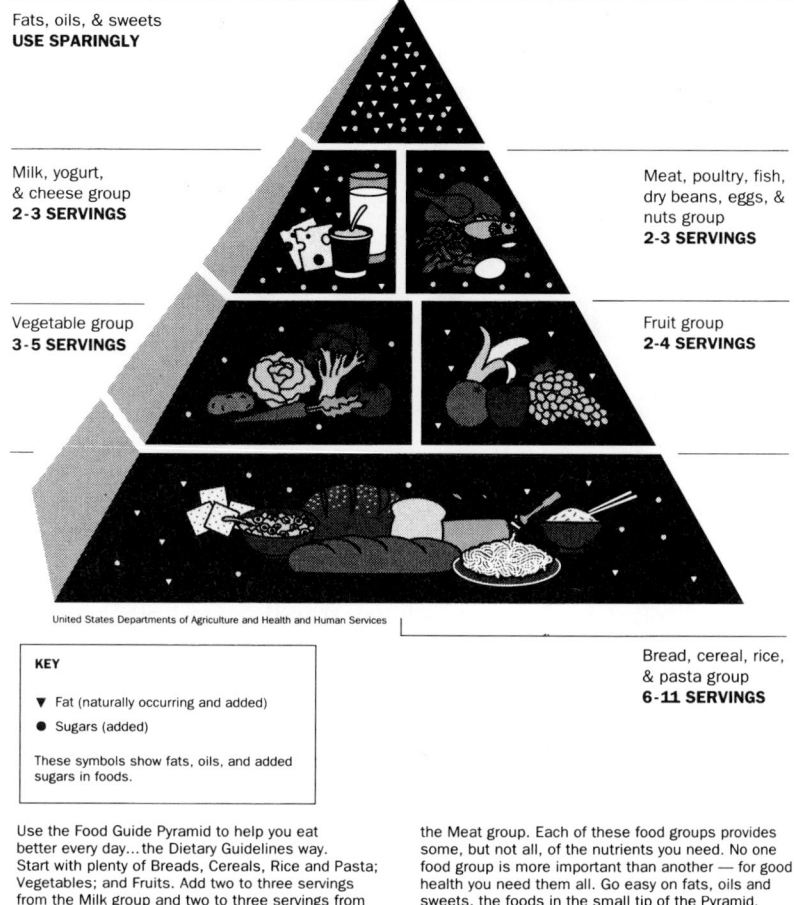

Fats, oils, & sweets
USE SPARINGLY

Milk, yogurt,
& cheese group
2-3 SERVINGS

Meat, poultry, fish,
dry beans, eggs, &
nuts group
2-3 SERVINGS

Vegetable group
3-5 SERVINGS

Fruit group
2-4 SERVINGS

United States Departments of Agriculture and Health and Human Services

Bread, cereal, rice,
& pasta group
6-11 SERVINGS

KEY

▼ Fat (naturally occurring and added)

● Sugars (added)

These symbols show fats, oils, and added
sugars in foods.

Use the Food Guide Pyramid to help you eat
better every day...the Dietary Guidelines way.
Start with plenty of Breads, Cereals, Rice and Pasta;
Vegetables; and Fruits. Add two to three servings
from the Milk group and two to three servings from
the Meat group. Each of these food groups provides
some, but not all, of the nutrients you need. No one
food group is more important than another — for good
health you need them all. Go easy on fats, oils and
sweets, the foods in the small tip of the Pyramid.

Figure 3.1   The food guide pyramid with a guide to daily food choices.

- **Milk:** one cup of milk or yoghurt, $1^1/_2$ ounces of natural cheese or 2 ounces of processed cheese;
- **Meat:** 2–3 ounces of cooked lean meat, poultry or fish, $^1/_2$ cup cooked dry beans, one egg, two tablespoons of peanut butter;
- **Fats:** one teaspoon of butter or margarine, one teaspoon of salad dressing or mayonnaise.

Figure 3.2 shows standardized serving sizes in the categories. Additional attention should be paid to the intake of alcohol and concentrated sources of sugar and fat (cookies, cakes, pies, candy, pastries, jelly, jams, sugar, sweetened sodas) which mainly provide calories but few nutrients.

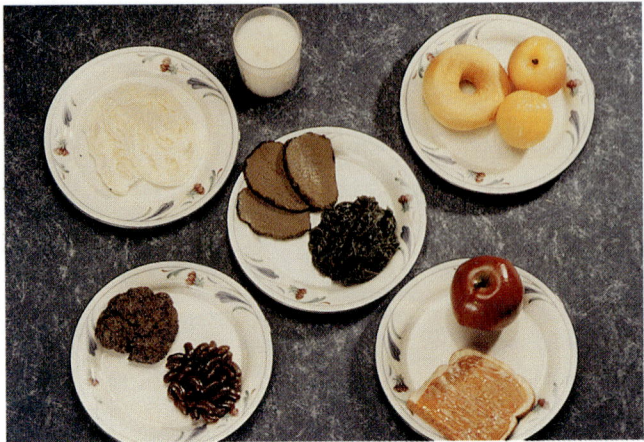

Figure 3.2   A guide to standardized serving portion sizes for the food guide pyramid.

OBJECTIVE

The objective parts of the nutritional assessment include the physical examination, anthropometrics, biochemical indices and other specialized tests.

The nutrition physical examination

The nutrition physical examination particularly concerns the epithelial tissues such as the skin, hair and oral tissues (Weinsier et al 1989, Weinsier & Morgan 1993). Since these epithelial tissues turn over rapidly, they are the sites in which signs of nutrient deficiency and excess are seen. Careful attention should also be paid to the general assessment of organs of the gastrointestinal tract. The physical findings of nutrient deficiency are cataloged in the sections on hair, mouth, eyes and skin. Nutrient deficiencies do not usually occur in isolation in the United States. Therefore, the presence of deficiency signs on the physical examination should alert the examiner to the possible presence of other signs.

Hair

- The flag sign (Fig. 3.3) is depigmentation of the hair in a linear stripe that corresponds to a time of nutritional stress, particularly protein calorie malnutrition of the protein type.
- Hair pluckability (Fig. 3.4) is the ability to pluck more than three hairs painlessly from the crown of the head. This physical finding is seen in dermatological disorders such as tellogen effluvium and is also seen in protein calorie malnutrition of the kwashiorkor type.

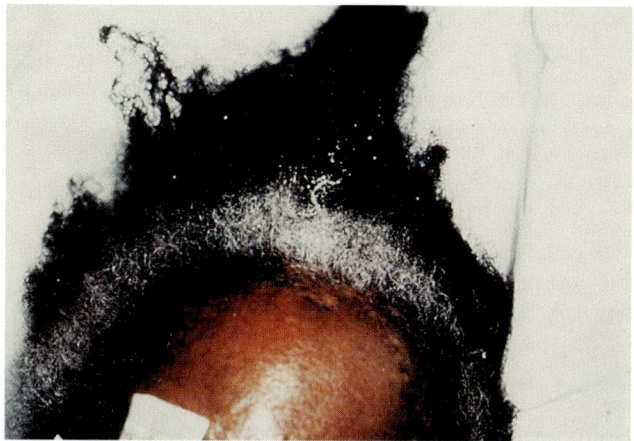

Figure 3.3   The flag sign.

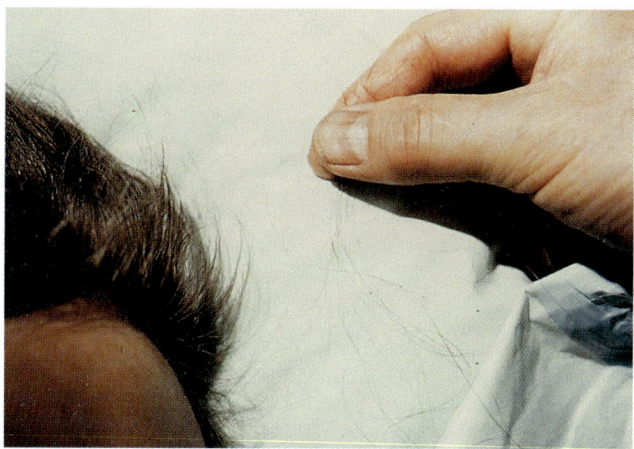

Figure 3.4   Easy hair pluckability (reproduced with permission from Mosby Year book, 1993).

- Corkscrew hairs and coiled hairs that have not emerged from a keratinized follicle (Fig. 3.5) are found in vitamin C deficiency or scurvy. Corkscrew hairs in affected individuals are generally found on the lower extremities and up to the umbilicus.

Mouth

Perioral tissues. Angular stomatitis or cheilosis is shown in Figure 3.6. The differential diagnosis of angular stomatitis includes pyridoxine deficiency, riboflavin deficiency and niacin deficiency.

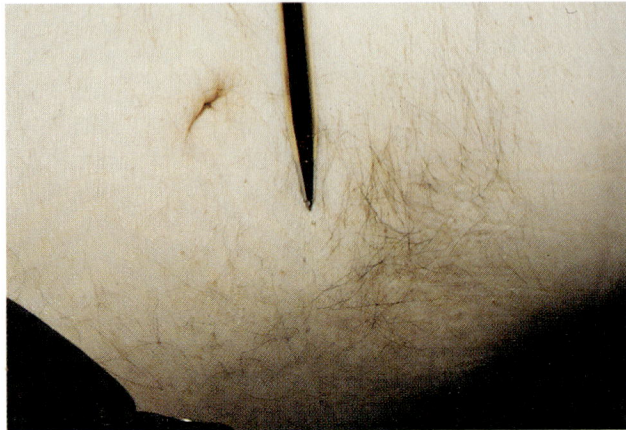

Figure 3.5 Coiled hairs in scurvy.

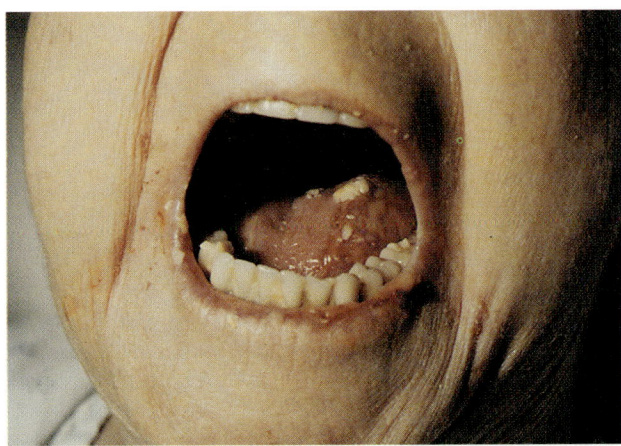

Figure 3.6 Angular stomatitis/cheilosis (courtesy of R. Endy, Reading Hospital and Medical Center, Reading, PA).

Tongue

A slick tongue or glossitis (Fig. 3.7) is the absence of papillae so that the underlying vascular bed of the tongue is exposed. This generally painful condition has a long differential diagnosis, but is seen in the nutritional states of vitamin B_{12}, folic acid and iron deficiency.

Teeth

• Enamel erosion (Fig. 3.8) occurs in patients with bulimia nervosa. The

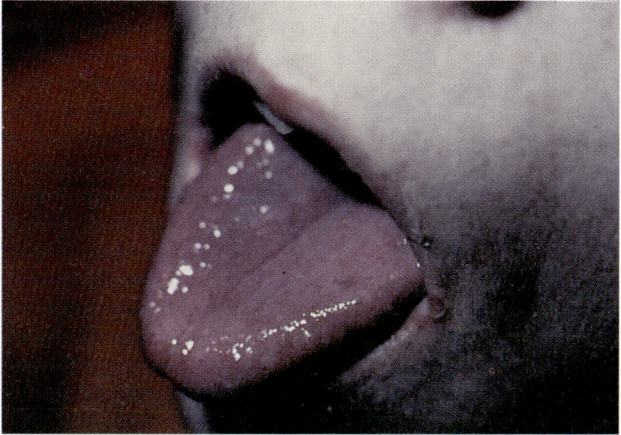

Figure 3.7 Glossitis.

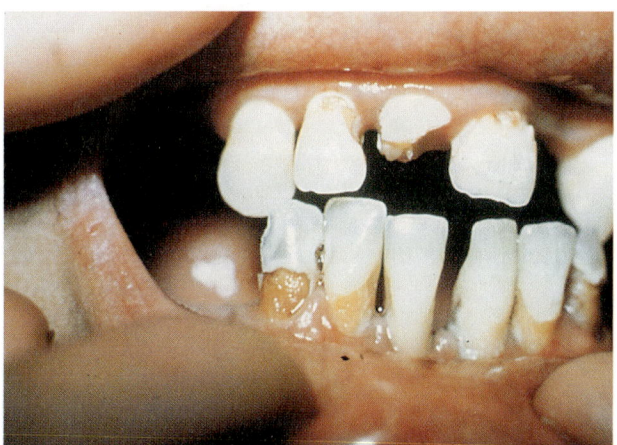

Figure 3.8 Enamel erosion in bulimia nervosa (reproduced with permission from Mosby Year book, 1993).

acid that is regurgitated during self-induced vomiting causes erosion of dental enamel. Extensive periodontal disease may also be seen.
- Scorbutic gingivitis with swollen, retracted and bleeding gums (Fig. 3.9) occurs in vitamin C deficiency only if there are teeth present in the mouth. Therefore, an edentulous person will not show the gum signs of scurvy even with biochemically documented vitamin C deficiency.

Eyes

- Xerophthalmia occurs in vitamin A deficiency. The changes that occur

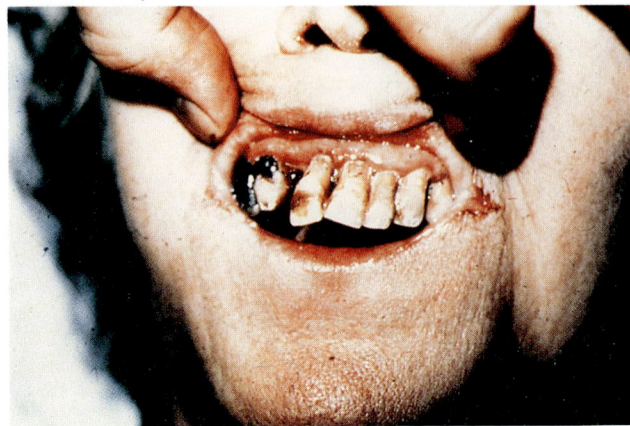

Figure 3.9 Scorbutic gingivitis (reproduced with permission from Mosby Year book, 1993).

in vitamin A deficiency include conjunctival xerosis, Bitot's spot with conjunctival xerosis, corneal xerosis, corneal ulceration with xerosis, keratomalacia, xerophthalmia fundus and corneal scars (Brown 1990).

Skin

- The perifollicular petechia (Fig. 3.10) is a pathognomonic sign of vitamin C deficiency.
- Purpura or bruising of the skin is seen in scurvy and vitamin K deficiency.

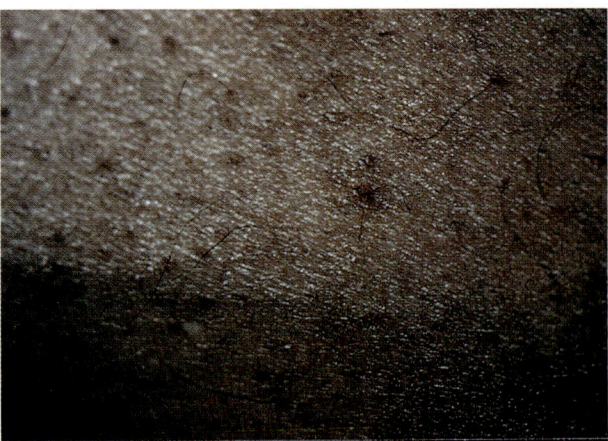

Figure 3.10 Perifollicular petechia in scurvy.

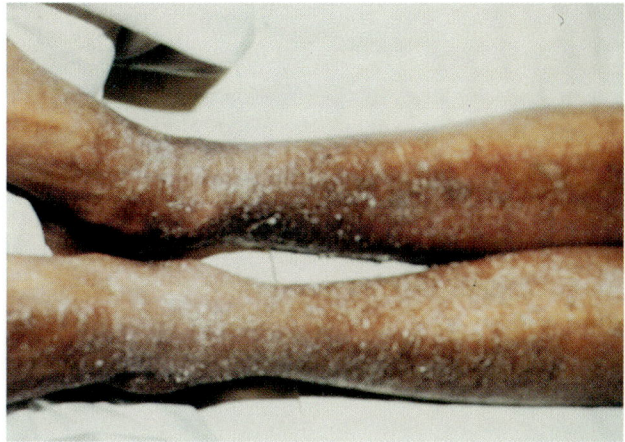

Figure 3.11 Dry scaly dermatitis of zinc and vitamin A deficiency (reproduced with permission from Mosby Year book, 1993).

- The differential diagnosis of scaly dermatitis (Fig. 3.11) is vitamin A deficiency and excess, zinc deficiency and essential fatty acid deficiency.
- Niacin deficiency or pellagra (Fig. 3.12) presents with the 3 Ds of diarrhea, dermatitis, dementia and ultimately death. Figure 3.12 shows the hand of a patient with alcoholism, diarrhea, dermatitis and dementia. Notice the prominent hypopigmentation as well as hyperpigmentation.

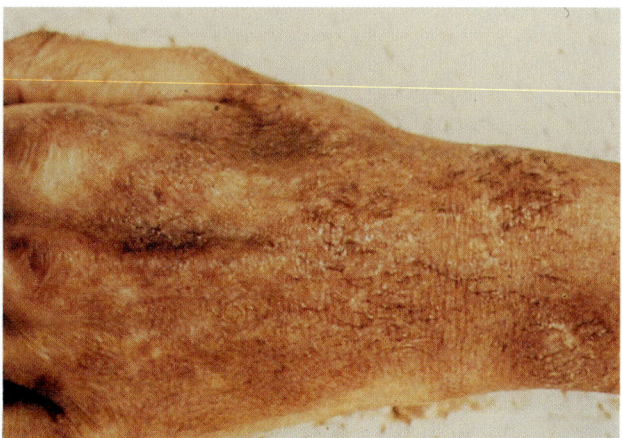

Figure 3.12 Pellagra (reproduced from Butterworth CE 1974 Nutrition Today March/April, 4–8, courtesy of Williams & Wilkins).

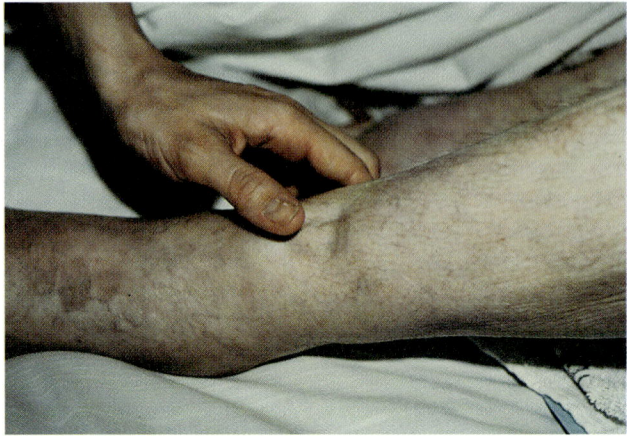

Figure 3.13   Pitting edema of protein calorie malnutrition.

- Pitting edema (Fig. 3.13) also has a nutritional differential, as it is one of the criteria used in making the diagnosis of kwashiorkor. Pitting edema indicates loss of intravascular colloid osmotic pressure.
- Flaky paint dermatitis (Fig. 3.14) occurs in protein calorie malnutrition, mainly of the kwashiorkor type. When there is protein malnutrition, there is loss of protein from all of the body compartments, including the dermis. Therefore the skin appears thin and cellophane-like with a variety of cracks. When this skin pattern is found on the physical examination, malnutrition must be considered.

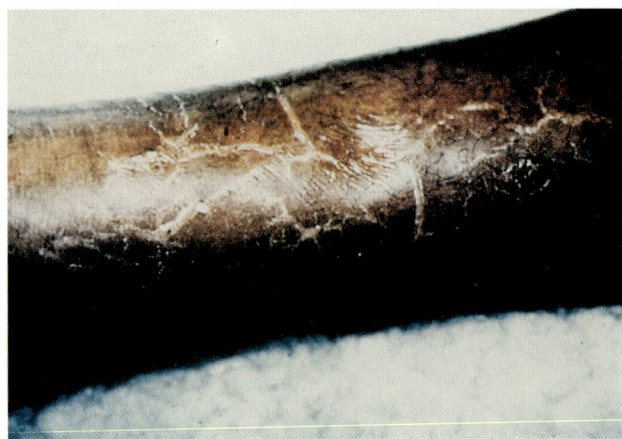

Figure 3.14   Flaky paint dermatitis.

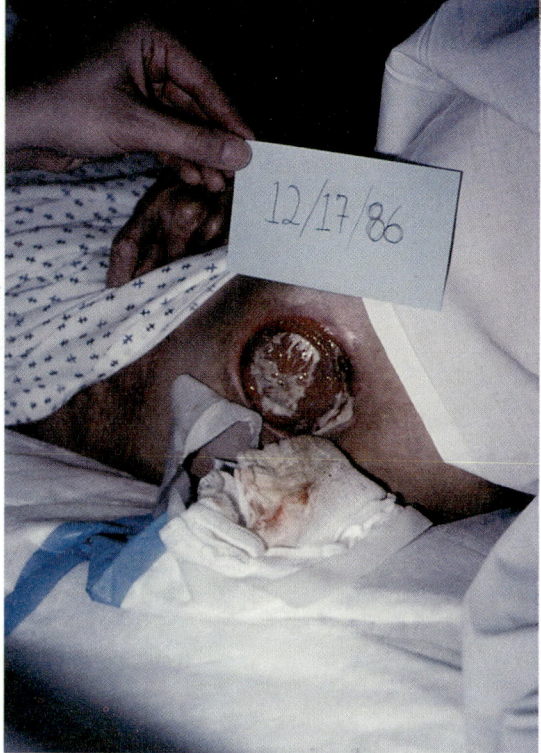

Figure 3.15 A decubitus ulcer in protein calorie malnutrition.

- Decubitus ulcer (Fig. 3.15) or skin breakdown is a classic consequence of protein calorie malnutrition of the kwashiorkor type. Delayed wound healing and wound dehiscence are also seen in kwashiorkor.
- Hypercarotenemia causes yellowing of the skin. This is differentiated from jaundice by the absence of scleral icterus.
- The loss of adipose tissue (Fig. 3.16) is also readily apparent on the physical examination and is characteristic of protein calorie malnutrition of the marasmus type which is predominantly calorie malnutrition. Similar physical signs are also seen in patients with anorexia nervosa.

Anthropometrics

Anthropometrics is the study of body measurements, typically involving measurement of skinfold thickness and limb circumferences (Frisancho 1990). Some of the most important anthropometric measurements for evaluation of nutritional status include weight in relation to height, triceps, suprailiac, abdominal and thigh skinfold thicknesses, and midarm

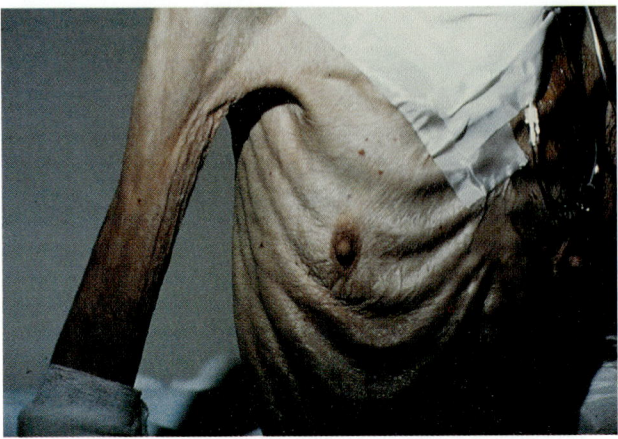

Figure 3.16   Loss of subcutaneous adipose tissue in marasmus.

and upper arm muscle circumferences. A variety of other anthropometric measurements are useful in nutritional assessment such as the waist and hip circumferences for the waist–hip ratio (Smith & Mullen 1991, Lee & Nieman 1993).

Weight and Height

Weight and height are two measurements that should be recorded for every patient. Optimal weight in relation to body height can be determined by using a table of reference weights in relation to heights such as the Metropolitan Life tables (Table 3.3) (Metropolitan Life Insurance 1959). The tables were revised in 1983 but they created a controversy because of a 5–10% increase in ideal body weights over that of the 1959 tables, which many health professionals believe is undesirable. Generally, individuals that are >20% above ideal body weight are considered overweight and individuals <20% of ideal body weight are considered underweight. Involuntary weight loss greater than 10% is usually associated with increased morbidity.

A simple rule of thumb for assessing ideal body weight without a table is as follows:

1. For men, allow 106 pounds for the first 5 feet of height and 6 pounds for every additional inch of height.
2. For women, allow 100 pounds for the first 5 feet of height and 5 pounds for every additional inch of height.
   Plus or minus 10% is allowed for body frame size.

Table 3.3 1959 Metropolitan Life Insurance company desirable weights for persons aged 25 and older (reproduced with permission from Metropolitan Life Insurance Company).

Males

Height		Small frame		Medium frame		Large frame	
in	cm	lb	kg	lb	kg	lb	kg
61	155	105–113	48–51	111–122	50–55	119–134	54–61
62	157	108–116	49–53	114–126	52–57	122–137	55–62
63	160	111–119	50–54	117–129	53–59	125–141	57–64
64	163	114–122	52–55	120–132	55–60	128–145	58–66
65	165	117–126	53–57	123–136	56–62	131–149	60–68
66	168	121–130	55–59	127–140	58–64	135–154	61–70
67	170	125–134	57–61	131–145	60–66	140–159	64–72
68	173	129–138	59–63	135–149	61–68	144–163	65–74
69	175	133–143	60–65	139–153	63–70	148–167	67–76
70	178	137–147	62–67	143–158	65–72	152–172	69–78
71	180	141–151	64–68	147–163	67–74	157–177	71–80
72	183	145–155	66–70	151–168	69–76	161–182	73–83
73	185	149–160	68–73	155–173	70–79	166–187	75–85
74	188	153–164	70–75	160–178	73–81	171–192	78–87
75	191	157–168	71–76	165–183	75–83	175–197	80–90

Females

Height		Small frame		Medium frame		Large frame	
57	145	90–97	41–44	94–106	43–48	102–118	46–54
58	147	92–100	42–45	97–109	44–49	105–121	48–55
59	150	95–103	43–47	100–114	45–51	108–124	49–56
60	152	98–106	45–48	103–115	47–52	111–127	50–58
61	155	101–109	46–50	106–118	48–54	114–130	52–59
62	157	104–112	47–51	109–122	49–55	117–134	53–61
63	160	107–115	49–52	112–126	51–57	121–138	55–63
64	163	110–119	50–54	116–131	53–59	125–142	57–65
65	165	114–123	52–56	120–135	54–61	129–146	59–66
66	168	118–127	54–58	124–139	56–63	133–150	60–68
67	170	122–131	55–60	128–143	58–65	137–154	62–70
68	173	126–136	57–62	132–147	60–67	141–159	64–72
69	175	130–140	59–64	136–151	62–68	145–164	66–75
70	178	134–144	61–65	140–155	64–70	149–169	68–77

Other information that may be calculated from height and weight includes the body mass index or Quetlet's Index. The index is calculated as: weight (kilograms)/height (meters²). The body mass index has been shown to correlate with body adiposity. However, this is only true if the excess body weight is adipose tissue. Indices between 20–25 kg/m² are generally considered as normal and with values above 25 kg/m² mortality and morbidity have been shown to increase (Garrow 1983, National Institutes of Health Development 1985, Lee & Nieman 1993).

Skinfold thickness measurements

Skinfold thickness measurements can be used to measure subcutaneous

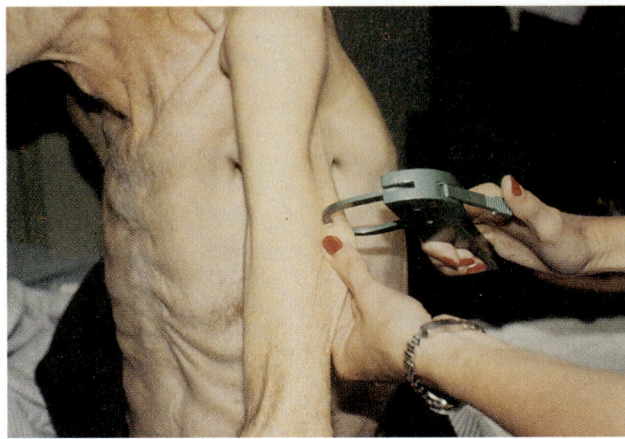

Figure 3.17 Measurement of the triceps skinfold with Lange skinfold calipers.

fat stores and to help with the estimation of body composition, particularly adipose tissues. Skinfold thickness measurements are taken using a caliper. Approximately 50% of body fat stores are subcutaneous. Therefore, a combination of skinfold measurements can be used to estimate total body adiposity. Other ways to measure body adiposity include underwater weighing, body impedance analysis and dual photon X-ray absorptiometry (DEXA); 13–17% of the mass of a 'normal' man is fat and 20–24% of that of a 'normal' woman is fat.

Triceps skinfold thickness

The thickness of the triceps skinfold is measured with a skinfold caliper in the flexed upper arm at the midpoint between the acromial process and the olecranon process and is reported in mm as the mean of three measurements. Figure 3.17 shows the measurement of a triceps skinfold. Tables 3.4 and 3.5 show reference values for the triceps skinfold thickness for Caucasian and African American males and females between the ages of 1 and 74 (Frisancho 1981, 1990).

Midarm muscle circumference and upper arm muscle area

The midarm muscle circumference (MAMC) and upper arm muscle area are used as estimates of skeletal muscle mass in the body. The MAMC is the muscle circumference of the biceps, brachialis and triceps at the midpoint between the acromion and the olecranon. Figure 3.18 shows the measurement of the circumference of the midarm.

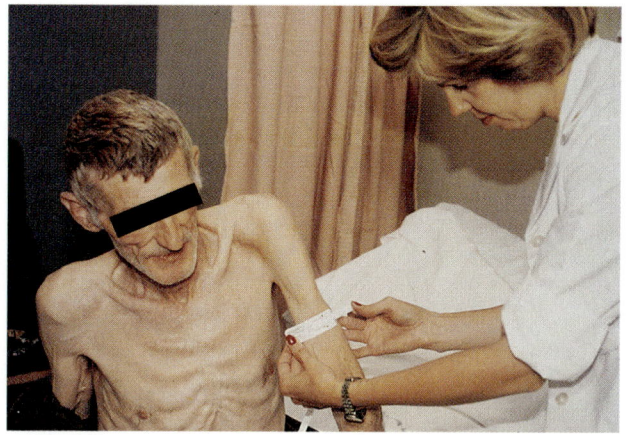

Figure 3.18 Measurement of the midarm muscle circumference.

Table 3.4 Triceps skinfold norms in African American males and females (reproduced from Frisancho 1990, courtesy of the University of Michigan Press)

Age (yrs)	N	Mean	SD	Percentiles									
				5	10	15	25	50	75	85	90	95
Males												
1.0–1.9	157	10.2	3.0	6.0	7.0	7.0	8.0	10.0	12.0	12.5	13.5	15.0
2.0–2.9	142	9.6	3.1	5.0	6.0	6.5	7.0	10.0	11.0	13.0	14.0	15.0
3.0–3.9	151	9.0	2.6	6.0	6.0	6.4	7.0	9.0	10.5	12.0	12.0	13.5
4.0–4.9	150	8.2	2.4	5.0	5.5	6.0	7.0	7.5	9.5	11.0	11.0	12.0
5.0–5.9	122	7.5	3.0	4.5	5.0	5.0	5.5	7.0	8.5	10.0	11.0	13.0
6.0–6.9	60	7.4	4.1	4.0	4.0	5.0	5.0	6.5	8.0	9.5	10.0	13.0
7.0–7.9	67	7.1	3.6	4.0	4.0	5.0	5.0	6.0	8.0	9.0	11.0	13.0
8.0–8.9	49	7.8	3.9	4.0	4.0	5.0	6.0	7.0	8.0	10.0	11.5	15.0
9.0–9.9	74	7.6	3.5	3.5	4.0	5.0	6.0	6.5	9.0	10.5	12.0	17.0
10.0–10.9	60	9.5	5.5	5.0	5.0	5.5	6.0	7.5	11.0	13.0	16.5	20.0
11.0–11.9	71	9.8	6.0	4.0	5.0	5.0	6.0	8.0	11.0	15.0	18.0	25.0
12.0–12.9	71	10.0	6.9	4.0	4.0	4.5	6.0	8.0	11.0	17.0	18.0	24.0
13.0–13.9	74	8.0	4.2	3.0	4.0	5.0	5.0	6.5	9.0	11.5	14.0	19.0
14.0–14.9	68	7.6	3.9	3.5	4.0	4.5	5.0	7.0	8.5	10.0	12.5	17.0
15.0–15.9	64	9.3	6.9	4.5	5.0	5.0	6.0	6.7	9.0	12.0	18.0	28.0
16.0–16.9	66	8.0	5.1	4.0	4.0	4.5	5.5	6.5	9.0	11.0	12.0	17.0
17.0–17.9	62	7.8	5.1	4.0	4.0	4.5	5.0	6.5	8.5	10.0	12.0	20.0
18.0–24.9	253	9.6	7.0	3.0	4.0	4.5	5.0	7.0	12.0	15.0	18.5	23.5
25.0–29.9	160	10.3	7.7	3.5	4.0	4.3	5.0	8.0	12.0	17.0	21.0	24.0
30.0–34.9	120	11.8	7.4	3.5	4.0	5.0	6.0	11.0	15.5	18.5	20.0	23.5
35.0–39.9	83	11.7	7.7	4.0	4.5	5.0	7.0	10.0	15.0	17.0	19.0	24.0
40.0–44.9	89	11.7	7.1	4.0	5.0	6.0	6.0	10.0	14.2	17.0	20.5	25.5
45.0–49.9	112	11.8	7.5	3.0	4.5	5.5	6.0	10.0	15.0	18.0	21.0	30.0
50.0–54.9	105	11.2	6.4	3.5	4.0	5.0	6.0	10.0	15.0	16.0	19.0	25.5
55.0–59.9	104	11.2	7.2	3.0	4.0	5.0	5.5	10.0	14.0	19.0	22.0	28.0
60.0–64.9	126	11.8	7.0	4.0	5.0	5.5	7.0	10.0	16.0	20.0	22.0	24.4
65.0–69.9	254	10.7	6.8	4.0	4.5	5.0	6.0	9.0	13.0	15.0	19.0	25.0
70.0–74.9	186	9.8	5.3	4.0	4.5	5.0	6.0	9.0	12.0	15.0	16.0	19.0

Table 3.4 Cont'd

Age (yrs)	N	Mean	SD	Percentiles								
				5	10	15	25	50	75	85	90	95
						Females						
1.0–1.9	134	10.2	2.9	6.0	6.0	7.0	8.0	10.0	12.0	13.0	14.0	15.0
2.0–2.9	119	9.8	2.7	6.0	6.5	7.0	8.0	10.0	11.0	12.0	13.0	16.0
3.0–3.9	127	9.4	3.2	5.5	6.0	7.0	7.0	9.0	11.0	12.0	13.0	15.0
4.0–4.9	147	9.4	3.2	5.0	6.0	6.5	7.0	9.0	11.0	12.0	13.5	16.0
5.0–5.9	163	9.6	4.0	5.0	5.5	6.5	7.0	8.5	11.5	13.0	15.0	18.0
6.0–6.9	72	9.1	3.9	4.5	5.5	6.0	7.0	8.0	10.0	12.0	12.0	18.5
7.0–7.9	81	10.0	4.4	5.0	6.0	6.5	7.5	9.0	12.0	13.0	15.0	18.0
8.0–8.9	54	10.4	4.5	5.0	6.0	7.0	7.0	9.0	12.0	15.0	17.5	19.0
9.0–9.9	71	11.1	5.7	5.5	6.0	6.5	7.0	10.0	13.0	17.0	20.0	21.0
10.0–10.9	61	13.0	7.0	5.5	6.5	7.5	8.0	10.0	17.5	19.5	22.0	24.5
11.0–11.9	67	13.6	7.7	5.0	6.5	7.5	8.0	11.5	17.5	22.0	23.0	30.0
12.0–12.9	71	14.7	7.6	6.0	7.0	7.0	9.0	12.5	19.0	25.0	26.0	31.0
13.0–13.9	82	16.3	8.1	6.0	8.0	8.5	10.5	15.5	20.5	24.0	25.0	34.0
14.0–14.9	79	15.5	7.7	6.5	8.0	9.0	10.5	13.5	19.0	24.0	27.0	32.0
15.0–15.9	73	16.1	8.8	6.0	8.0	9.0	10.0	14.0	20.0	23.0	27.5	40.0
16.0–16.9	54	18.9	7.5	8.0	11.0	11.5	12.0	18.5	24.0	26.0	31.0	33.0
17.0–17.9	66	15.9	6.9	7.0	9.0	9.0	12.0	14.0	20.0	24.0	27.0	28.0
18.0–24.9	473	19.3	8.9	8.0	9.0	10.5	12.5	17.0	25.0	30.0	32.0	36.0
25.0–29.9	275	22.8	10.2	8.5	10.5	12.0	15.0	22.0	29.0	32.2	35.0	40.5
30.0–34.9	236	25.0	11.0	8.0	10.0	13.0	16.0	24.0	32.0	35.5	40.0	45.0
35.0–39.9	235	26.6	10.7	10.0	12.0	15.0	18.0	26.0	33.5	37.0	40.8	46.0
40.0–44.9	231	26.8	10.0	11.0	14.0	15.5	20.0	27.0	35.0	37.0	40.5	42.0
45.0–49.9	125	27.1	11.7	10.0	12.0	14.0	19.0	26.0	34.0	40.0	42.0	50.0
50.0–54.9	135	29.5	10.9	10.0	13.5	16.5	22.0	30.5	37.5	41.0	42.5	46.0
55.0–59.9	119	28.7	12.0	8.5	13.0	15.0	20.0	28.0	37.5	41.0	43.0	50.0
60.0–64.9	152	27.7	10.1	12.0	15.0	17.0	21.0	27.0	34.5	39.5	40.5	46.0
65.0–69.9	282	25.6	9.6	10.0	13.0	15.5	18.5	25.5	31.0	35.0	38.0	44.0
70.0–74.9	196	24.3	9.3	10.0	13.0	15.0	17.0	24.0	30.0	33.0	37.0	40.5

Table 3.5 Triceps skinfold norms in white males and females (reproduced from Frisancho 1990, courtesy of the University of Michigan Press)

Age (yrs)	N	Mean	SD	Percentiles								
				5	10	15	25	50	75	85	90	95
						Males						
1.0–1.9	508	10.5	2.8	6.5	7.0	7.5	8.5	10.0	12.0	13.5	14.0	15.5
2.0–2.9	513	10.1	2.8	6.0	7.0	7.0	8.0	10.0	12.0	13.0	14.0	15.0
3.0–3.9	541	10.1	2.7	6.5	7.0	7.5	8.0	10.0	12.0	13.0	14.0	15.0
4.0–4.9	547	9.6	2.7	6.0	7.0	7.0	8.0	9.0	11.0	12.0	13.0	14.5
5.0–5.9	535	9.3	3.0	5.5	6.5	6.5	7.0	8.5	10.5	12.0	13.0	14.5

Table 3.5 Cont'd

Age (yrs)	N	Mean	SD	Percentiles								
				5	10	15	25	50	75	85	90	95
6.0–6.9	231	9.3	3.6	5.0	6.0	6.0	6.5	8.5	10.5	12.0	13.0	16.0
7.0–7.9	240	9.6	4.0	5.0	6.0	6.0	7.0	9.0	11.0	13.0	15.0	17.5
8.0–8.9	240	9.9	4.3	5.0	6.0	6.0	7.0	9.0	11.5	13.0	16.0	18.5
9.0–9.9	242	11.1	5.3	5.5	6.0	6.5	7.0	10.0	13.0	16.5	17.0	21.0
10.0–10.9	269	12.0	5.7	5.5	6.0	7.0	8.0	10.5	14.5	18.0	20.0	24.0
11.0–11.9	248	13.2	7.1	5.5	6.0	7.0	8.0	11.5	16.0	20.0	24.0	30.0
12.0–12.9	272	12.8	6.7	5.5	6.0	7.0	8.0	11.0	14.5	20.0	23.0	28.5
13.0–13.9	268	11.9	7.0	5.0	5.5	6.5	7.0	10.0	14.0	18.5	22.0	26.0
14.0–14.9	286	11.1	6.9	4.5	5.0	6.0	6.6	9.0	14.0	16.0	20.0	24.0
15.0–15.9	286	10.0	6.5	5.0	5.0	5.0	6.0	7.5	11.5	15.0	18.0	22.0
16.0–16.9	279	10.4	6.1	4.0	5.0	6.5	6.5	8.5	12.5	15.5	18.5	24.0
17.0–17.9	266	9.3	5.2	4.5	5.0	5.5	6.0	7.5	11.5	14.0	16.0	19.0
18.0–24.9	1463	11.6	6.3	4.5	5.0	6.0	7.0	10.0	15.0	18.0	20.0	24.0
25.0–29.9	1070	12.5	6.5	5.0	5.5	6.0	7.5	11.0	16.0	19.0	21.0	25.0
30.0–34.9	794	13.4	6.5	5.0	6.0	7.0	8.5	12.0	16.5	20.0	22.0	25.5
35.0–39.9	732	13.1	6.0	5.0	6.0	7.0	8.5	12.0	16.0	19.0	21.0	24.5
40.0–44.9	722	13.2	6.4	5.0	6.0	7.0	8.5	12.0	16.0	19.0	22.0	26.0
45.0–49.9	745	13.1	6.2	5.5	6.5	7.0	9.0	12.0	16.0	19.0	21.0	24.5
50.0–54.9	764	12.8	6.0	5.5	6.5	7.5	8.5	12.0	15.5	19.0	20.5	25.0
55.0–59.9	694	12.6	5.7	5.0	6.0	7.0	8.5	11.5	15.0	18.0	20.5	24.0
60.0–64.9	1120	12.6	5.9	5.0	6.5	7.0	8.5	11.5	15.5	18.0	20.0	23.5
65.0–69.9	1489	12.4	5.8	5.0	6.0	6.5	8.0	11.5	15.0	18.0	20.0	23.0
70.0–74.9	1051	12.4	5.7	5.0	6.0	7.0	8.0	11.5	15.0	18.0	20.0	23.0
Females												
1.0–1.9	470	10.5	3.1	6.0	7.0	7.5	8.0	10.0	12.0	13.5	15.0	16.5
2.0–2.9	482	10.7	2.9	6.5	7.0	8.0	9.0	10.5	12.5	14.0	15.0	16.0
3.0–3.9	509	10.6	2.8	6.5	7.0	8.0	8.5	10.5	12.0	13.0	14.0	16.0
4.0–4.9	522	10.5	2.9	6.0	7.0	7.5	8.5	10.0	12.0	13.0	14.0	15.5
5.0–5.9	504	10.6	3.3	6.0	7.0	8.0	8.5	10.0	12.0	14.0	15.0	16.5
6.0–6.9	218	10.8	3.6	6.0	7.0	7.5	8.0	10.5	12.0	13.5	15.0	17.0
7.0–7.9	244	11.4	4.0	6.0	7.0	8.0	9.0	11.0	13.0	15.0	17.0	19.0
8.0–8.9	221	12.5	5.5	6.5	7.0	8.0	9.0	11.5	15.0	17.0	18.0	22.5
9.0–9.9	248	14.1	5.8	7.0	8.0	8.5	10.0	13.0	16.5	19.5	22.0	25.5
10.0–10.9	266	14.2	5.9	7.0	8.0	8.0	10.0	13.0	17.5	20.0	22.5	27.0
11.0–11.9	229	15.4	6.6	7.0	8.5	9.0	11.0	13.0	18.5	21.5	24.5	29.0
12.0–12.9	247	15.2	5.9	8.0	9.0	9.5	11.0	14.0	18.0	20.5	23.0	27.0
13.0–13.9	275	16.4	7.2	7.0	8.0	9.5	11.0	15.0	20.0	24.0	25.0	30.0
14.0–14.9	287	17.5	7.1	9.0	10.0	10.5	12.0	17.0	21.0	23.5	27.0	31.0
15.0–15.9	234	17.6	6.8	8.5	10.0	11.0	12.5	17.0	20.5	23.0	26.0	32.0
16.0–16.9	284	19.4	6.9	10.5	12.0	13.0	14.5	18.0	22.5	26.0	29.0	32.5
17.0–17.9	223	20.0	8.1	10.0	11.5	12.0	14.0	19.0	24.0	26.5	30.0	35.0
18.0–24.9	2058	20.2	8.1	10.0	11.0	12.0	14.5	19.0	24.5	28.0	31.0	35.5
25.0–29.9	1608	21.5	8.5	10.0	12.0	13.0	15.0	20.0	26.0	30.5	33.5	38.0
30.0–34.9	1362	23.5	8.8	11.0	13.0	15.0	17.0	22.5	29.0	32.5	35.0	40.0
35.0–39.9	1194	24.3	9.0	12.0	13.5	15.5	18.0	23.0	30.0	34.0	36.0	40.5
40.0–44.9	1136	24.7	8.7	12.0	14.0	16.0	18.5	24.0	30.0	34.0	36.5	40.0
45.0–49.9	826	25.9	8.9	12.5	15.0	16.5	20.0	25.5	31.0	35.5	37.5	42.0
50.0–54.9	858	26.1	8.6	12.0	15.5	17.5	20.5	25.5	31.5	35.5	37.5	40.5
55.0–59.9	754	26.3	8.8	12.0	15.0	17.0	20.5	26.0	32.0	35.0	37.5	42.0
60.0–64.9	1223	26.5	8.7	13.0	16.0	17.5	20.5	26.0	32.0	35.5	38.0	42.0
65.0–69.9	1644	25.0	8.3	12.0	15.0	16.0	19.0	24.5	30.0	33.0	35.5	39.0
70.0–74.9	1260	24.0	8.3	11.5	14.0	15.5	18.0	24.0	29.5	32.0	34.5	38.0

The MAMC is calculated by the following equation:

MAMC = arm circumference in cm − [3.14 × triceps skinfold in cm]

Table 3.6 gives reference values for the MAMC from the National Health and Nutrition Examination Study (Frisancho 1981, 1990).
The upper arm muscle area is calculated from the formula:

Upper muscle area (m^2) =
$$\frac{[\text{midarm circumference in mm} - (\pi - \text{triceps skinfold in mm})]^2}{4\,\pi}$$

The use of the upper arm muscle area is felt to be more sensitive than circumference in detecting changes in body composition. Tables 3.7 and 3.8 give reference values for upper arm muscle areas for Caucasian and African Americans (Frisancho 1981, 1990). The upper arm muscle area equations can be corrected by subtracting a factor that accounts for bone, vascular tissue and nerves in the upper arm (Heymsfield et al 1982).

Corrected arm muscle area:
Females =
$$\frac{[\text{midarm circumference in mm} - (\pi \times \text{triceps skinfold in mm})]^2 - 6.5}{4\,\pi}$$

Males =
$$\frac{[\text{midarm circumference in mm} - (\pi \times \text{triceps skinfold in mm})]^2 - 10}{4\,\pi}$$

Laboratory data

Laboratory data are essential to nutritional assessment. Many of the tests commonly performed on patients also have nutritional implications (Labbé & Veldee 1993, Weinsier et al 1989, Weinsier & Morgan 1993).

Assessment of body muscle compartments

There are two major muscle compartments in the body, visceral muscle tissue and skeletal muscle. The visceral muscle compartment includes proteins such as albumin, prealbumin, transferrin, retinol binding protein,

Table 3.6 Midarm muscle circumference norms in white males and females (reproduced from Frisancho 1981, courtesy of the American Journal of Clinical Nutrition)

				Percentiles			
Age	5	10	25	50	75	90	95
				Males			
1–1.9	110	113	119	127	135	144	147
2–2.9	111	114	122	130	140	146	150
3–3.9	117	123	131	137	143	148	153
4–4.9	123	126	133	141	148	156	159
5–5.9	128	133	140	147	154	162	169
6–6.9	131	135	142	151	161	170	177
7–7.9	137	139	151	160	168	177	190
8–8.9	140	145	154	162	170	182	187
9–9.9	151	154	161	170	183	196	202
10–10.9	156	160	166	180	191	209	221
11–11.9	159	165	173	183	195	205	230
12–12.9	167	171	182	195	210	223	241
13–13.9	172	179	196	211	226	238	245
14–14.9	189	199	212	223	240	260	264
15–15.9	199	204	218	237	254	266	272
16–16.9	213	225	234	249	269	287	296
17–17.9	224	231	245	258	273	294	312
18–18.9	226	237	252	264	283	298	324
19–24.9	238	245	257	273	289	309	321
25–34.9	243	250	264	279	298	314	326
35–44.9	247	255	269	286	302	318	327
45–54.9	239	249	265	281	300	315	326
55–64.9	236	245	260	278	295	310	320
65–74.9	223	235	251	268	284	298	306
				Females			
1–1.9	105	111	117	124	132	139	143
2–2.9	111	114	119	126	133	142	147
3–3.9	113	119	124	132	140	146	152
4–4.9	115	121	128	136	144	152	157
5–5.9	125	128	134	142	151	159	165
6–6.9	130	133	138	145	154	166	171
7–7.9	129	135	142	151	160	171	176
8–8.9	138	140	151	160	171	183	194
9–9.9	147	150	158	167	180	194	198
10–10.9	148	150	159	170	180	190	197
11–11.9	150	158	171	181	196	217	223
12–12.9	162	166	180	191	201	214	220
13–13.9	169	175	183	198	211	226	240
14–14.9	174	179	190	201	216	232	247
15–15.9	175	178	189	202	215	228	244
16–16.9	170	180	190	202	216	234	249
17–17.9	175	183	194	205	221	239	257
18–18.9	174	179	191	202	215	237	245
19–24.9	179	185	195	207	221	236	249
25–34.9	183	188	199	212	228	246	264
35–44.9	186	192	205	218	236	257	272
45–54.9	187	193	206	220	238	260	274
55–64.9	187	196	209	225	244	266	280
65–74.9	185	195	208	225	244	264	279

Table 3.7 Upper arm muscle area norms in African American males and females (reproduced from Frisancho 1990, courtesy of the University of Michigan Press)

Age (yrs)	N	Mean	SD	Percentiles								
				5	10	15	25	50	75	85	90	95
Males												
1.0–1.9	157	13.2	2.5	9.0	10.3	10.8	11.5	13.2	14.7	15.6	16.6	17.4
2.0–2.9	142	14.1	2.5	10.4	11.1	11.8	12.6	13.9	15.7	16.3	17.0	19.1
3.0–3.9	151	15.3	2.8	11.9	12.2	12.7	13.5	14.9	16.8	17.9	18.9	20.4
4.0–4.9	149	16.4	2.8	11.7	13.0	13.7	14.7	16.3	18.0	19.0	20.0	21.3
5.0–5.9	122	18.5	2.9	14.8	15.2	15.8	16.4	18.4	20.3	21.5	22.3	23.5
6.0–6.9	60	20.5	4.8	15.3	16.2	16.4	17.8	19.3	22.8	24.4	25.0	26.3
7.0–7.9	67	21.9	5.4	16.4	16.7	17.5	18.9	21.1	23.7	25.3	27.2	28.8
8.0–8.9	49	22.5	3.3	18.1	18.4	19.2	19.8	22.1	25.1	26.1	26.9	28.5
9.0–9.9	74	24.9	5.5	18.5	19.3	20.3	22.5	23.9	27.4	28.8	29.9	32.2
10.0–10.9	60	27.0	5.2	19.7	21.3	22.0	23.6	26.1	29.7	31.2	32.4	35.1
11.0–11.9	71	29.4	6.9	21.0	23.0	24.0	25.1	27.7	32.2	34.8	36.9	40.2
12.0–12.9	71	32.8	8.5	22.7	25.1	25.7	27.3	30.4	36.7	39.9	41.2	49.7
13.0–13.9	74	38.0	11.4	24.8	26.5	27.5	30.4	35.2	44.0	47.4	50.9	58.5
14.0–14.9	68	43.2	9.7	28.6	31.7	32.7	34.9	42.8	47.5	51.2	53.9	59.4
15.0–15.9	64	48.9	9.7	33.3	36.6	39.7	42.2	49.4	54.9	57.2	59.1	65.6
16.0–16.9	66	55.2	9.3	42.0	44.4	46.1	49.5	54.7	57.9	63.7	66.9	70.5
17.0–17.9	62	54.0	10.0	38.9	42.3	44.9	46.9	52.8	59.3	63.7	66.1	71.7
18.0–24.9	253	52.0	11.8	35.5	38.3	40.1	44.2	51.0	59.4	63.1	65.3	73.0
25.0–29.9	160	56.9	12.6	36.9	40.9	44.3	48.8	55.6	63.2	68.7	74.5	81.1
30.0–34.9	120	60.3	14.0	42.9	45.8	47.7	50.1	57.3	67.1	73.6	76.7	80.0
35.0–39.9	83	61.6	13.6	39.3	41.8	46.0	52.8	61.2	70.8	77.3	80.5	85.4
40.0–44.9	89	59.6	13.8	36.9	41.2	44.2	50.3	59.0	68.4	74.5	79.4	83.7
45.0–49.9	112	58.8	13.7	39.0	42.7	46.5	49.4	56.8	66.9	72.8	75.0	82.5
50.0–54.9	105	60.6	17.1	39.1	41.3	44.7	47.7	60.1	69.3	72.7	81.3	88.8
55.0–59.9	104	58.7	13.4	36.6	42.0	44.6	50.8	57.6	66.8	73.6	76.5	80.6
60.0–64.9	126	55.5	12.3	34.4	39.6	45.1	48.3	55.0	62.7	66.3	70.7	77.0
65.0–69.9	254	53.1	14.3	33.4	36.9	40.4	43.2	51.0	62.2	67.5	71.4	80.1
70.0–74.9	186	50.2	13.2	30.7	34.3	37.7	41.2	48.9	58.9	63.2	67.1	72.3
Females												
1.0–1.9	134	12.2	2.3	8.1	9.8	10.3	10.8	12.3	13.7	14.5	15.2	16.7
2.0–2.9	119	13.6	2.5	9.9	10.4	10.8	12.0	13.3	14.8	16.2	17.1	18.3
3.0–3.9	126	14.4	2.3	11.2	11.5	11.8	12.8	14.2	15.9	16.5	17.2	18.8
4.0–4.9	147	15.7	2.8	11.4	12.4	12.8	13.8	15.6	17.6	18.3	18.9	19.9
5.0–5.9	163	17.0	3.5	12.0	13.5	14.1	14.8	16.6	18.3	19.3	22.4	23.5
6.0–6.9	72	19.0	5.2	14.0	14.8	15.2	15.9	18.2	20.2	22.3	22.9	27.5
7.0–7.9	80	19.7	3.5	14.4	16.0	16.4	17.3	19.1	21.4	22.9	24.1	25.5
8.0–8.9	54	20.7	3.8	15.7	16.6	17.9	19.2	20.6	23.0	23.7	25.4	27.2
9.0–9.9	71	22.5	3.8	16.9	18.7	19.2	20.1	21.4	25.5	26.9	27.9	28.3
10.0–10.9	61	26.0	6.2	18.9	19.8	20.6	21.9	24.7	29.5	31.3	32.2	34.0
11.0–11.9	67	29.0	6.3	22.2	22.9	23.2	24.9	27.5	31.7	33.2	35.7	42.1
12.0–12.9	71	30.6	8.6	18.0	20.9	22.0	23.6	30.8	35.8	39.6	40.1	40.8
13.0–13.9	82	32.0	5.7	24.5	25.1	26.0	27.8	31.2	36.2	37.6	39.3	42.8
14.0–14.9	79	34.6	9.0	23.3	25.2	27.6	29.2	33.0	37.1	40.6	44.2	57.2
15.0–15.9	73	35.3	7.2	25.3	27.5	27.8	30.2	33.5	40.0	43.5	46.9	49.1
16.0–16.9	54	37.9	9.7	26.5	28.1	29.2	31.7	35.5	41.0	44.9	48.6	61.6
17.0–17.9	66	37.2	8.2	26.1	28.4	29.7	32.3	35.5	40.0	46.3	49.2	52.6
18.0–24.9	473	32.3	9.8	21.0	23.0	24.2	25.8	30.2	35.9	40.3	43.6	49.4
25.0–29.9	275	34.6	10.5	21.8	23.5	25.6	27.4	33.0	40.3	44.6	47.6	53.2

Table 3.7 Cont'd

Age (yrs)	N	Mean	SD	Percentiles								
				5	10	15	25	50	75	85	90	95
30.0–34.9	236	37.3	11.2	22.8	24.6	27.3	29.9	35.0	42.9	47.1	51.5	58.3
35.0–39.9	235	40.2	13.8	23.4	27.1	28.4	31.2	37.7	44.9	51.6	56.7	68.0
40.0–44.9	231	41.5	18.6	23.9	26.5	28.2	30.9	38.5	48.4	53.3	56.5	70.8
45.0–49.9	125	41.6	15.3	27.3	28.9	30.4	32.6	37.2	43.4	52.0	60.1	65.8
50.0–54.9	134	41.9	12.9	23.9	27.9	29.0	32.6	40.2	48.7	51.6	56.2	68.9
55.0–59.9	119	43.4	18.9	24.6	26.5	29.7	33.1	41.2	47.3	53.9	62.1	65.7
60.0–64.9	152	40.6	12.1	23.1	26.0	29.3	32.3	38.7	47.0	50.1	56.8	63.7
65.0–69.9	282	40.0	11.9	22.6	25.6	28.7	32.5	39.6	46.6	50.5	53.6	58.1
70.0–74.9	196	37.6	11.3	21.9	24.4	26.6	29.2	36.3	44.7	48.4	51.3	55.5

Note: Values for males and females aged 18 years and older have been adjusted for bone area by subtracting 10.0 cm^2 and 6.5 cm^2 respectively from the calculated mid upper arm muscle area.

Table 3.8 Upper arm muscle area norms in white males and females (reproduced from Frisancho 1990, courtesy of the University of Michigan Press)

Age (yrs)	N	Mean	SD	Percentiles								
				5	10	15	25	50	75	85	90	95
						Males						
1.0–1.9	508	13.1	2.3	9.7	10.4	10.8	11.6	12.9	14.5	15.4	16.3	17.1
2.0–2.9	508	14.1	3.5	10.1	10.9	11.2	12.2	13.8	15.6	16.5	16.9	18.4
3.0–3.9	539	15.2	3.2	11.1	12.0	12.6	13.5	15.1	16.4	17.4	18.1	19.2
4.0–4.9	547	16.3	2.7	12.0	12.8	13.5	14.5	16.2	18.0	18.8	19.8	20.9
5.0–5.9	534	17.6	3.9	13.0	14.0	14.5	15.3	17.4	19.2	20.5	21.4	23.1
6.0–6.9	231	19.0	3.8	14.1	15.1	15.5	16.3	18.5	21.3	22.5	23.2	24.9
7.0–7.9	240	20.8	4.2	15.1	16.0	16.8	18.5	20.5	22.4	24.2	24.9	27.3
8.0–8.9	240	22.1	4.4	16.2	17.4	18.2	19.5	21.4	23.9	25.5	26.6	29.4
9.0–9.9	242	24.4	5.1	18.1	19.3	20.3	21.6	23.5	26.7	28.7	30.4	33.1
10.0–10.9	268	26.6	6.1	19.6	20.6	21.4	22.8	25.5	29.0	32.2	34.2	36.6
11.0–11.9	248	28.6	6.7	20.9	21.7	22.7	24.5	27.7	31.5	33.4	35.9	41.4
12.0–12.9	272	31.7	7.1	22.2	23.9	24.9	26.8	30.7	35.8	39.0	40.8	44.1
13.0–13.9	268	36.5	8.2	24.4	26.8	28.1	30.4	36.0	41.2	44.6	47.8	51.5
14.0–14.9	286	42.2	9.0	28.5	30.9	33.1	36.3	41.2	47.4	51.3	54.0	56.8
15.0–15.9	286	46.3	9.4	31.8	34.6	35.8	40.1	45.9	52.6	56.1	57.3	61.5
16.0–16.9	279	51.9	10.1	36.2	40.7	41.8	44.9	51.0	57.8	63.6	66.2	69.9
17.0–17.9	266	54.9	10.6	40.2	42.7	44.3	48.3	53.5	60.6	64.6	67.9	73.2
18.0–24.9	1463	50.5	11.4	34.5	37.4	39.6	42.6	49.2	56.7	61.7	65.0	71.6
25.0–29.9	1069	53.8	11.7	36.7	40.0	42.4	45.8	52.8	61.2	65.8	68.5	73.5
30.0–34.9	793	55.2	11.4	38.1	40.9	43.4	47.3	54.3	62.6	67.2	70.3	74.8
35.0–39.9	732	56.3	11.9	39.7	43.0	44.9	47.8	54.7	63.3	68.8	71.7	76.7
40.0–44.9	722	56.3	11.2	39.0	42.2	45.3	48.7	55.6	63.8	67.6	70.3	74.4
45.0–49.9	745	55.6	12.0	37.3	41.2	43.6	47.8	55.1	62.6	67.7	71.3	75.5
50.0–54.9	764	54.3	11.6	36.0	40.0	42.7	46.5	53.4	62.0	65.5	68.9	75.3
55.0–59.9	694	54.2	11.4	36.3	40.8	42.7	46.4	53.8	61.6	65.1	68.1	73.3
60.0–64.9	1120	52.6	11.6	34.5	38.7	41.1	44.5	51.8	59.7	64.4	67.2	71.4
65.0–69.9	1488	49.3	11.1	31.3	35.6	38.3	42.1	48.9	56.7	60.4	63.0	67.5
70.0–74.9	1050	47.4	11.1	29.7	33.8	35.9	40.1	46.8	54.3	58.5	61.7	66.1

Table 3.8 Cont'd

Age (yrs)	N	Mean	SD	Percentiles								
				5	10	15	25	50	75	85	90	95
Females												
1.0–1.9	470	12.4	2.2	8.9	9.7	10.1	10.8	12.3	13.8	14.6	15.3	16.1
2.0–2.9	482	13.3	2.2	10.1	10.6	11.0	11.8	13.2	14.7	15.5	16.2	17.1
3.0–3.9	509	14.3	2.5	10.6	11.3	11.8	12.6	14.3	15.7	16.7	17.5	18.7
4.0–4.9	521	15.3	2.9	11.2	12.2	12.7	13.6	15.1	16.9	17.8	18.5	19.7
5.0–5.9	503	16.6	3.0	12.5	13.2	13.8	14.7	16.3	18.4	19.4	20.6	21.3
6.0–6.9	218	17.6	3.3	13.5	14.1	14.4	15.4	17.3	19.1	20.4	21.8	24.0
7.0–7.9	244	19.2	4.2	14.2	15.1	15.6	16.5	18.8	21.1	22.5	23.9	24.7
8.0–8.9	220	21.1	5.0	15.2	15.8	16.7	18.1	20.6	23.3	24.7	26.5	28.1
9.0–9.9	247	23.0	4.8	17.0	17.7	18.6	19.8	22.2	25.6	27.6	29.2	31.4
10.0–10.9	266	23.9	5.3	17.5	18.3	19.1	20.7	23.4	26.8	28.5	29.8	32.9
11.0–11.9	229	27.3	6.7	19.1	20.2	21.3	22.9	26.1	30.0	33.5	36.8	38.8
12.0–12.9	247	29.5	5.8	21.0	22.4	23.8	25.8	29.0	32.5	35.1	37.2	39.1
13.0–13.9	275	31.9	7.9	22.7	24.3	25.2	26.9	30.5	34.9	38.2	40.4	44.2
14.0–14.9	287	33.7	7.4	24.3	26.4	27.1	29.0	32.8	36.9	39.8	42.0	47.1
15.0–15.9	234	33.4	6.8	24.3	25.4	27.0	29.1	32.6	36.6	39.1	41.1	43.2
16.0–16.9	284	34.3	7.6	24.7	26.5	28.1	29.7	33.5	37.6	39.8	42.7	46.6
17.0–17.9	223	35.6	8.7	25.9	27.4	28.6	30.5	33.9	39.5	43.2	44.4	49.5
18.0–24.9	2058	29.3	8.0	19.2	21.4	22.5	24.3	28.0	32.7	35.7	38.0	42.2
25.0–29.9	1608	30.5	8.7	20.2	21.7	22.9	24.8	29.1	34.2	37.6	40.4	45.8
30.0–34.9	1362	32.1	10.1	21.0	22.8	24.0	25.9	30.1	35.8	39.9	42.9	49.5
35.0–39.9	1194	33.0	10.6	21.0	23.1	24.4	26.8	31.1	37.1	41.6	44.6	50.9
40.0–44.9	1135	33.9	11.7	21.2	23.1	25.1	27.1	31.5	38.2	43.2	47.4	52.8
45.0–49.9	825	34.0	10.8	21.3	22.8	24.4	27.0	32.0	38.4	44.2	47.5	54.0
50.0–54.9	857	34.7	10.4	21.8	24.4	25.5	27.8	32.9	39.1	43.1	47.9	54.1
55.0–59.9	753	36.0	11.9	22.4	24.7	26.1	28.4	33.9	41.4	46.1	50.8	58.0
60.0–64.9	1223	35.8	11.1	22.3	24.5	26.1	29.1	34.0	40.6	44.8	48.3	53.0
65.0–69.9	1644	35.7	11.1	21.9	24.4	26.0	28.5	33.9	40.5	45.2	48.5	55.8
70.0–74.9	1260	35.8	10.7	22.1	24.4	25.9	28.7	34.1	41.1	45.9	48.7	54.6

Note: Values for males and females aged 18 years and older have been adjusted for bone area by subtracting 10.0 cm^2 and 6.5 cm^2 respectively from the calculated mid upper arm muscle area.

immunoglobulins and transfer proteins. The skeletal muscle compartment includes the structural proteins of the body. Various biochemical tests help in the assessment of the size of these compartments (Young et al 1990, Spiekerman 1993).

Visceral muscle assessment. A variety of visceral proteins including albumin, transferrin, prealbumin and retinol binding protein are commonly assayed (Smith & Mullen 1991, Lipkin & Bell 1993). The visceral proteins all have different half-lives. The half-life of albumin is approximately 14–21 days, the half-life of transferrin is 7 days, the half-life of prealbumin is 2–3 days and the half-life of retinol binding protein is 12 hours. This information is useful because the longer the half-life, the longer it takes for the protein to increase when positive nitrogen balance is established. Therefore, a labile protein such as retinol binding protein rises more rapidly during nutritional support than does serum albumin. Serum albumin is the visceral protein most commonly monitored. Normal values range from 40 to 60 g/L. Serum albumin levels are a poor measure of acute stress but they can be used as an indicator of long-term status. A value of <28 g/L is one of the criteria used in making the diagnosis of kwashiorkor. Increasing values of albumin during nutritional support indicate positive nitrogen balance.

One of the problems with albumin as an indicator of nutritional status is that it is not particularly specific since many other disease processes besides malnutrition can contribute to a low serum albumin level. Other causes of a low serum albumin level include increased losses, diminished production and dilution. It is possible to have a normal serum albumin level despite the presence of malnutrition on the clinical exam. This occurs in patients who have had infusions of albumin or blood products. Therefore, it is useful to be able to measure levels of other visceral proteins with shorter half-lives.

Transferrin is another visceral protein that can be assayed. Transferrin levels and total iron binding capacity are linearly related. Normal values for transferrin are 1.7–3.7 g/L. The interpretation of transferrin and total iron binding capacity levels is similar to that of albumin. However, iron deficiency can cause an elevated transferrin and total iron binding capacity level in the face of malnutrition.

Prealbumin and retinol binding protein are more labile visceral proteins that may be used to monitor nutritional status in the acutely ill. However, in renal failure, prealbumin and retinol binding protein levels are poor indicators of visceral protein status.

Skeletal muscle compartment. A 24-hour urine collection for creatinine is a laboratory test that can help to assess the size of the skeletal muscle mass (McMahon & Bistrian 1990). Creatine phosphate, a high energy compound present in muscle, is non-enzymatically dephosphorylated and excreted in the urine. Therefore, the amount of creatinine in the urine depends upon the size of the body skeletal mass. A low value for a 24-hour urine creatinine is an indicator of depleted lean body mass. The creatinine height index is the actual 24-hour urine for creatinine divided by the ideal 24-hour urine for creatinine:

$$\text{Creatinine height index} = \frac{\text{actual 24-hour urine for creatinine (mg)}}{\text{ideal 24-hour urine for creatinine (mg)}}$$

A value that is 60–80% of that predicted shows moderate depletion of skeletal muscle mass and a value that is <60% of standard shows severe depletion. The ideal 24-hour urine excretion can be estimated from a reference table of 24-hour urine creatinine excretion as shown in Table 3.9

Table 3.9 Normal values for 24-hour urinary creatinine excretion (reproduced from Blackburn et al 1977, courtesy of the Journal of Enteral and Parenteral Nutrition)

Men*			Women**		
Height		Predicted creatinine (mg/24 h)	Height		Predicted creatinine (mg/24 h)
5'2"	157.5 cm	1288	4'10"	147.3 cm	830
5'3"	160.0 cm	1325	4'11"	149.9 cm	851
5'4"	162.6 cm	1359	5'0"	152.4 cm	875
5'5"	165.1 cm	1386	5'1"	154.9 cm	900
5'6"	167.6 cm	1426	5'2"	157.5 cm	925
5'7"	170.2 cm	1467	5'3"	160.0 cm	949
5'8"	172.7 cm	1513	5'4"	162.6 cm	977
5'9"	175.3 cm	1555	5'5"	165.1 cm	1006
5'10"	177.8 cm	1596	5'6"	167.6 cm	1044
5'11"	180.3 cm	1642	5'7"	170.2 cm	1076
6'0"	182.9 cm	1691	5'8"	172.7 cm	1109
6'1"	185.4 cm	1739	5'9"	175.3 cm	1141
6'2"	188.0 cm	1785	5'10"	177.8 cm	1174
6'3"	190.5 cm	1831	5'11"	180.3 cm	1206
6'4"	193.0 cm	1891	6'0"	182.9 cm	1240

*Creatinine coefficient (men) = 23 mg/kg of ideal body weight/24 hours
**Creatinine coefficient (women) = 18 mg/kg of ideal body weight/24 hours

(Blackburn et al 1977). The ideal value depends upon sex and height. It should be stressed that the ideal 24-hour creatinine excretion levels in tables may not reflect some segments of the population such as the elderly. If a table is not available, the ideal 24-hour urine for creatinine can be estimated as 20–26 mg/kg/day for a male and 14–22 mg/kg/day for a female.

Nitrogen balance

The 24-hour urine for urine urea nitrogen (UUN) aids in estimation of protein balance. The 24-hour UUN in grams plus 4 g (as a factor for non-urinary nitrogen losses) multiplied by 6.25 yields the protein loss in grams. When the protein loss estimated from the UUN is subtracted from the protein intake, it yields the protein balance:

Protein balance = protein intake – (24-hour UUN (g) + 4) 6.25

It is important to remember that a 24-hour urine for UUN is a balance procedure and should always be evaluated in relation to the level of the dietary protein intake. If a 24-hour urine for UUN is done in a fasting individual, it more closely approximates obligate protein needs. A 24-hour urine for UUN in a non-stressed individual who is not eating a large amount of protein is generally less than 5 g per day. Thus the 24-hour UUN is also an estimate of the catabolic stress of a patient. As a patient is more highly stressed, the 24-hour urine UUN value will be higher. If an approximately constant amount of protein is fed over a period of time and the UUN decreases, this indicates that the stress of the patient is abating.

In some situations the 24-hour UUN levels may not correspond to the clinical assessment of the degree of malnutrition. A 24-hour UUN will be falsely low during the onset of renal failure or if there is an incomplete urine collection. A 24-hour urine UUN will be falsely elevated during corticosteroid therapy and in active diuresis during a time that the BUN level is decreasing and if the urine is collected for longer than 24 hours. The 24-hour urine for UUN can be corrected for changes in BUN and body weight by the calculation of urinary nitrogen appearance rate or UNA (Weinsier et al 1989):

$$UNA = \frac{UUN + (\Delta BUN \times 10)\,(W_m)\,(BW) + (BUN_m \times 10)(\Delta W)}{1000}$$

where:
ΔBUN = BUN at the end of the collection − BUN at the beginning of the collection
BUN_m = mean BUN (mg/dL) during the urine collection
ΔW = weight at the end of the urine collection − weight at the beginning of the urine collection
W_m = mean weight in kg during the urine collection
BW = assumed body water (L/kg body weight). The normal value is 0.5 for women and 0.6 for men. 0.05 is subtracted for marked obesity and dehydration and 0.05 is added for leanness and edema.

Other laboratory tests with nutritional significance

Other tests which have significance in nutritional assessment include BUN, hematology profiles and vitamin and mineral assays.

The complete blood count

The differential diagnosis of anemia includes anemias of nutritional origin. The nutritional anemias can be stratified by diagnosis using the mean corpuscular volume. The major nutritional causes of a microcytic anemia are iron and pyridoxine deficiency. The major nutritional cause of a normocytic anemia is kwashiorkor. This type of anemia is also called an anemia of chronic disease. The nutritional causes of a macrocytic anemia are vitamin B_{12} and folic acid deficiency.

Total lymphocyte count

The total lymphocyte count can also be used as an indicator of malnutrition, since both cellular and humoral immunity are impaired in malnutrition. A total lymphocyte count $<1500 \times 10^6/L$ is associated with kwashiorkor. Other causes of a low total lymphocyte count include corticosteroid administration, renal failure and cancer of the colon. The total lymphocyte count can be elevated despite frank malnutrition in patients with infections, leukemia, myeloma, cancers of the stomach and breast and in adrenal insufficiency.

Prothrombin time

The prothrombin time is a functional assay for vitamin K status. The prothrombin time depends upon the integrity of the vitamin K-dependent clotting factors II, VII, IX and X of the extrinsic pathway. A prolonged prothrombin time may indicate vitamin K deficiency. Confounding factors include severe liver disease and anticoagulant therapy.

Vitamin and mineral assays

Vitamin and mineral assays will not be discussed in depth; information about specific assays may be obtained from other sources (Jacob & Milne 1993). Vitamin and mineral assays can be done in a variety of tissues, such as plasma, serum, cells and urine.

The delayed hypersensitivity skin test

The delayed hypersensitivity skin test is a measure of cell-mediated immunity. Anergy is seen in protein calorie malnutrition and may be reversed with adequate nutritional therapy.

Other specialized tests for the assessment of body composition

A variety of other specialized tests can be used in the assessment of body composition (Lusaki 1987, Lee & Nieman 1993, Lipkin & Bell 1993). However, at the present time many of these tests are mainly research tools.

Underwater weighing

Underwater body weighing is used to determine the degree of adiposity of the body. Underwater body weighing is based on Archimedes' principle that the volume of an object submerged in water is equal to the volume of the water displaced. Since density = mass/volume, the percent body fat can be calculated using specific equations.

Electrical conductance

Electrical conductance measures the impedance of an electrical current. Fat and cell membranes are non-conducting compared to a fat-free mass. Bioelectrical impedance analysis uses this principle to measure total body water and then to estimate body fat and fat-free mass. Total body conductivity operates on the principle that the degree to which an object interrupts an electromagnetic field is related to the amount of fat-free mass. Machines such as TOBEC (total body electrical conductivity) are used to measure total body water and from this total body fat and fat-free mass are calculated.

Dual energy X-ray absorptiometry

Dual energy X-ray absorptiometry (DEXA) uses an X-ray source (a dose less than a chest X-ray) within a table and counts the photon attenuation rates of the different tissues. It involves a three-compartment model of body composition because it can measure bone mineral content of the skeleton, lean body mass and fat mass. It can also be used to measure regional body composition in the arms, legs and trunk.

ASSESSMENT

The synthesis of information from nutritional evaluation is used to determine whether a patient has evidence of micronutrient deficiencies and has normal or abnormal body composition. The two most frequent diagnoses of malnutrition in the hospitalized patient are marasmus and kwashiorkor. Table 3.10 shows the criteria for the diagnoses of marasmus and kwashiorkor (Weinsier et al 1989, Weinsier & Morgan 1993).

Marasmus

Marasmus, the predominantly calorie form of protein calorie malnutrition, takes months to years to occur in complete form. The characteristics of a patient with marasmus are a starved appearance, low weight for height and triceps skinfold and midarm muscle circumference less than the 5th

Table 3.10   Criteria for the diagnosis of marasmus and kwashiorkor (reproduced with permission from Mosby Year book, 1993)

Disease	Clinical setting	Time course to develop	Clinical features	Laboratory findings	Clinical course	Mortality
Marasmus	↓ Calorie intake	Months or years	Starved appearance Weight <80% standard for height Triceps skinfold <3 mm Midarm muscle circumference <15 cm	Creatinine-height index <60% standard	Reasonably preserved responsiveness to short-term stress	Low, unless related to underlying disease
Kwashiorkor	↓ Protein intake during stress state	Weeks	Well-nourished appearance Easy hair pluckability Edema	Serum albumin <2.8 g/dL Total iron binding capacity <200 μg/dL Lymphocytes <1500/mm^3 Anergy	Infections Poor wound healing, decubitus ulcers, skin breakdown	High

percentile. Laboratory findings, such as low visceral protein levels, are generally not present. The minimum criteria for a diagnosis of marasmus are a midarm muscle circumference and triceps skinfold less than the 5th percentile.

The marasmic patient has simple starvation without superimposed stress. The physiological response of a patient with marasmus is a normal response to starvation. Such patients have decreased metabolic rates and low levels of insulin, catecholamines, glucagon and cortisol. After an obligate period of protein breakdown, the rates of proteolysis and gluconeogenesis diminish because of a shift to fatty acid utilization and ketone production. Patients with marasmus have a relatively good response to short-term stress and their mortality is low unless they are refed improperly.

Kwashiorkor

Kwashiorkor, the predominantly protein form of protein calorie malnutrition, can occur in an extremely short period of time. Kwashiorkor occurs in stressful states such as infection, surgery or trauma. Patients with kwashiorkor often do not look malnourished and may appear obese. The physical findings of kwashiorkor are easy hair pluckability, skin breakdown and pitting edema (either central or peripheral). The laboratory findings of kwashiorkor are an albumin <28 gm/L (other visceral protein levels are also low) and a lymphocyte count $<1500 \times 10^6$/L. The minimum criteria for a diagnosis of kwashiorkor are an albumin <28 gm/L and one of the following: poor wound healing, easy hair pluckability and edema. The clinical course of patients with kwashiorkor is complicated by impaired immunocompetence, poor wound healing and infectious complications.

The patient with kwashiorkor is hypermetabolic. There are elevated levels of insulin, glucagon and catecholamines. There is elevated gluconeogenesis with resultant proteolysis and urea excretion. These patients also metabolize fatty acids, but there is no shift to ketone metabolism as in marasmus. Kwashiorkor represents an abnormal response to starvation. The mortality in such patients is high if they are left untreated.

PLAN
Calorie and protein goals

Calorie needs of patients may be estimated using the Harris Benedict equation. The value that is calculated is called the basal energy expenditure (BEE). The height, weight and age in years are entered into the equation. For patients with marasmus, it is recommended that feedings start at $0.8 \times$ BEE and ultimately be increased to $2.0 \times$ BEE. For patients with kwashiorkor, feeding in the range of 1.2–1.5 × BEE is generally sufficient. The Harris Benedict equation is useful up to a weight of 100 kg.

Women: BEE $= 655.10 + 9.56$ (W) $+ 1.85$ (H) $- 4.68$ (A)
Men: BEE $= 66.47 + 13.75$(W) $+ 5$(H) $- 6.76$(A)
where W = weight in kg, H = height in cm and A = age in years

Indirect calorimetry is another way to estimate caloric needs. By evaluation of oxygen consumption and CO_2 production, the respiratory quotient and estimated resting energy expenditure can be determined.

For an estimation of protein requirements, the 24-hour urine for UUN can be used as a guide. When no UUN is available, in patients with normal hepatic and renal function a reasonable estimate is 1.0–1.5 g of protein per kilogram per day. Patients undergoing hemodialysis generally require 1.0–1.4 g/kg ideal body weight/day and patients undergoing peritoneal dialysis generally require 1.2–1.5 g/kg ideal body weight/day. Serial visceral protein levels also help in the determination of nitrogen balance.

Refeeding

Refeeding should take into consideration the metabolic and physiological consequences of the depletion, repletion and shifts in fluid, electrolytes and vitamins and minerals as patients with malnutrition are provided with nutrients. Table 3.11 shows a summary of the approach to refeeding patients with marasmus and kwashiorkor.

Refeeding and marasmus

The refeeding of a patient with marasmus can be complicated by repletion heart failure and hypophosphatemia. Repletion heart failure may occur because the atrophy of the heart parallels the loss of lean body mass.

Table 3.11 Selective approaches to nutritional support (reproduced with permission from Mosby Year book, 1993)

Patient type	Aim	Nutritional support	Risks of overfeeding	Error likely
Hypometabolic, starved	Rebuild	Cautious, with portion of fuel as fat	Hypophosphatemia, repletion heart failure	Commission (overzealous support)
Hypermetabolic, stressed	Replace	Aggressive but not excessive	$\uparrow O_2$ consumption and CO_2 production	Omission (inadequate support)

During the reintroduction of calories and fluid, metabolic rate rises along with plasma volume and afterload. If fluid and electrolytes are not carefully controlled, repletion heart failure may follow.

Hypophosphatemia is another threat in improper feeding of a patient with marasmus (Weinsier & Krumdieck 1981). Patients with marasmus utilize fatty acids and ketones as their major body fuels and may be depleted in electrolytes such as phosphorus. The metabolism of glucose (present in parenteral and enteral feedings) requires phosphorus in its intermediary metabolism. If sufficient phosphorus is not added to such feedings, patients may become profoundly hypophosphatemic with altered myocardial function, hemolysis, acute ventilatory failure and neuromuscular compromise.

The correct strategy for refeeding patients with marasmus is to start feeding slowly and aim for repletion of lost body stores. Generally such patients are fed at 0.8 times the BEE for the first several days, carefully watching fluid balance and electrolytes. Total calories are then slowly increased to BEE $\times$ 1.0, BEE $\times$ 1.2, and BEE $\times$ 1.5 as patients' tolerance permits. Ultimately, the goal in such patients should be twice the BEE.

Refeeding and kwashiorkor

The patient with kwashiorkor requires aggressive support to provide adequate calories and protein. However, overly aggressive support of such patients, particularly with high carbohydrate concentrations, can increase O_2 consumption and CO_2 production (Askanazi et al 1980). The correct approach to refeeding patients with kwashiorkor is to provide adequate calories and protein fairly quickly (i.e. within 1 to 2 days). The strategy is to be aggressive but not excessive. For most patients the caloric needs can be estimated as 1.2–1.5 $\times$ the BEE.

Routes of support

Enteral nutrition includes oral feeding, tube feeding and feeding through a variety of enterostomies. Parenteral nutrition involves feeding through an intravenous route, either peripherally or centrally. Parenteral and enteral routes can be used concurrently. If the gut works, it should be used. Enteral nutrition does not involve the hazards of central line placement and infection and is much cheaper than parenteral nutrition.

FOLLOW-UP AFTER NUTRITIONAL ASSESSMENT

Nutritional assessment and planning are the first steps in the nutritional care of the patient. Follow-up monitoring includes evaluation of changes in body composition and biochemical indices.

FURTHER READING

Askanazi J, Carpentier Y A, Elwyn D H et al 1980 Influence of total parenteral nutrition on fuel utilization in injury and sepsis. Annals of Surgery 191: 40–46

Blackburn G L, Bistrian B R, Maini B S, Schlamm H T, Smith M F 1977 Nutritional and metabolic assessment of the hospitalized patient. Journal of Parenteral and Enteral Nutrition 1: 11–22

Brown M L (ed) 1990 Present knowledge in nutrition. International Life Sciences Institute/ Nutrition Foundation, Washington DC.

Floch M H 1981 Nutrition and diet therapy in gastrointestinal disease. Plenum Medical Book Company, New York

Frisancho A R 1981 New norms of upper limb fat and muscle areas for assessment of nutritional status. American Journal of Clinical Nutrition 34: 2540–2545

Frisancho A R 1990 Anthropometric standards for the assessment of growth and nutritional status. University of Michigan Press, Ann Arbor

Garrow J S 1983 Indices of adiposity. Nutrition Abstracts and Reviews 53: 697–708

Gleeson M H, Dowling R H, Peters T J 1972 Biochemical changes in intestinal mucosa after experimental small bowel by-pass in the rat. Clinical Science 43: 743–757

Heymsfield S B, McManus C, Smith J, Stevens V, Nixon D W 1982 Anthropometric measurement of muscle mass: revised equations for calculating bone-free arm muscle area. American Journal of Clinical Nutrition 36: 680–690

Heymsfield S B, Waki M 1991 Body composition in humans: advances in the development of multicompartment chemical models. Nutrition Reviews 49: 97–108

Jacob R A, Milne D B 1993 Biochemical assessment of vitamins and trace minerals. Clinics in Laboratory Medicine 13: 371–385

Labbé R F, Veldee M S 1993 Nutrition in the clinical laboratory. Clinics in Laboratory Medicine 13: 313–327

Lee R D, Nieman D C 1993 Nutritional assessment. Brown & Benchmark, Madison, Wisconsin

Levin G M, Deren J J, Steiger E, Zinno R 1974 Role of oral intake in maintenance of gut mass and disaccharide activity. Gastroenterology 76: 975–982

Lipkin E W, Bell S 1993 Assessment of nutritional status. The clinician's perspective. Clinics in Laboratory Medicine 13: 329–352

Lusaki H C 1987 Methods for the assessment of human body composition: traditional and new. American Journal of Clinical Nutrition 46: 537–556

McMahon M M, Bistrian B R 1990 The physiology of nutritional assessment and therapy in protein-calorie malnutrition. Disease-a-Month 7: 375–415

Metropolitan Life Insurance Company 1959 New weight standards for men and women. Statistical Bulletin of the Metropolitan Life Insurance Company 40: 1–3

National Institutes of Health Development Conference Statement Panel 1985 Health implications of obesity. Annals of Internal Medicine 103: 1073–1077

Roe D A 1985 Drug-induced nutritional deficiencies. AVI Publishing Co, Westport

Roe D A 1989 Diet and drug interactions. Van Nostrand Reinhold, New York

Roubenoff R, Kehayias J J 1991 The meaning and measurement of lean body mass. Nutrition Reviews 49: 163–175

Sampson L 1985 Food frequency questionnaires as a research instrument. Clinical Nutrition 4: 171–178

Smith L C, Mullen J L 1991 Nutritional assessment and indications for nutritional support. Surgical Clinics of North America 71: 449–457

Sorenson A W, Calkins B M, Connolly M A, Diamond E 1985 Comparison of nutrient intake determined by four dietary intake instruments. Journal of Nutrition and Education 17: 92–99

Spiekerman A M 1993 Proteins used in nutritional assessment. Clinics in Laboratory Medicine 13: 353–369

Steiner M, Bourges H R, Freedman L S, Gray S J 1986 Effect of starvation on the tissue composition of the small intestine in the rat. American Journal of Physiology 215: 75–77

Stuff J E, Garza C, O'Brian Smith E, Nichols B L, Montandon C M 1983 A comparison of dietary methods in nutritional studies. American Journal of Clinical Nutrition 37: 330–336

Weinsier R L, Krumdieck C L 1981 Death resulting from overzealous total parenteral nutrition: the refeeding syndrome revisited. American Journal of Clinical Nutrition 34: 393–399

Weinsier R L, Morgan S L 1993 Fundamentals of clinical nutrition. C V Mosby, St Louis, Mo

Weinsier R L, Heimburger D C, Butterworth C E 1989 Handbook of clinical nutrition. C V Mosby, St Louis

Young V R, Marchini S, Cortiella J 1990 Assessment of protein nutritional status. Journal of Nutrition 120: 1496–1502

4

Endoscopy

J. Christensen   R. W. Summers

THE INSTRUMENTS

Endoscopy in gastroenterology, the direct inspection of the lining of the gastrointestinal tract through its natural orifices, makes use of complex flexible instruments. Two forms of flexible endoscopes are currently in use, the first developed fiberoptic endoscopes and those which have almost replaced them, the video endoscopes. Rigid endoscopes – formerly used for the examination of the upper gut, are not used any more but the rigid sigmoidoscope remains in use for a limited examination of the anorectum.

In fiberoptic endoscopes, the fiberoptic bundle of thousands of flexible glass fibers transmits a coherent image though a long flexible cable which can be inserted into the gut. An end-viewing lens fused to the distal end of the bundle captures the image for transmission through the bundle. A second lens fused to the bundle at the proximal end magnifies the image for presentation to the observer's eye which is applied directly to the instrument. The illumination of the imaged mucosa comes from an external source of light which passes through the instrument through a second fiberoptic bundle. The fiberoptic instrument also contains tubes or channels that allow the injection of air to distend the viscus, the passage of instruments of various kinds and the injection of water to wash the distal viewing lens and the mucosa itself. Long braided steel cables activated by knobs allow the deflection of the tip of the instrument left and right and up and down in order to show the entire internal surface of the organ being examined.

In the videoscope, the image is transmitted through the flexible cable electrically and displayed on a video monitor. Light to illuminate the interior of the viscus passes from an external source through a fiberoptic bundle. Channels for washing the distal lens and mucosa, for inflation of the viscus and for the passage of instruments are all present as well, just as in the fiberoptic instruments.

The video endoscopes have so many advantages that they have nearly supplanted the fiberoptic instruments. They are much easier to use, project a high-resolution image, induce less operator fatigue, allow many observers to see the same view simultaneously, allow for rapid video photographic documentation and cost less to maintain since they are less subject to damage. These advantages outweigh a higher initial cost.

Both kinds of flexible endoscope accept the wide variety of instruments useful and necessary to fully exploit endoscopic technology. Biopsy forceps and grasping forceps in a variety of sizes and designs, cytology brushes and many designs of wire-loop snares provide various ways to biopsy or to remove lesions for histological evaluation. Flexible needles for injection, tubes for aspiration, heat-generating probes and electro-cautery devices for inducing hemostasis, pneumatic balloons for the dilatation of strictures and calibrated rules for measurement all find frequent use. The utility of such newly developed accessories as the Doppler ultrasound probe remains to be established.

Although all flexible endoscopes have the same general designs and capabilities, those intended to be passed through the mouth differ in some ways from those meant to be passed through the anus. Endoscopes meant to visualize the esophagus, stomach and duodenum, for example, are somewhat shorter and narrower than those intended to allow inspection of the colon. A recently devised enteroscope, designed to allow inspection of the small intestine, has still other dimensions. The instrument used for retrograde cannulation of the sphincter of Oddi requires special features as well. Instruments of special dimensions for use in children provide still other variations. Each kind of instrument requires accessories of appro-priate dimensions. The fully equipped gastrointestinal suite must possess a large number of different instruments for different uses, along with appropriate accessories, if it is to provide the full range of benefits possible from the use of diagnostic and therapeutic gastrointestinal endo-scopy.

The potential for the transmission of enteric bacteria and viruses, and bloodborne pathogens when biopsy is done, mandates rigorous attention to cleaning and disinfection of endoscopes. The totally immersible instruments and accessories should receive a brushing and perfusion of all channels with a detergent solution followed by immersion and perfusion with such bactericidal-viricidal solutions as glutaraldehyde or peroxy-acetic acid. Some experts advocate the wider use of autoclaving (for accessories only) and gas sterilization with ethylene oxide. Practices will undoubtedly evolve, but a rigorous modern program of disinfection must be maintained carefully. The time required for thorough disinfection necessitates the duplication of instruments in order to maintain a continuous operation of reasonable size. A 'disposable' endoscope has been devised in which a reusable optic portion is incorporated into a disposable sheath which includes the air, water and biopsy channels. Although it appears to function appropriately and probably prevents transmission of pathogens from patient to patient, it has not been widely adopted in practice because of its relatively high cost.

UPPER GASTROINTESTINAL ENDOSCOPY
Indications for diagnosis

The upper gastrointestinal endoscopic examination is prompted by symptoms suggesting disease of those organs which are accessible to that endoscope – the oropharynx, esophagus, stomach and duodenum. The indications are essentially the same as those for the radiographic examination of the upper gastrointestinal tract.

The two kinds of examination, endoscopy and radiography, were once believed to be equivalent and equally effective ways of doing the same job, but this is not so. The endoscopic examination gives much more detailed and convincing information about the state of the mucosa than does the X-ray and the endoscope allows biopsies or other specimens to be collected. In many situations it also permits definitive therapy to be done in addition to its diagnostic capabilities. The radiographic examination, on the other hand, provides a superior view of gross structure, revealing details about such gross lesions as diverticula, hernias, malrotations, dilatations and obstructions better than the endoscope can. Careful observation with video fluoroscopy also provides much more information about motor function and flow than does endoscopy. However, it is purely diagnostic and has no therapeutic potential. Thus, radiographic and endoscopic techniques are complementary and the choice of one or both depends upon the differential diagnosis that a detailed analysis of the clinical history and physical examination generates.

Most indications for upper gastrointestinal endoscopy fall within one of the following five broad categories. That is, a clinical history prominently displaying some aspect of one of these five categories of complaints is an indication for endoscopic examination of the oropharynx, esophagus, stomach and duodenum.

1. *Dysphagia* for solid boluses and *odynophagia* more commonly reflect mucosal disease than a gross structural abnormality and so endoscopy usually constitutes the better first study. In one case, oropharyngeal dysphagia, a radiographic study seems to be better as the first approach, because the complaint so often reflects a gross functional abnormality characterized by disturbed movement of the pharyngeal musculature and disturbed flow of pharyngeal contents. For the same reason, when esophageal dysphagia seems, from analysis, to arise from an esophageal motor disorder, radiographic study seems the appropriate first diagnostic step since the endoscope gives a poor idea of the pattern of esophageal contractions. Of course, a radiographic study can reveal the commoner causes of esophageal dysphagia, strictures and rings, but it can miss such lesions when they are small or incipient. Endoscopy with biopsy offers better sensitivity and specificity when the analysis of the symptom suggests an organic obstruction rather than a motor abnormality.

2. *Pyrosis* and *heartburn*, two terms that seem to denote the same sensation, reflect mucosal inflammation mainly in the esophagus, sometimes in the stomach, often in both organs. For this reason, upper gastrointestinal endoscopy constitutes the usual first approach to diagnosis.

3. *Chest* and *epigastric pains* of gastrointestinal origin are usually caused by severe inflammation, ulceration or infiltration of the wall by tumors. Upper gastrointestinal endoscopy is most useful not only to observe the lesion directly, but to obtain specimens for specific diagnoses by brushing, biopsy or electrocautery snare.

4. *Dyspepsia* and *indigestion*, two terms that seem to denote the same sensation, seem to reflect mucosal inflammation mainly in the stomach, sometimes in the duodenum, often in both. Thus, the greater selectivity and specificity of endoscopy recommend it as the best first approach to diagnosis. These symptoms are frequently ill-defined, however, and often poorly understood. It is not uncommon for the endoscopist to fail to find mucosal and motor abnormalities which would clearly explain these two symptoms.

5. *Upper gastrointestinal bleeding* is commonly inferred from the occurrence of occult gastrointestinal blood loss or the black tarry stools that constitute melena. Hematemesis, of course, always means bleeding from this region. Since, in almost all cases, upper gastrointestinal bleeding occurs from lesions located rostral to the ligament of Treitz, either radiography or upper gastrointestinal endoscopy may be used to identify the source. Radiographic demonstration of a lesion does not establish that it is the source of bleeding. The nearly universal preference for endoscopy reflects its greater sensitivity and specificity as well as the potential it offers for therapy through the several methods available for hemostasis. Thus, bleeding esophageal varices can be injected with an agent to induce clotting, a technique called sclerotherapy. Bleeding from non-variceal sources, such as ulcers, ectatic vessels or arteriovenous malformations, often slows or stops after the injection of the bleeding site with 1:10 000 epinephrine or a sclerosant solution, after the application of thermocautery with an accessory device called the heater probe, after electrocoagulation with appropriate monopolar or dipolar electrode probes or after laser photocoagulation with a laser delivery catheter. Endoscopy performed early in upper gastrointestinal bleeding has greatly reduced the need for emergency operation for this indication and it has greatly reduced the number of operations done for non-malignant lesions of the esophagus, stomach and duodenum.

Indications for therapy

Upper gastrointestinal endoscopy also finds many applications when the diagnosis is already known. Thus, it may be done for confirmation of a radiographic diagnosis by direct inspection, photography or biopsy but the usual reason for endoscopy in a situation of known diagnosis is for therapy. The control of bleeding from a known source is a common therapeutic indication. Foreign body removal is another, since appropriately designed forceps or graspers allow easy removal of coins, safety pins and the many other kinds of solid objects sometimes swallowed by depressed, psychotic or careless persons.

The endoscope facilitates the dilatation of non-malignant strictures with balloon dilators or wireguided bougies. The physician can use the endoscope to locate the balloon properly and to place the guidewire correctly. The endoscope also allows the operator to evaluate the results of dilatation immediately. Another use of the endoscope with a wireguided balloon is for dilatation of the lower sphincter in achalasia. The balloon used for this purpose is of a large diameter (35, 40 or 45 mm) and it actually produces a controlled tear of the esophageal sphincter muscle.

Another important therapeutic indication for endoscopy is the need for the placement of a percutaneous endoscopic gastrostomy tube or a jejunostomy tube. The description of the technique is beyond the scope of this chapter but the technique allows for long-term gastrointestinal feeding in situations where the use of the oral route is not possible.

Sometimes various stents are endoscopically placed in malignant esophageal strictures. They do not prolong life but they provide relief of dysphagia and improve nutrition. In some cases tumors can be vaporized endoscopically using lasers or coagulated using an electrocautery device called a tumor probe.

Preparation of the patient

In the preparation of the patient for upper gastrointestinal endoscopy, the endoscopist must always begin with a review of the history and the physical examination to satisfy himself of the appropriateness of the indications and the absence of contraindications and to discover reasons for special precautions. That is, a request for a diagnostic or therapeutic upper gastrointestinal endoscopic examination is a request for professional and expert consultation and it should be treated as such by all parties if error and waste are to be minimized. In particular, the upper gastrointestinal endoscopist must concern himself with situations that might enhance the likelihood of the three major risks of the procedure: aspiration, perforation and bleeding.

The examination requires that the patient have an empty stomach both for optimal viewing and to minimize the risk of vomiting and aspiration. For this reason the physician orders an overnight fast before the examination. In emergencies or situations not allowing much delay, one can demand no solid foods for at least 6 hours and/or no liquids except small sips of water for 4 hours. Patients suspected or known to have achalasia, gastric outlet obstruction or gastroparesis can be expected to retain solids beyond the usual time of fasting required for endoscopy. Gastric or esophageal lavage with a large-bore tube, an Ewald or Levacuator tube, should be done first in cases where obstruction or retention is known to be present.

Informed consent and risks in upper gastrointestinal endoscopy

The risks in upper gastrointestinal endoscopy constitute anesthetic/sedative risks, perforation and bleeding. The actual incidence of such complications has not been reported recently, but the estimate is less than one-tenth of 1% for each of them, overall. Some kinds of patient groups are more at risk than others. Thus, patients with severe cardiac or pulmonary disease seem to be unusually susceptible to the anesthetic/sedative risks. Similarly, those taking anticoagulant drugs and those with bleeding disorders suffer more risk of bleeding. And patients with such gross structural lesions as Zenker's hypopharyngeal diverticulum, esophageal diverticula, achalasia, paraesophageal hiatal hernia and malignant strictures all seem likely to be at higher risk for perforation. Complications can be minimized, as in all surgical procedures, by the exercise of complete preendoscopy assessment and good clinical judgement. Careful attention to drug dosages and to monitoring can minimize the risks of drug-related complications. The risk of perforation probably declines with the experience of the endoscopist. Bleeding can be minimized if the use of anticoagulant drugs is suspended for a time (if possible) and if biopsies are done judiciously. Written and oral informed consent must be obtained before the endoscopic examination (and before sedation). The patients must be completely informed of the potential for adverse reactions to medications, for bleeding and for perforation even though serious complications are rare.

Premedication, anesthesia, sedation, antibiotic prophylaxis and monitoring

Drugs are used in the upper gastrointestinal endoscopic examination (a) to anesthetize the oropharyngeal mucosa, (b) to diminish gastrointestinal motility and secretion, and (c) to reduce anxiety and discomfort. Many patients can tolerate upper gastrointestinal endoscopic examination just with a spray of a local anesthetic applied to the pharyngeal mucosa, without premedication or sedation, but few willingly accept the examination under such conditions, at least in the United States. Accordingly, most patients receive sedative agents orally or intravenously.

A little time before the examination begins, anesthesia of the oropharyngeal mucosa is achieved with a gargle or a spray of a local anesthetic such as dyclonine HCl, xylocaine or a similar agent. Just before the introduction of the endoscope, many endoscopists give atropine sulfate intravenously, 0.6 mg, and follow that with a benzodiazepine, meperidine or both in intravenous doses titrated to achieve the desired level of sedation.

Not all examiners use atropine routinely. Those who do use it justify its use on the grounds that it prevents reflex bradycardia in response to gastric distension and that it reduces the volume of saliva and gastric secretions which can interfere with the examination. Those who do not use atropine say that these benefits are unimportant to them. Atropine, of course, can and should be avoided in patients with glaucoma and bladder neck obstruction.

Many experts believe that endoscopy requires the continuous monitoring of blood pressure, pulse rate and blood oxygen saturation (by pulse oximetry) even though it has not been proved that monitoring reduces the incidence of important complications. The direct observation of respiration and of the level of consciousness is essential, regardless of the use of monitoring equipment, regardless of the depth of sedation achieved and especially when no sedation is used at all.

After the examination, whether or not sedation is used and regardless of the depth of sedation achieved, a period of observation is required. This should continue as long as the responsible nurses and physicians judge it to be needed, but about 1 hour seems a reasonable estimate of the average minimum. Antagonists to opiates and benzodiazepines may be used to hasten recovery or to treat the consequences of overdosage. Patients who have received sedatives must be forbidden to drive or undertake tasks requiring anything more than simple judgements or simple physical activities for 24 hours. Such advice is best given both as written instructions and as oral advice to responsible accompanying persons.

It is essential to appreciate the degree of amnesia which follows sedation. Even after apparent complete recovery, discussions with the patient are frequently not recalled 24 hours later. Descriptions of the findings or instructions regarding therapy must be given in the presence of an accompanying person, communicated in writing or repeated at a later time if they are to be remembered.

The appropriate use of prophylactic antibiotics before upper endoscopy constitutes an area of controversy. Patients with previous subacute bacterial endocarditis or prosthetic heart valves absolutely require antibiotic prophylaxis to prevent endocarditis. Those with valvular heart disease or mitral valve prolapse may or may not benefit from such use of antibiotics (an area of controversy).

Introduction of the endoscope

There are three methods for introducing an instrument such as the endoscope into the esophagus: the indirect method using finger guidance, the direct vision method and the method of blind tip manipulation. All three have advantages and disadvantages and the endoscopist is well advised to know all three techniques. In all, the endoscopist begins with the patient on the left side, though other body positions are feasible if necessary.

The *indirect method using finger guidance* involves the guidance of the instrument into the esophagus by the endoscopist. Its passage is detected by the fingers feeling the tip of the instrument traverse the upper esophageal sphincter. The instrument, with the mouthpiece slipped over the shaft, is held with the dominant hand placed about 12–15 inches from the tip. At the same time, the index and middle fingers of the subordinate hand are inserted into the patient's mouth. The endoscopist says to the patient, 'I need to feel the back of your throat' as two fingers are inserted so that the fingertips lie deep in the oropharynx with the knuckles at the level of the patient's incisor teeth. The endoscopist separates the two fingers, pulling the middle finger forward to draw the posterior tongue forward and pressing the index finger against the posterior pharyngeal wall in the midline (palpable as the ridge formed by the anterior surface of the vertebral column). In this position, the middle finger usually touches the epiglottis. Some endoscopists use only the index finger to manipulate the instrument to the bottom of the pharynx. With the two-finger technique, the index finger protects the gag receptors from excitation by the endoscope and tells the operator where the midline is located. The two fingers spread the pharynx anteroposteriorly and pull the opening to the airway more directly in line.

The endoscopist introduces the tip of the scope in the midline using the pad at the tip of the index finger to curve it. In the correct position, the instrument advances 15–18 cm from the incisors with no sense of resistance. If, at this point, the endoscope encounters some resistance, the scope should be pressed very gently forward while the patient swallows. The resistance vanishes when the patient swallows and the operator feels the instrument escape into the esophagus. If the placement of the instrument is exactly right it passes into the esophagus with absolutely no hang-up at the upper sphincter and no need for the patient to swallow. The advantage of this method lies in its speed and therefore its safety. Ideally, it achieves esophageal entry in less than about 2 seconds and so obviates or minimizes significant gagging, coughing, choking and aspiration. The use of this method also assures the quick peroral passage of esophageal bougies, ultrasound probes, electrodes (in cardiology), large-bore Ewald and Levacuator tubes and Levine or other small-bore tubes for gastric aspiration or feeding. The principal risk of the method, perforation through the pyriform sinuses, is prevented if the operator never presses the instrument forward with more than slight force and if he observes that the tip of the instrument advances 15–18 cm from the incisor teeth before any resistance is felt. The upper esophageal sphincter lies at this depth while the pyriform sinuses are reached at something less, 10–14 cm. Accidental intubation of the airway with this technique very rarely occurs. Such intubation is immediately apparent and immediately reversible.

In the *direct vision method*, the endoscopist advances the endoscope through the tubular mouthpiece which is held between the patient's teeth while looking through the endoscope or observing the image it projects on the video monitor screen. The openings to the trachea and to the closed upper esophageal sphincter can be seen. The instrument is pressed against the sphincter gently as the patient is asked to swallow. As the esophageal sphincter opens, the tip of the endoscope slips into the esophagus. The endoscopist cannot perforate the pyriform sinuses, be bitten by the patient or intubate the airway when using this method. Its disadvantages are that it usually takes longer than the indirect method and the instrument moves freely against the midline of the posterior pharyngeal wall where the gag receptors are located. Hence, gagging, coughing, choking and aspiration are more likely to occur.

In the method of *blind tip manipulation*, the endoscope is introduced through the mouthpiece which the patient holds between the incisors. The instrument is advanced while it is steered over the tongue only by manipulation of the controls until it reaches a point of resistance at 15–18 cm. With a little pressure, the endoscopist then asks the patient to swallow. The resistance to the instrument disappears and it is felt to enter the esophagus. With this method, perforation through the pyriform sinuses and intubation of the airway are both possible. Also, gagging, coughing, choking and aspiration are frequently encountered. For these reasons this method is not encouraged. It is mainly useful for introduction of the side-viewing endoscope by an operator who does not know the indirect method using finger guidance.

The steps in systematic upper gastrointestinal endoscopy

The upper gastrointestinal endoscopic examination may be prompted by the clinical suspicion of a specific lesion at a specific site, but the procedure requires a thorough and systematic inspection of all accessible organs. For that reason, a fixed or routine order of procedure should be followed to ensure a complete examination in all cases.

Once the end of the endoscope has entered the esophagus, the examiner should inject 30–50 cc of water into the esophagus. This washes the distal esophagus removing the foamy saliva often trapped there and, flowing into the stomach, dilutes the thick, foamy fluid or bile refluxate usually accumulated there. This fluid can be aspirated easily a few moments later when the endoscope enters the stomach. The endoscopist quickly surveys the whole esophagus looking for any abnormalities of the mucosa and the squamocolumnar junction and noting any narrowing or irregularities of the lumen before passing on to the stomach. The fluid collected in the fundus is aspirated and the tip of the instrument is advanced to the pylorus, the endoscopist simply noting any abnormalities without delaying much. The end of the endoscope is placed against the pylorus and pressed into the duodenum, proceeding caudad as far as possible. This is normally the third part of the duodenum. The logic prompting this wish to achieve maximum penetration quickly is that the intubation of the duodenum is the most uncomfortable part of the examination. The operator should aim to examine the duodenum early in the process while the effect of the sedative is maximal rather than later when the sedative is wearing off.

Having achieved the maximum penetration, the endoscopist withdraws the instrument slowly, reinserting it, rotating it and retroflexing it as necessary to see all parts. A special effort must be made to inspect all of the duodenal bulb because the bulb is a difficult place to see and lesions there are easily missed. Likewise, the technique of retroflexion of the endoscope with the endoscope tip placed in the antrum must be applied with the expenditure of enough time and effort to ensure the complete visualization of the gastric fundus and body. In the esophagus, the presence of a Schatzki ring or of inflammation at the gastroesophageal mucosal junction can be best revealed if the patient inhales and then exhales deeply and slowly while the endoscopist observes the esophagogastric junction carefully from a few centimeters above. The whole esophagus dilates briefly with such a deep respiration, revealing the area of the mucosal junction in detail. The location of the diaphragm, the lower esophageal sphincter and the squamocolumnar junction should be carefully noted by determining the distance from the gums using the calibration rings inscribed on the outer surface of the endoscope. Lesions and areas of special interest are best photographed and biopsied as they are encountered in this systematic inspection during withdrawal. The endoscopist may easily return to a deeper point at the end of the systematic study to confirm an opinion or to repeat a photograph or a biopsy.

Role of the endoscopic assistant

Specially-trained nurses, called gastrointestinal endoscopic assistants, now have an essential role in these procedures. They take major responsibility for the preparation of patients, for the administration of most if not all drugs used during the procedure, for monitoring procedures and for the postendoscopic observation. Also, they participate directly in the examination itself, in watching the image on the video screen, in handling accessories and specimens and, in some cases, in sharing the actual handling of the endoscope.

The role of the endoscopic assistant in the use of the endoscope varies. Some endoscopists manipulate the instrument entirely by themselves, using one hand to operate the controls and the other to advance, withdraw and rotate the instrument. Others keep both hands on the controls and ask the endoscopic assistant to advance, withdraw and rotate the instrument. In either case, the process works best if the examination is a team effort with shared responsibility, constant verbal communication, mutual trust and mutual respect.

Costs

Upper gastrointestinal endoscopy involves expensive equipment, expensive facilities and highly-trained personnel. The costs are correspondingly high. As economic pressures force changes in medicine, the wish to restrict the use of costly procedures, replacing them with less costly methods for diagnosis, will increase. The specificity and selectivity of endoscopy make this procedure so powerful, both in diagnosis and therapy, that it must continue as a mainstay of gastroenterology. It can, however, be overused and it certainly is. As in all of medicine, clinical judgement and clinical wisdom determine the outcomes of diagnosis and therapy far more than the number of tests and procedures done. Costs, however, being easily measurable, have become the easiest way to regulate medical practice and the yardstick of cost is likely to be applied without regard to issues of quality. In the long run, the most accurate diagnostic tool is usually the cheapest one because accuracy helps to prevent error and error is costly. The ability to obtain tissue and to perform definitive therapy greatly increases the value of endoscopy over other imaging techniques.

COLONOSCOPY AND FLEXIBLE SIGMOIDOSCOPY

Colonoscopy and flexible sigmoidoscopy, the examination of the whole colon or only its distal part, respectively, use instruments that differ principally in length. Flexible sigmoidoscopy, which involves much less preparation, risk and time, finds application when only the distal colon needs examination and when no electrocautery is to be used. Its principal usefulness lies in screening, as part of a general physical examination that involves a survey for colorectal polyps and cancer.

Indications for diagnosis and therapy

In general, the endoscopic examination of the colon has the same broad range of indications as the radiographic examination, the 'barium enema', but not exactly. Endoscopy is superior to the barium enema in evaluating the mucosa, but it does not reveal gross morphology well. The barium enema is better than the colonoscope in showing such gross features of the colon as size, disposition, herniation, diverticula and so on. Also, the colonoscope sometimes will not pass through parts of the colon fixed in place by adhesions from irradiation or operations, whereas barium does. Thus, the two examinations, colonoscopy and barium enema, are not competing but complementary.

The use of one or the other depends upon a thoughtful choice made by the physician according to the differential diagnosis. In cases of suspected mucosal disease, inflammation or tumor, colonoscopy usually wins because of its sensitivity and specificity. The ability to obtain biopsies and to remove polyps immediately enhances its value further. In making the choice, no matter what the indication, the physician must always consider both the greater risks of colonoscopy (risks of medication, perforation and bleeding) and the greater discomfort of the double contrast barium enema which is usually done without medication, includes the insufflation of air and requires the cooperation of the patient.

1. *Occult gastrointestinal blood loss with or without iron deficiency anemia* probably constitutes the commonest indication for the endoscopic examination of the colon. Since the patients may be bleeding also from the upper tract, colonoscopy and upper gastrointestinal endoscopy are often done at the same session.

2. Gross bleeding from the anus, *hematochezia*, also commonly prompts endoscopic examination first, usually flexible sigmoidoscopy because the commonest sources for gross hematochezia lie in the rectoanal region or in the sigmoid colon. This is especially relevant when the blood is bright red, is found on the surface of the stool or on the toilet tissue or is noted by the patient to drip into the toilet bowl or to appear in the underclothing following passage of the stool. All those signs suggest a source in the anal canal. The failure to find a source at flexible sigmoidoscopy requires colonoscopy and some physicians use that first in the interest of avoiding an extra examination. The choice between immediate colonoscopy or flexible sigmoidoscopy depends on the exact differential diagnosis arrived at by the careful consideration of details from the history and clinical examination.

3. *Chronic or long-standing recurrent diarrhea*, in many cases, reflects inflammatory disease of the colon and/or terminal ileum, both regions being accessible to the colonoscopist. Thus, colonoscopy is clearly the single most useful diagnostic test in establishing or refuting such inflam-

mation as causative. Clearly, however, the choice for colonoscopy in any single case must follow a thoughtful analysis of details from the history and clinical examination. Such an analysis might obviate the risk and expense of colonoscopy in cases where the existence of other common causes such as disaccharide intolerance, the chronic use of laxative substances, pancreatic insufficiency or small intestinal malabsorption actually explains the diarrhea.

4. *Polyps and other mass lesions* known to be present from an antecedent barium enema or a flexible sigmoidoscopy commonly prompt a referral for colonoscopy. A full colonoscopy is necessary in all such cases in order to detect any other such lesions that may have been missed because of the lesser sensitivity or extent of the other examination. Also colonoscopy is necessary to biopsy or to remove all the lesions discovered.

5. *Cancer surveillance* increasingly brings patients for endoscopic examination of the colon. There are various justifications for endoscopic examination of the colon in asymptomatic subjects as a part of a cancer surveillance program. A strong family history of cancer or a specific family history of colon polyps or cancer are common reasons. Age is another factor. Some experts advocate a program of routine regular flexible sigmoidoscopy in all persons past a specific age, 50, 55 or 60, but certainly only a small fraction of persons actually follow that practice even though presumably it reduces the mortality and morbidity of colon cancer.

6. *Altered bowel habit*, a sudden and persistent change in the frequency, size, shape or consistency of stools without reasonable explanation, is a frequent indication for colonoscopic examination of the colon because such changes frequently occur early in the course of colorectal cancer. That being the case, colonoscopy seems to be the clear first choice among possible next steps in the evaluation.

Non-indications for colonoscopy

The wide distribution of colonoscopes and colonoscopists, the lucrative nature of the practice and the eagerness with which some people subject themselves to dangerous and costly procedures that are paid for by others has led, without doubt, to the use of colonoscopy to try to explain complaints that actually arise elsewhere than the colon. To be specific, colonoscopy should rarely be prompted by solitary complaints of abdominal pain, bloating, chronic nausea, back pain or chronic constipation in the absence of any of the indications listed in the preceding section. In many such cases, a barium enema constitutes a sufficient and appropriate study. In all cases, the thoughtful construction of a differential diagnosis from a detailed analysis of the history and the physical examination is the only way to arrive at a satisfactory justification for the risks and costs of endoscopic examination of the colon.

Preparation of the patient

As explained above for endoscopic examination of the upper gastro-intestinal tract, the endoscopist who is to examine the colon must treat this task as a consultation. That is, the endoscopist must review all details of the clinical examination to assess fully the indications, to assure the absence of contraindications and to be prepared for exigencies.

Colonoscopy, but not flexible sigmoidoscopy, requires the presence of an empty stomach, achieved by a fast of at least 6 hours, and the presence of an empty colon. The fact that so many programs to achieve the latter requirement exist in various institutions only means that no one scheme has proved universally superior to all others, just as is true of the preparation for a barium enema. The endoscopist, in contrast to the radiologist, can compensate for a little residual liquid in the colon by aspirating it. All patients, however, must have undergone some procedure to empty the colon before endoscopic examination.

For flexible sigmoidoscopy, one or two small-volume tapwater or phosphate enemas usually suffice to evacuate the distal colon, often up to a level near the splenic flexure. These enemas should precede the examination by less than 1 hour. If only the anal canal and rectal mucosa concern the examiner and if the patient has defecated within 3–4 hours, flexible sigmoidoscopy often may be done successfully without any preparation of the colon.

For full colonoscopy, it is useful to discontinue any use of iron or bismuth preparations by the patients because of the black stools that these agents produce. Any residual black stool confuses the examiner. Likewise, anticoagulant drugs, including salicylates, should be stopped if possible to obviate bleeding after biopsy. The evacuation of the colon seems to be best accomplished by purging with a balanced electrolyte solution, 4–6 L being taken by mouth 6–18 hours beforehand. Some patients cannot manage the taste or the required volume of such solutions. Giving a little metoclo-pramide at the start to prevent gastric retention or giving the solution by nasogastric tube seems to help. For still others, a 3-day liquid diet with the interval ingestion of osmotic purges seems preferable. The use of hyper-tonic solutions containing mannitol or other poorly absorbed carbohy-drates is forbidden since they promote hydrogen generation by colonic bacteria, an obvious risk for explosion in the use of electrocautery. Although a recipe for bowel preparation must be tailored to each case, the high-volume orally administered flush with a balanced isotonic electrolyte solution seems, overall, to be the most satisfactory.

Premedication, sedation, the use of antibiotics and monitoring are the same as they are for upper gastrointestinal endoscopy, described above.

Informed consent and risks

The risks for colonoscopy are essentially the same as those for upper gastrointestinal endoscopy: cardiovascular risks, sedative/analgesia risks, perforation and bleeding. These must be discussed with the patient when obtaining informed consent in written form.

Colonoscopy, even more than upper gastrointestinal endoscopy, causes considerable physiological stress such that cardiac dysrhythmias and hypotension are likely, especially in those with cardiovascular disease. Thus, the procedure is contraindicated by recent myocardial infarction. The risks of overreaction to sedation with consequent hypotension and hypoxemia exist in all patients but they are greater in those with chronic cardiopulmonary disease. Such patients must be treated with special caution.

The risk of perforation is intrinsically greater in colonoscopy than in upper gastrointestinal endoscopy. The likelihood is increased during difficult examinations and in those patients who have diseases in which the colonic wall is thinned or weakened, in severe inflammation and in tumors that extend transmurally. Therapeutic maneuvers certainly increase the risk of perforation and probably aggravate bacteremia. Overall, the reported rate of perforation in colonoscopy is one in 700 with a mortality of one in 10 000.

The risk of significant bleeding, present even in those with normal clotting function, seems to be about twice that of perforation.

Other less common complications exist as well. Asymptomatic pneumoperitoneum can occur. Surgeons who open the abdomen soon after colonoscopy often report finding subserosal and mesenteric tears and hematomas. The existence of such asymptomatic trauma should not surprise the endoscopist who has watched the procedure fluoroscopically. The extreme looping and bending of the instrument that occurs during an apparently straightforward colonoscopic examination might well be expected to produce such trauma.

Introduction of the colonoscope and the flexible sigmoidoscope

The examinations can be and are done with the patient in a variety of positions, including the prone, supine, left and right lateral decubitus, lithotomy, knee–chest and knee–elbow positions. The choice seems to rest on the endoscopist's habit and on finding out what works best in each case. Although the choice is idiosyncratic, it should be tailored to each case. Many endoscopists start the examination with the patient lying on the left side. Changes in patient position during the exam can assist the endoscopist to get blood or other fluids to flow out of the visual field where they obscure the view and also to facilitate passage of the instrument through various segments of the colon.

The endoscopist always performs a digital examination of the anal canal first in order to discover any abnormality in the anal canal or distal rectum through palpation (anal stricture, tumor) and to dilate and lubricate the anal canal. The tip of the endoscope is then inserted by supporting it with the tip of the index finger and pressing the tip of the instrument obliquely against the opening.

Advancing the instrument

The technique for advancing the colonoscope or the flexible sigmoido-scope must be learned by direct observation and practice because it is too complex to describe adequately in writing. The technique involves all of a variety of possible maneuvers, pushing the instrument in or pulling it out, rotating it left or right, the insufflation or aspiration of air, compressing the abdomen and changing the position of the patient. The goal is the advancement of the tip of the instrument to the apex of the cecum as easily as possible. An experienced endoscopist working with an ideal patient can often do this in 5–10 minutes. Ease rather than speed, however, is the object. The risk of perforation seems likely to be greater when the passage is difficult or the examiner is in haste.

The steps in the examination

The principal objective in the forward passage of the instrument is usually to reach the cecal apex. In order to ensure that the entire colon has been examined it is important to identify the appendiceal orifice, the ileocecal valve, the characteristic triangular cecal folds and the blind cecal cul-de-sac. In cases where visualization of the ileum is desirable, this can be ventured before withdrawal of the colonoscope begins, with success in about four out of five cases. Abnormalities may be seen during forward passage of the instrument through the colon and their positions should be noted but the endoscopist should wait until the withdrawal of the colonoscope to deal definitively with them. Since the advancement of the instrument is far more uncomfortable than its withdrawal, advancement needs to be completed early in the allotted time while sedation and analgesia are maximal.

After the cecal apex is reached and positively identified from the characteristic landmarks, the instrument is withdrawn very slowly with rotation and transient readvancement as needed to allow the examiner to inspect all surfaces of the lumen at all levels of the colon. Sometimes a change of body position or abdominal compression is necessary to get full visualization. Any abnormalities encountered are best dealt with as they are encountered with the use of biopsy, snare cautery, photography or other appropriate techniques. Retroflexion of the tip of the instrument is possible at many places in the colon and it may help to visualize difficult areas. It is routinely done in the rectum in order to give a view of the inner end of the anal canal which cannot otherwise be seen well.

Therapeutic procedures

Besides its diagnostic abilities, the colonoscope allows for a variety of treatments. Since most of these treatments involve the generation of heat, this therapeutic potential does not apply in flexible sigmoidoscopy where the usual preparatory enema does not ensure the absence of the explosive gases generated by colonic bacteria. The commonest therapeutic procedure at colonoscopy is polypectomy, either by the use of snare cautery or, for small polyps, cauterizing forceps. Electrocoagulation, laser photocoagulation and injection therapy of vascular lesions are all routine. Laser ablation of tumors is possible. Also, tube or stent placement is possible and balloon dilation of strictures can be done transcolonoscopically.

Role of the assistant in colonoscopy

As in upper gastrointestinal endoscopy, a highly-trained assistant is essential to the optimal performance of colonoscopy and flexible sigmoidoscopy. The assistant normally takes the major responsibility for the preparation of the patient, the administration of nearly all drugs, the monitoring of the procedure, the handling of accessory instruments and the handling of biopsy specimens. The assistant can play a key role in successfully passing the instrument to the cecum by the application of abdominal pressure to prevent or minimize the formation of loops. This is very important because further insertion with a loop present will painfully expand the loop without transmitting forward force at the tip. Some endoscopists also ask the assistant to help directly with the examination, advancing, withdrawing or rotating the scope as the endoscopist uses both hands to manipulate the controls. With modern video endoscopes, the assistant also provides valuable service in the continuous observation of the video monitor. Two observers are better than one and a constant dialogue between observers about the screen image makes for a complete and satisfying examination.

RIGID PROCTOSIGMOIDOSCOPY

Although limited in its use, rigid proctosigmoidoscopy has a definite place in the assessment of hemorrhoids and rectal lesions. The examination should extend up to the rectosigmoid junction but not go beyond it.

Negotiation of the rectosigmoid junction is the most uncomfortable part of the examination which should be avoided. Flexible instruments are not suitable for this assessment because the administration of an enema prior to the examination may produce minimal hyperemia which mimics grade I proctitis. Also, lesions in the lower rectum are more liable to be missed with the flexible instruments (see also Ch. 18, pp. 413–414).

ENDOSCOPIC RETROGRADE CHOLANGIOPANCREATO- GRAPHY AND ACCESSORY PROCEDURES

Instrumentation

The technique of endoscopic retrograde cholangiopancreatography (ERCP) and related procedures developed as an extension of upper gastrointestinal endoscopy. The endoscopic instrument usually used, a side-viewing flexible endoscope, possesses an 'elevator', a manipulatable lever which facilitates the steering of a catheter passed through the endoscope into the ampulla of Vater. In a few cases, ordinary end-viewing endoscopes prove satisfactory or even superior. The technique of visualization of the biliary and pancreatic duct systems involves the injection of a radioopaque fluid into the systems through these catheters. The visualization of these ducts requires an appropriate high-quality radiographic instrument with an image intensifier and a video monitor. A variety of injection catheters (varying in size and configuration), cytology brushes, papillotomes and drainage catheters provide for the range of techniques needed to investigate and manage pancreatobiliary disease by ERCP.

Indications for ERCP

The commonest use for ERCP is in the diagnostic approach to suspected biliary tract or pancreatic diseases. The cardinal symptoms of such diseases, jaundice and abdominal pain, do not constitute a full indication by themselves. Rather the decision for ERCP rests on the presence of suspected disease of these organ systems as prominent parts of a differential diagnosis which in turn reflects a thoughtful analysis of the history and clinical examination and the results of previous laboratory investigations and other imaging techniques.

ERCP also finds prominent use in the therapy of known or established pancreatobiliary disease. Today with judicious use of preprocedural tests, the majority of procedures are therapeutic rather than diagnostic. Thus, ERCP must be done before endoscopic papillotomy, biliary and/or pancreatic drainage and transductal balloon dilatation of duct strictures. Also, ERCP is sometimes helpful to provide mapping of the duct systems before surgical operations undertaken to treat chronic pancreatitis or pancreatic pseudocysts.

Preparation of the patient

As is true in other kinds of endoscopic procedures, the endoscopist must treat a request for ERCP as a consultation. This requires that the consultant review all of the available clinical and laboratory data in order to confirm the presence of an indication for the study and the absence of contraindications and to prepare for exigencies or to take special precautions.

The patient must be fasted for at least 6 hours to ensure an empty stomach. The endoscopist must ask about the symptoms of conditions that might impede the passage of the instrument, for the side-viewing instrument is passed 'blind'. It should not be passed if there is any reason to suspect obstruction, stricture or any other major morphological abnormality (major herniation or malrotation) in the proximal gastro-intestinal tract. The examiner must also ask about sensitivity to iodine because radiographic contrast media contain iodine.

The exact procedure must be explained by the endoscopist to the patient, as is now required by modern rules for informed consent. This must include a discussion of risks and precautions.

Premedication, anesthesia, sedation, antibiotic prophylaxis and monitoring procedures are the same as described for upper gastro-intestinal endoscopy above. Since much of the work takes place in the darkened X-ray room, special attention to the monitoring of cardio-vascular function is required. In the presence of ductal obstruction, antibiotics must be given to avoid cholangitis and other serious infections.

The procedure

Either the side-viewing duodenoscope or, rarely, the end-viewing upper gastrointestinal endoscope is introduced with the patient in the left lateral decubitus position. It must be introduced by the indirect method using finger guidance as described above (p. 106) and passed to the stomach where the pylorus must be brought into view by the insufflation of air and the rotation of the instrument. Its subsequent passage through the pylorus is partially blind, but the endoscopist recognizes passage by a change in the resistance to advancement of the instrument and a change in the appearance of the mucosa. The location of the ampulla of Vater is discovered by advancement and rotation of the endoscope. The endoscopist must be prepared for considerable variation in the position of this structure. Cannulation of one or the other of the two ducts that enter into the ampulla can be achieved selectively by repeated attempts with the cannula directed to the correct portion of the ampulla.

A scout film must be taken at the outset, before cannulation. After cannulation, the radioopaque fluid is injected and the filling of the duct system is visualized by fluoroscopy with films being taken as appropriate for the record and for detailed study. At some point, the patient must be put prone since radiographs are most easily read and interpreted when they are taken with the patient in that position. But the patient can and often must be rotated to one side or the other to get optimal filling and visualization of one part of the duct system or another.

The technique allows for therapeutic maneuvers immediately after diseases are demonstrated. For example, manometry of the sphincter of the ampulla can be done immediately and, if symptoms compatible with sphincter dysfunction prompted the study, hypertensive sphincters can be cut by the sphincterotome. Likewise, the finding of common duct stones can lead to prompt sphincterotomy and stone removal. The dilatation of strictures, the placement of stents, the removal of stones and a variety of other therapeutic procedures can be done at the first or later sessions as allowed by time, the drugs administered and other factors.

Risks

The principal risk of ERCP, acute pancreatitis, occurs after one-half to two-thirds of pancreatograms, to judge from studies of serum pancreatic enzyme levels. Clinically significant pancreatitis is much less common, following only 0.7–7.4% of examinations. Severe necrotizing pancreatitis occurs in only about 0.1%.

Another common risk is bacterial infection of the duct systems. The risk is so high in patients with suspected partial obstruction by stones, tumors or strictures that ERCP must be delayed in those situations until the availability of endoscopic or surgical drainage promptly after an obstruction is demonstrated. The use of antibiotics and prompt drainage reduces the risk of serious bacterial cholangitis to less than 1%.

With sphincterotomy and stone removal, the principal risks are bleeding and perforation. Significant bleeding occurs in less than 2% of cases and is only rarely problematic. Perforations occur in up to 1.1% of cases, the risk being higher in patients with juxtapapillary diverticula.

After endoprosthesis (stent) placement, acute bacterial cholangitis, the greatest risk, can be ameliorated by the use of antibiotics. Still, using the combination of sphincterotomy with stent placement, a procedure most often done in patients with malignant obstructions, the risk of infection is 2–6%. Eventually all stents become obstructed and thus are a cause of serious infections. When this occurs, emergency removal of the stent with antibiotic therapy and the placement of a new stent are required. Bleeding and perforation are no more common with a stent placement than after sphincterotomy alone.

FURTHER READING

Baillie J 1992 Gastrointestinal endoscopy: basic principles and practice. Butterworth-Heinemann, Oxford

Blackstone M O 1984 Endoscopic interpretation. Raven Press, New York

Cotton P B, William C B 1990 Practical gastrointestinal endoscopy, 3rd edn. Blackwell Scientific Publications, Oxford

Katon R M, Keeffe E B, Melynk C S 1985 Flexible sigmoidscopy. Grune and Stratton, Orlando

Shinya H 1982 Colonoscopy: diagnosis and treatment of colonic diseases. Igaku-Shoin, New York

Silvis S E 1984 Therapeutic gastrointestinal endoscopy. Igaku-Shoin, New York

Sivak M V 1987 Gastroenterologic endoscopy. W B Saunders, Philadelphia

Waye J, Geenen J, Fleicher D, Venu R P 1987 Techniques in therapeutic endoscopy. W B Saunders, Philadelphia

5

Laparoscopic surgery

D. B. Jones N. J. Soper

INTRODUCTION

In 1901 Kelling performed the first endoscopic exploration of the abdominal cavity using a cystoscope inserted under local anesthesia (Kelling 1901, Stellato 1992). Later laparoscopists learned to insufflate the abdominal cavity with a gas to create a working space. Modified surgical instruments introduced through specialized ports with airtight valves allowed manipulation of organs and therapeutic interventions. Today, laparoscopy is invaluable as a diagnostic technique, especially when combined with intraoperative ultrasonography and endoscopic guided biopsy. This chapter will describe minimally invasive techniques of abdominal exploration and tissue sampling as well as discussing common anatomical findings, indications, contraindications and risks using this approach.

Advantages

Diagnostic laparoscopy has many potential advantages over other diagnostic studies and traditional 'open' laparotomy (Table 5.1). Compared with other imaging modalities, diagnostic laparoscopy most realistically characterizes the lesion's color and contour. Enhanced resolution and magnification may detect lesions <1 mm in size, a size usually missed by CT scan and MRI. Furthermore, overall cost of the procedure may be less than that of multiple non-invasive tests. Compared to exploratory laparotomy, postoperative pain and intestinal ileus are less after diag-

Table 5.1 Potential advantages of diagnostic laparoscopy

Over CT scan, MRI and ultrasonography
- Accuracy of diagnosis
- Directed biopsy
- Reduced complications of hemorrhage
- Enhanced resolution ($\leq$ 1 mm size lesions)

Over laparotomy
- Reduced pain
- Decreased hospital stay and costs
- Rapid return to work and full activity

---

nostic laparoscopy. Small trocar puncture sites are also more appealing cosmetically than large laparotomy incisions. By avoiding the morbidity of a laparotomy, otherwise healthy patients can usually be discharged from the hospital within 24 hours after a diagnostic laparoscopy and return to 'normal' activity within a few days.

Disadvantages

Diagnostic laparoscopy also has several disadvantages. Patients should be acceptable candidates for general anesthesia. Even if laparoscopy is performed under local anesthesia, inadvertent perforation of a viscus or uncontrolled hemorrhage may occur and require formal laparotomy. Two-dimensional video systems lack depth perception, distort anatomical relationships and hinder task performance. The elongated laparoscopic instruments have diminished tactile feedback and structures in the abdomen and retroperitoneum may not be palpated. Instead, the laparoscopist mainly relies on visualizing the surfaces within the abdominal cavity. Therefore, surgeons and physicians performing these procedures must be skillful in laparoscopic techniques, must perform laparoscopy routinely and should achieve formal credentialing. Some patients are not suitable candidates for laparoscopy because of intraabdominal adhesions which are too extensive to allow visual exploration via a laparoscope. Adequate pneumoperitoneum and exposure of the operative field may be difficult to maintain because of continuous air leaks, unrecognized perforated viscera or excessive irrigation. Intraoperative complications are also more challenging to manage laparoscopically than during open surgery, especially the control of brisk hemorrhage, and the laparoscopy suite should be equipped to deal with these rare emergencies. Still, the major concern with diagnostic laparoscopy is whether the surgeon is overlooking pathology. To minimize this problem, just as with conventional laparotomy, the surgeon needs to develop a systematic approach to the examination of the entire abdomen.

Technological advances may solve many of the current limitations of laparoscopy. Three-dimensional video systems restore depth perception, perhaps enhancing the safety and accuracy of laparoscopic examination and biopsies compared to two-dimensional systems. Intraoperative laparoscopic ultrasonography permits directed evaluation of the organ parenchyma beyond the visible surface. Mechanical and robotic camera holders free the laparoscopist's hands to perform other tasks (Sackier & Wang 1994). Alternatively, pneumoperitoneum with its potential risks can be avoided using various abdominal retractors (Banting et al 1993, Smith et al 1993, 1994). In the ensuing discussion, we review the current status of diagnostic laparoscopy, focusing on preoperative, intraoperative and postoperative considerations.

General indications

Diagnostic laparoscopy should only be performed if patient management is likely to be affected. The current indications for laparoscopy in management algorithms are evolving, but diagnostic laparoscopy has a role in the assessment of abdominal masses, abdominal pain and trauma (Table 5.2). Laparoscopic guided liver biopsy may be performed under local anesthesia. Staging of abdominal malignancy will determine whether patients receive adjuvant therapy or undergo a major therapeutic operation. Some patients will be found to have unresectable cancer due to local invasion or metastasis and these patients can avoid unnecessary laparotomy. Likewise, supposedly 'surgical' abdominal pain may be discovered at laparoscopy not to be operable at all. Pelvic inflammatory disease may mimic appendicitis, for example, and be managed non-operatively.

At select centers, diagnostic laparoscopy is used to evaluate blunt and penetrating trauma either in the emergency room or in the operating room before deciding on the need for laparotomy (Berci et al 1983, 1991, Cuschieri et al 1988, Sosa et al 1992, 1993).

Depending on the findings during diagnostic laparoscopy and the patient's overall medical status, therapeutic interventions are commonly performed laparoscopically. When diagnostic laparoscopy is performed by the surgeon, many of the therapeutic interventions may be done at the time of diagnosis rather than being referred to a surgeon for a second laparoscopic procedure. The proper role of therapeutic laparoscopy is still being defined. To date, laparoscopic cholecystectomy has clearly emerged as the 'gold standard' treatment of cholelithiasis (Soper et al 1992b). Procedures that are gaining acceptance include appendectomy, exploration of the common bile duct, operations for control of gastroesophageal reflux, repair of inguinal hernia, colon resection, acid-reducing procedures

Table 5.2 Common indications for diagnostic laparoscopy

Accepted
- Assessment of liver
- Acute abdominal pain in women
- Ascites of unknown etiology

Gaining acceptance
- Staging of malignancy
- Blunt and penetrating trauma
- Vague abdominal pain in children
- Chronic abdominal pain

Anecdotal experience
- ICU setting
- Fever of unknown origin
- Second look procedure

for peptic ulcer disease, and splenectomy (Soper et al 1994). Other procedures that are being performed include adrenalectomy, gastrojejunostomy, cholecystojejunostomy and pancreatic resection. Procedures under investigation include aortofemoral bypass, splenorenal shunt and pancreaticoduodenectomy.

Therapeutic laparoscopy is beyond the scope of this chapter, but randomized prospective studies to evaluate long-term outcome of most of these operations and formal credentialing of laparoscopic surgeons both still need to be done before minimally invasive operations can be recommended to patients without reservation. Diagnostic laparoscopy, on the other hand, is a well-accepted procedure that has been performed safely by gastroenterologists, hepatologists and surgeons.

Absolute and relative contraindications

Preoperative evaluation should determine the presence of confounding medical problems which may adversely affect the outcome of laparoscopy. Absolute contraindications to laparoscopy include the following (Table 5.3): inability to tolerate general anesthesia, uncorrectable coagulopathy, a 'frozen' abdomen or a hemodynamically unstable patient. Relative contraindications are as dependent on the experience of the laparoscopist as on any particular attribute of the patient (Table 5.3). With experience, most of these conditions can be successfully managed. For example, morbidly obese patients may require longer trocars to traverse the anterior abdominal wall and higher insufflation pressures to obtain an adequate working space. Appendicitis and cholecystitis may occur during pregnancy and diagnostic laparoscopy is often helpful for diagnosing and treating this subset of patients with vague abdominal pain in whom additional radiological studies are undesirable. Although laparoscopic

Table 5.3 General contraindications to laparoscopy

Absolute
- Uncorrected coagulopathy
- Poor risk for general anesthesia
- Inability to tolerate a laparotomy
- Hemodynamically unstable

Relative
- Prior abdominal surgery
- Peritonitis
- Obesity
- Pregnancy
- Unreducible abdominal/inguinal hernia
- Umbilical abnormalities
- Severe pulmonary disease
- Intestinal obstruction

cholecystectomies have been performed safely during pregnancy (Soper et al 1992a), the prolonged exposure to carbon dioxide pneumoperitoneum may have untoward effects on the fetus. Hyperventilation and monitoring of end-tidal carbon dioxide minimize maternal hypercarbia and fetal acidosis. Insufflation pressures are kept low, preferably below 12 mmHg, to obviate respiratory problems and monitoring of fetal heart sounds should be done in consultation with an obstetrician (See & Soper 1994). Based on our experience, women in their reproductive years are not denied laparoscopy; however, the novice laparoscopist may wish to refer these complex cases to more experienced laparoscopy centers.

In the gastrointestinal suite, laparoscopy has been used mainly to evaluate the liver's surface and to accurately diagnose hepatic lesions (Kalk 1929). Laparoscopy under local anesthesia allows the patient to help localize intraabdominal sources of pain (Salky 1993). Likewise, traumatologists have introduced the laparoscope under local anesthesia in the emergency room to evaluate the severity of traumatic wounds (Berci et al 1983, 1991, Cuschieri et al 1988). In properly selected patients the mortality is <0.5% in several large series (Easter et al 1992, Kalk 1929, Salky 1993). In the future, as technology advances and the skills of the laparoscopist improve, more and more procedures will undoubtedly be performed under local or regional anesthesia by minimally invasive techniques.

TECHNIQUE OF LAPAROSCOPIC ABDOMINAL EXPLORATION

Preoperative care and anesthesia

Ideally, patients are fasted from midnight before the operation. Patients without other major medical problems are admitted to the hospital on the morning of operation and given preoperative sedatives. If the possibility of intraoperative contamination exists, a single dose of intravenous antibiotics is administered. Gastric distension is diminished by administering both intravenous metoclopramide and a H_2 receptor antagonist. Sequential compression stockings are placed on both legs to avoid pooling of blood in the lower extremities. In patients with known malignancy and in those at risk for venous thromboembolism, minidose subcutaneous heparin may be used. After the induction of anesthesia, a bladder catheter and orogastric tube may be placed to decompress these hollow organs before inserting laparoscopic trocars. For more emergency exploration, such as for trauma, the orogastric tube is placed and the stomach drained before induction to prevent aspiration. The abdomen is prepared and draped sterilely.

Local anesthesia

Bupivacaine (0.5%) is injected at the initial port site and is used to a maximum dose of approximately 2.5 mg/kg. The skin and peritoneum surrounding the site of incision should be adequately infiltrated with anesthetic before inserting the laparoscopic trocar. All patients receive oxygen by nasal cannula or mask. As an adjunct, intravenous sedation and/or inhaled nitrous oxide may be added. Intravenous agents for sedation and amnesia may include a benzodiazepine, commonly midazolam, and a short-acting opioid such as fentanyl. Nitrous oxide also has analgesic properties, but inhalational agents are contraindicated if the patient has eaten within 6 hours of operation because of the high risk of aspiration with pneumoperitoneum. Routine patient monitoring should include blood pressure, pulse oximetry and EKG. Nord & Boyd (1994) reported 357 patients examined by diagnostic laparoscopy under local anesthesia. None required intubation, general anesthesia or ventilatory support. Transient vasovagal reactions occurred in 3% of patients, but hypotension generally responded promptly to atropine. Because local anesthesia is safe for most patients, cost containment issues will probably encourage more procedures to be performed under local anesthesia as an outpatient rather than under general anesthesia in the operating room.

General anesthesia

Although diagnostic laparoscopy can be performed with local or regional anesthesia, we prefer inhalational anesthesia and controlled ventilation. General anesthesia allows pain-free probing of inflamed tissues, biopsy of peritoneal lesions and, if need be, facilitates rapid conversion to an open laparotomy. Adequate depth of anesthesia, complete muscle relaxation and administration of antiemetics are important considerations for the optimal anesthetic management. Patient monitoring during laparoscopy using general anesthesia includes electrocardiography, pulse oximetry, blood pressure, precordial stethoscope, airway pressure and capnography. Invasive monitoring with arterial lines and Swan–Ganz catheters may be indicated in selected high-risk individuals (Gravenstein et al 1989, Monk & Weldon 1994). Postoperative pain is lessened by preincisional subcutaneous injection at the port sites with a long-acting local anesthetic, such as 0.5% bupivacaine (Tverskoy et al 1992).

Room set-up

Instrumentation and set-up for laparoscopy require consideration. The laparoscope used may be 2–10 mm in diameter and with a forward-viewing (0°) or obliquely angled lens. Smaller laparoscopes are more commonly used in the emergency room setting. Larger laparoscopes have the advantage of supplying more light and a wider visual field. The 30–45° angled lenses diminish illumination but permit a more thorough

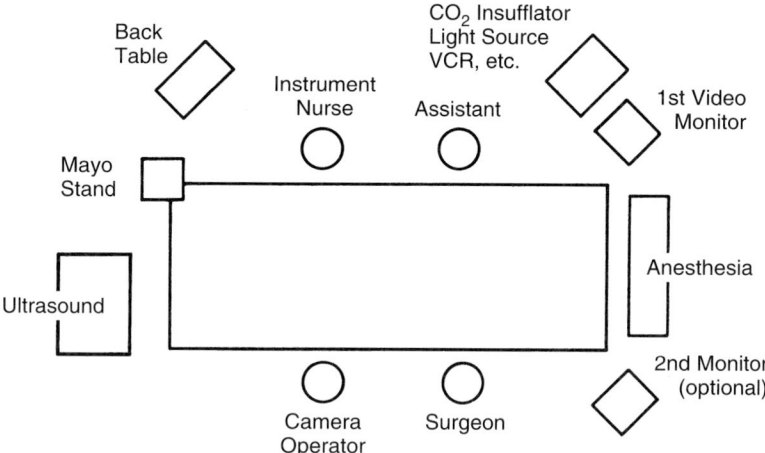

Figure 5.1 Room set-up. The patient's head is to the right. The surgeon stands on the patient's left and the assistant is to the patient's right. Video equipment is placed on carts and monitors are positioned for clear visualization by the entire surgical team.

examination of the extremes of the peritoneal cavity whereas a straight scope only views objects straight ahead. Other standard instruments for diagnostic laparoscopy include scissors, grasping devices, liver retractor, blunt probe, Babcock clamp, hook cautery, cupped forceps, biopsy forceps, uterine retractor and a hollow suction/irrigator probe. If reusable instruments are used, proper cleansing and sterilization techniques are important to minimize the risk of infection.

Room set-up will vary by the preferences of the laparoscopist (Fig. 5.1). The patient is monitored by an anesthesiologist or nurse anesthetist at the head of the table. The patient lies supine or in lithotomy stirrups on a table which is capable of multiplanar movement to maximize gravitational retraction of intraabdominal organs. Electrocautery and suction/irrigation tubes are draped off the patient's left shoulder. The instrument stand is at the foot of the operating table. One video system and monitor are positioned across from the laparoscopist and a second monitor is usually placed across from the assistant. The intraoperative ultrasound monitor is aligned next to the laparoscopic video screen unless the sonogram image is already channeled into the video monitor with a dual image display.

Access and pneumoperitoneum

A working space (pneumoperitoneum) in the abdominal cavity is established by insufflating gas using a high-flow insufflator. The pneumoperitoneum is established by either a closed or an open technique.

Closed technique

First, the Veress needle should be checked to ensure that the spring-loaded stylet is functioning properly and that the lumen is patent to the injection of water. The patient is then placed in a 10–15° Trendelenburg position and a 10 mm incision is made into the subcutaneous tissue of the infraumbilical skinfold. In patients who have had previous abdominal surgery, an alternative site distant from previous incisions is chosen for initial access. With an upper midline scar, a right or left lower quadrant insertion site is chosen two-thirds of the distance from the umbilicus to the iliac crest lateral to the rectus sheath. Adhesions from a lower midline scar may be avoided by an initial puncture in the right or left upper abdomen at the lateral edge of the rectus muscle. The positions of the liver, spleen and bladder relative to the port site must be ascertained before needle insertion to avoid iatrogenic injury.

The lower abdominal wall is grasped to elevate the fascia safely away from the intraabdominal organs before needle puncture. The Veress needle is then inserted at a right angle to the abdominal wall, usually at a 45° angle off the vertical axis toward the pelvis but away from the aortic bifurcation and iliac arteries. Two or three 'clicks' of the obturator may be heard as the needle passes through the fascia and peritoneum into the peritoneal cavity. Absence of blood, urine or stool on aspiration and a positive drop test corroborate the correct needle position. A drop test is confirmatory if sterile saline flows rapidly by gravity into the peritoneal cavity. Elevating the lower abdominal wall during the drop test will decrease intraabdominal pressure and enhance free flow. The abdominal cavity is then insufflated with the appropriate gas to a pressure of 8–15 mmHg beginning at a flow rate of 1 liter per minute.

After the abdominal cavity is distended, the Veress needle is removed and a trocar is inserted carefully into the abdominal cavity while manually exerting countertraction on the abdominal wall. The resistance of the fascia and peritoneum is apparent as the trocar slowly penetrates the abdominal wall. The sharp inner trocar is removed and the sheath may be secured with adhesive patches, screw threads, internal balloons or suture. Bloodstained fluid or frank blood after trocar insertion are ominous signs. If trocar insertion is followed by brisk return of blood and hemodynamic compromise, a laparotomy should be performed immediately while leaving the trocar in place. Delay in converting to formal laparotomy has resulted in several deaths from injury to a major blood vessel.

Open technique

The closed technique is applicable in most patients, but for patients with previous abdominal surgery, pregnancy or distended bowel we generally use the open technique.

Open port insertion is similar to the cut-down procedure used for catheter insertion during diagnostic peritoneal lavage. A vertical or horizontal 1.5 cm skin incision is made in the infraumbilical skinfold. Blunt dissection of the subcutaneous tissue is performed deep to the skin until the fascia is clearly visible. Kocher clamps are applied to both sides of the midline of the linea alba and a small vertical incision is made into the peritoneal cavity. A finger or curved Kelly clamp is carefully introduced into the incision and any loose adhesions may be swept away. A blunt-tipped (Hasson) port is then placed under direct vision through the fascial incision into the peritoneal cavity. The pneumoperitoneum is established only after ensuring safe access. The Hasson port is secured with two sutures on both sides of the fascial incision. Alternatively, standard ports can be secured with two concentric purse-strings around the fascial incision. The purse-string sutures are tightened down using a section of red rubber catheter similar to a vascular tourniquet.

Open techniques take a few minutes longer than the closed technique for initial port insertion; however, open insertion is especially advantageous in patients with previous abdominal incisions or whenever the Veress needle position is in doubt. At conclusion of the operation, all trocar entry sites >5 mm should be closed to avoid the risk of postoperative herniation (Jones et al 1995).

Gases

For diagnostic laparoscopy, several gases may be used to create the pneumoperitoneum. Many laparoscopists use nitrous oxide during short cases or those performed with local anesthesia because it is inexpensive and associated with a lower incidence of cardiac arrhythmias than carbon dioxide. Nitrous oxide also does not irritate the peritoneum (as does CO_2) and when absorbed does not cause metabolic abnormalities. However, nitrous oxide will support combustion and is therefore contraindicated when the use of electrocautery is anticipated (Gunatilake 1978). Nitrous oxide is also less soluble in blood than carbon dioxide and may be more likely to cause gas embolism. Carbon dioxide, on the other hand, is commonly used during therapeutic laparoscopy because it is non-combustible. Carbon dioxide is eliminated rapidly from the systemic circulation and will not form gas emboli under experimental conditions unless infused into a systemic vein at a rate greater than 1 liter per minute (Graff et al 1959). However, carbon dioxide absorption may lead to hypercarbia and respiratory acidosis in patients with chronic obstructive pulmonary disease (Fitzgerald et al 1992). Carbon dioxide may also cause postoperative discomfort due to referred diaphragmatic pain as it is converted on the moist peritoneal surfaces to carbonic acid.

During insufflation and throughout the case, the patient must be closely monitored. Gas embolism may cause right ventricular outflow obstruction signaled by a fall in end-tidal carbon dioxide, hypotension or a 'millwheel' heart murmur. When this life-threatening complication is suspected, the patient is placed immediately in Trendelenburg position with the left side down and the gas is promptly aspirated through a central venous catheter (Beck & McQuillan 1994). Other problems encountered during laparoscopy include hypotension because of decreased venous return and diminished cardiac output, bradycardia due to vagal reactions and acidosis secondary to hypercarbia. Fortunately, most of these complications improve by deflating the pneumoperitoneum through an open port. These complications may be circumvented altogether by external retraction devices which create a working space without pneumoperitoneum (Smith el al 1994).

Visualization

After access is established, the laparoscope is introduced. A video system then digitizes, enhances and transmits images to a color monitor screen for the entire operating team to view. Careful abdominal inspection may detect pathology or iatrogenic injury. The camera operator must maintain the proper orientation of the camera and scope, center the operative field on the video monitor, follow instruments as they enter and exit the ports and wipe off condensation or blood that may cloud the lens. Anti-fog solution should be applied to the lens and the laparoscope tip should be warmed to 38°C in sterile water prior to introduction into the abdominal cavity to minimize condensation.

Intraoperative ultrasonography

In the past, a criticism of diagnostic laparoscopy was that only the surfaces of organs could be visualized and parenchymal disease was overlooked. Intraoperative laparoscopic ultrasonography improves the sensitivity of abdominal exploration when performed by laparoscopists skilled in sonographic interpretation (Goletti et al 1994). This technology has proven particularly useful in the staging of malignancy (Goletti et al 1994, Spinelli & Difelice 1991). At our institution, the radiologist plays an integral role in intraoperative sonography. Images are transmitted from the operating room to the radiologist's reading room in real time to clarify any ambiguities. The radiologist and laparoscopist communicate via an intercom and additional views are obtained as necessary. With experience, laparoscopists have become quite adept with this technology and we are using ultrasonography for more and more applications.

Endoscopic transillumination

Laparoscopically-assisted panenteroscopy has been performed in select patients. Patients with obscure gastrointestinal bleeding or inaccessible small bowel lesions, who would otherwise require open laparotomy, may benefit from this novel approach. With the help of the laparoscopist, the endoscopist can very quickly advance an enteroscope for intraluminal examination. In an animal model, Bleau et al (1994) used laparoscopically-assisted panenteroscopy to reach the ileocecal valve in about 30 minutes without perforation. Moreover, distension and endoscopic transillumination of the bladder, stomach and colon can sometimes aid in diagnosis during laparoscopy (Anderson 1937). Transillumination of the duodenum and small bowel delineates tumors, arteriovenous malformations and other lesions which may be present.

Tissue sampling

Ruddock (1937) established the importance of tissue sampling during diagnostic laparoscopy. Laparoscopic-directed biopsy of lesions is more accurate than blind percutaneous biopsy. Nord (1982), in a review of several studies, found a false negative rate of 24% (range 1–67%) for blind percutaneous biopsy of the liver and an average false negative rate of only 9% (range 4–18%) for laparoscopic-guided biopsy. Directed trans-abdominal sonographic-guided biopsy is comparable to laparoscopy in focal and diffuse disease of the liver; however, ultrasound and CT scan are relatively insensitive to metastatic disease (Nord & Boyd 1994). Just as with percutaneous biopsy, the patient should have normal blood coagulation parameters on preoperative assessment. Occasionally, patients will require vitamin K therapy or transfusions with fresh frozen plasma or platelets to correct underlying coagulopathies. We routinely check complete blood count and prothrombin time in any patient with a history of a bleeding tendency.

For most solid hepatic tumors a Tru-cut biopsy is sufficient to make the diagnosis. Several biopsy instruments are available which can be passed under laparoscopic guidance through the abdominal wall or introduced through an accessory port. Bleeding is usually controlled by direct pressure. Most small exophytic lesions are ideally suited for the punch forceps. This instrument has a cup-shaped blade which will biopsy a small tissue sample without tearing adjacent structures.

If larger tissue samples are required, an incisional biopsy is made and the specimen retrieved in an entrapment sac. Control of hemostasis should be considered prior to biopsy. Good exposure should be achieved and hemostatic agents (Avitene©, Neu-Knit©, Surgicel© and thrombin) should be readily available. Most surface bleeding is controlled by electrocautery. Laparoscopic suturing may be necessary and the laparoscopist should develop expertise in both intracorporeal and extracorporeal suturing techniques.

Advanced laparoscopic procedures may be indicated during diagnostic laparoscopy. For large tissue specimens, morcellation of an organ may be performed in order to retrieve the tissue through a small skin incision. The spleen, for example, after laparoscopic splenectomy may be placed in a sac and divided into smaller fragments until the contents can be retrieved through a 10 mm incision. Morcellation destroys tissue margins and therefore, its use for malignancy is limited.

Cysts may be needle aspirated, but at the risk of determining that the lesion is in fact a hemangioma. These lesions are notorious for uncontrolled hemorrhage after biopsy of any kind. Needle aspiration may also be used to confirm gallbladder cancer by cytologic examination of bile. One method to prevent contamination of the peritoneal cavity is to introduce the needle through the liver rather than by direct puncture of the gallbladder.

The laparoscopic suction/irrigator is designed to aspirate fluid. Large quantities of ascitic fluid are easily collected by this means. Similarly, peritoneal washing may be done by injecting 200–300 cc of sterile saline and then aspirating the contents into a sterile container.

Postoperative care

Patients are either observed in the hospital overnight or discharged later the same day following diagnostic laparoscopy. Common problems encountered in the immediate postoperative period include urinary retention and nausea. Antiemetics and analgesics are given as needed. Most patients tolerate clear liquids in the immediate postoperative period and resume a regular diet the next day. Nausea and mild shoulder pain due to diaphragmatic irritation may occur in the early postoperative period (Albala & Clayman 1994). Patient activity is not restricted and abdominal tenderness usually subsides by the second or third post-operative day. Patients discharged home the same day should be advised about these problems and live relatively near the hospital, preferably with another person, should there be any unexpected problems. Within 1 week patients usually feel ready to return to their normal activity.

ABDOMINAL INSPECTION

Whenever a laparoscope is inserted into the abdomen, the entire abdominal cavity and pelvis should be explored systematically and thoroughly. For diagnostic exploration most laparoscopists recommend a 5 mm laparoscope, while for therapeutic laparoscopy a larger 10 mm laparoscope is usually inserted into the abdomen through a periumbilical port. Commonly, a second trocar is inserted in the flank and adhesions divided to facilitate a thorough exploration. A third port may be necessary to allow a second working instrument to help retract, 'run' the bowel or biopsy. A minimum of three ports is usually required if therapeutic intervention is anticipated. After accessing the abdomen, the abdominal viscera and retroperitoneum immediately posterior to the initial port are first viewed to ensure that there is no injury as a result of inserting the trocar or sheath. If access is uneventful, the abdomen is examined systematically. The following discussion highlights just a few of the more common findings the laparoscopist encounters during abdominal inspection.

Pelvis

The pelvic viscera are examined for pathologic abnormalities before evaluating the upper abdomen. In women, the ovaries, fallopian tubes and uterus should be inspected. If pelvic pathology is expected, a uterine manipulator is used to elevate the uterus and increase access to the adnexa, cul-de-sac and bladder. Mature ovaries are white and almond-shaped and usually measure about 2 × 3 × 3 cm. Benign functional cysts have a characteristic appearance and may be left alone as they will resolve spontaneously (Fig. 5.2), while other cysts are neoplastic and may require oophorectomy. If an ovarian malignancy is suspected, peritoneal washings are generally required. The fallopian tubes may be red and

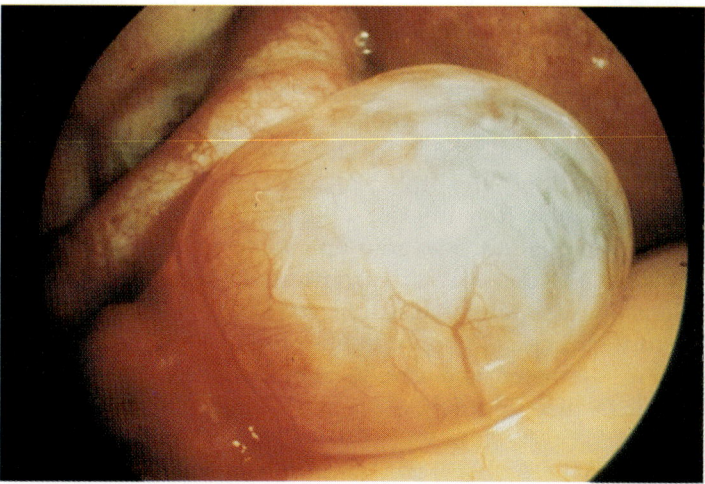

Figure 5.2   Ovarian cyst. Removal of this cyst proved it to be benign (courtesy of the Society of American Gastrointestinal Endoscopic Surgeons).

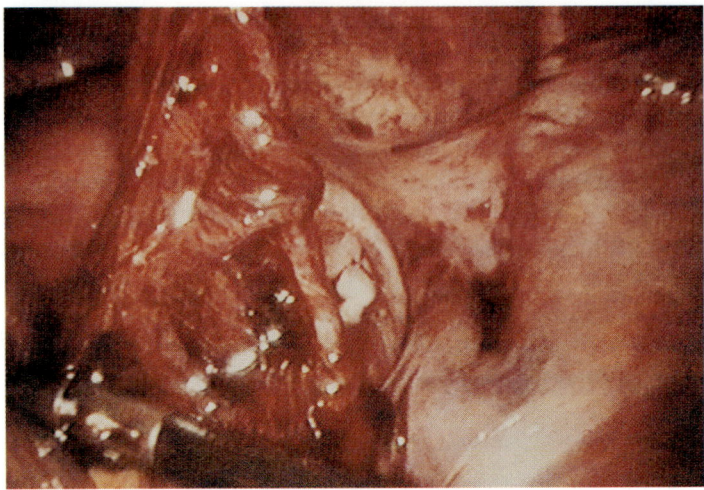

Figure 5.3 Ectopic pregnancy. At laparoscopy the fallopian tube had ruptured secondary to an ectopic pregnancy. Unilateral oophorectomy was performed (courtesy of the Society of American Gastrointestinal Endoscopic Surgeons).

inflamed from salpingitis or an early ectopic pregnancy. During the first 2–6 weeks of an ectopic pregnancy the tubes are dilated to 3–4 cm and if unrecognized at that time, may later rupture, causing life-threatening hemorrhage (Fig. 5.3). Uterine leiomyomata may be painful and are common, occurring in one in four women during reproductive life. Leiomyomata are usually gray, firm masses that may be microscopic in size or fill the abdominal cavity. If the ovary, fallopian tube or uterus is abnormal at laparoscopy, we generally request the presence of a gynecologist to assist in diagnosis. Whenever gynecological problems are suspected by history and physical examination, diagnostic laparoscopy is preferably performed by a gynecologist.

The pelvic floor should be inspected for inguinal hernias as well as tumors of the bladder and colon. An indirect hernia appears as an outpouching lateral to the inferior epigastric vessels, whereas a direct hernia defect is medial to the inferior epigastric vessels (Fig. 5.4). Bowel or bladder attached to this area may represent an incarcerated hernia or tumor extension. The sigmoid colon may reveal diverticular disease, abscess or tumor. Typically, diverticula are herniations 1 mm to several centimeters in diameter and are located between the mesenteric and antimesenteric taeniae (Fig. 5.5).

Midabdomen

The anterior surfaces of the intestines, omentum and stomach are

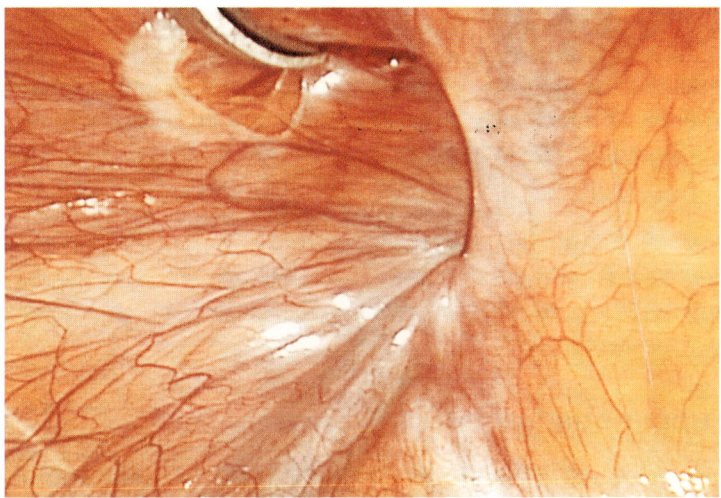

Figure 5.4 Inguinal hernia. A small, indirect inguinal hernia is present to the left of the inferior epigastric vessels (reproduced with permission from Soper et al 1994).

examined for abnormalities. Following the taeniae of the cecum proximally will locate the appendix. With early appendicitis, the appendix is erythematous with engorged surface vessels or covered by a fibrino-purulent material; later, green-black foci of necrosis typify gangrenous

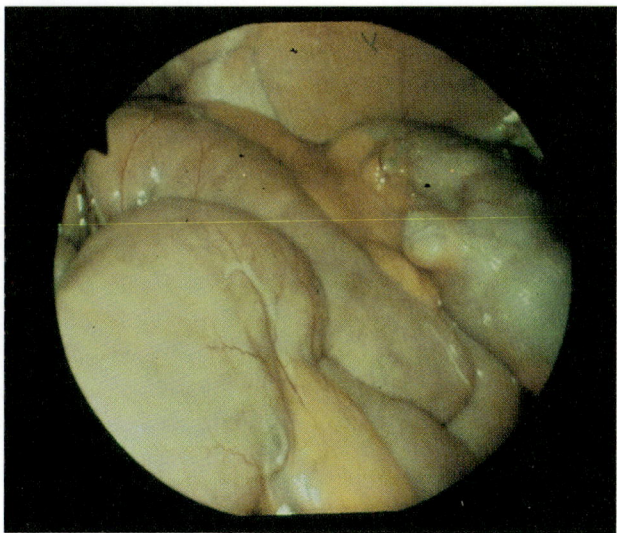

Figure 5.5 Diverticular disease. A diverticulum is present in the wall of the sigmoid colon. Small bowel loops appear normal (courtesy of the Society of American Gastrointestinal Endoscopic Surgeons).

appendicitis and herald impending perforation. Crohn's disease generally occurs in sharply demarcated segments of bowel that have a rubber-hose consistency surrounded by creeping fat. The duodenum may have a sealed patch of omentum covering a perforated ulcer which may be missed altogether by cursory examination. If portal hypertension is present, the veins of the omentum and abdominal wall will be dilated. Intestine may be ischemic and appear blue because of volvulus or vascular infarction. With intestinal obstruction, the proximal bowel is generally distended and the bowel distal to the obstructive lesion decompressed, especially with a complete obstruction secondary to an adhesive band from a previous operation.

Right upper quadrant

To examine the right upper abdomen the patient is placed in a reverse Trendelenburg position of 30–40° while the table is rotated to the patient's left by 15–20°. This maneuver allows the colon and duodenum to fall away from the liver's edge. Normal liver is reddish-brown and has a smooth surface. The falciform ligament and both lobes of the liver are closely examined for pathology. Adhesions on the anterior liver surface may be due to inflammation from Fitz-Hugh–Curtis syndrome (Fig. 5.6). Primary carcinoma of the liver may appear as small nodular lesions with

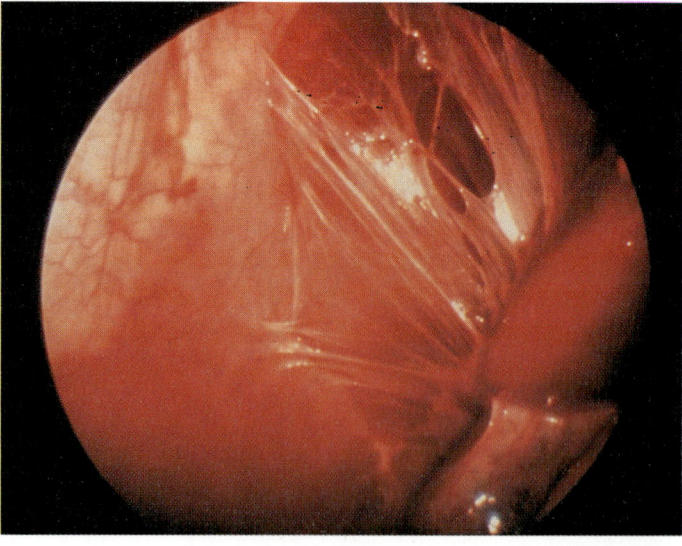

Figure 5.6 Fitz-Hugh–Curtis syndrome, secondary to previous gonococcal pelvic inflammatory disease, results in peritonitis and adhesions of the liver capsule (courtesy of the Society of American Gastrointestinal Endoscopic Surgeons).

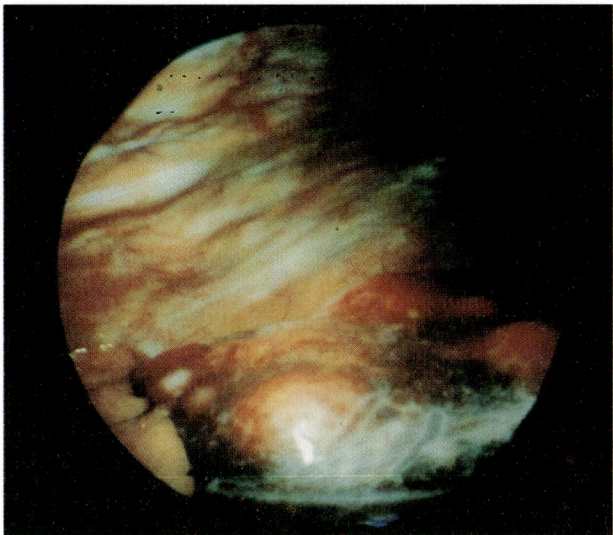

Figure 5.7 Primary liver malignancy. Multiple orange nodules are present in the right hepatic lobe. Extensive metastases have caused intrahepatic venous stasis as evident by the dark blue color of the liver (courtesy of the Society of American Gastrointestinal Endoscopic Surgeons).

widespread peritoneal metastasis (Fig. 5.7). Fatty degeneration imparts a yellow color to the liver, while nodularity of the liver suggests cirrhosis (Figs 5.8 and 5.9). Extrahepatic biliary obstruction from periampullary cancer may cause cholestasis and the liver will generally be tense and appear greenish due to bile discoloration (Fig. 5.10). Most metastatic liver lesions appear as yellow, gray or white nodules that feel solid (Fig. 5.11). Metastatic melanoma appears as brownish-black spots (Fig. 5.12). Solid masses should be biopsied with a cutting needle, cupped forceps or cautery scissors or needle aspirated in order to determine histology and cytology. Bluish cystic hepatic lesions, however, should never be biopsied as hemangiomas can cause severe bleeding which may be difficult to control laparoscopically (Figs 5.13 and 5.14). Hepatic, pancreatic and other suspicious lesions may be further evaluated by laparoscopic ultrasonography (Fig. 5.15).

The inferior margin of the liver is visualized to determine the location of the gallbladder; usually, the gallbladder can be seen protruding beyond the edge of the liver, but sometimes it is not visible without carefully elevating the liver and/or taking down adhesions. The normal gallbladder has a shiny bluish-green color. In acute cholecystitis the gallbladder may be tense, edematous, fiery red and covered with a fibrinosuppurative exudate. Extensive adhesions surrounding a thickened, gray-white, tough gallbladder wall are usually due to chronic inflammation. Distal extra-

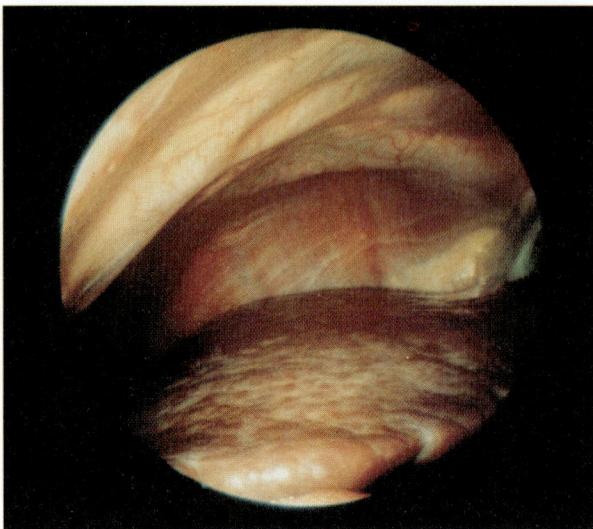

Figure 5.8 Chronic active hepatitis and early cirrhosis. Rounding of the inferior margin of the lobe is indicative of intrahepatic disease. The irregular surface and small nodules characterize fibrosis and early cirrhosis of the liver (courtesy of the Society of American Gastrointestinal Endoscopic Surgeons).

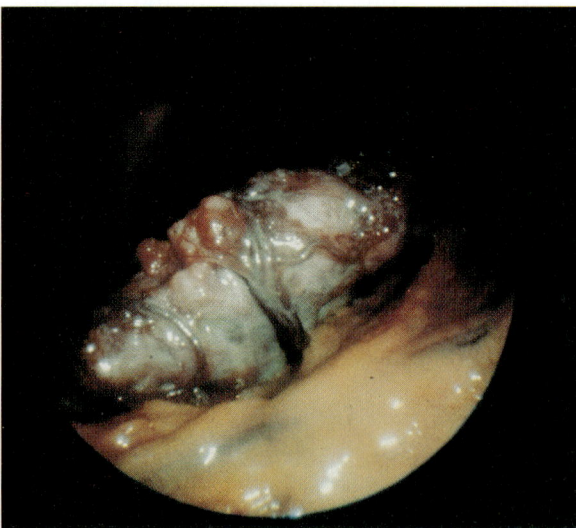

Figure 5.9 Hepatoma with cirrhosis. Hepatic parenchyma has been replaced by pinkish-white nodules, characteristic of hepatocellular carcinoma. Safe biopsy is difficult because of the large blood vessels on the surface (courtesy of the Society of American Gastrointestinal Endoscopic Surgeons).

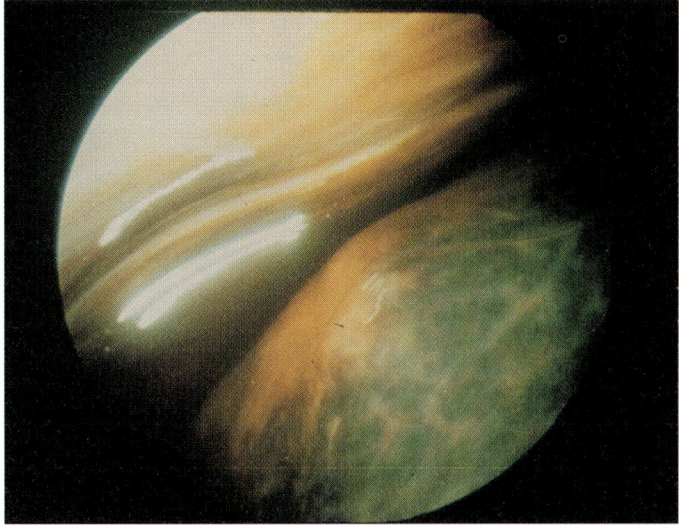

Figure 5.10 Cholestasis. Hepatic parenchyma appears cholestatic due to extrahepatic obstruction. Umbilicated metastasis is also present in the right hepatic lobe. The combination of these two findings is typical of cancer of the pancreas or common bile duct (courtesy of the Society of American Gastrointestinal Endoscopic Surgeons).

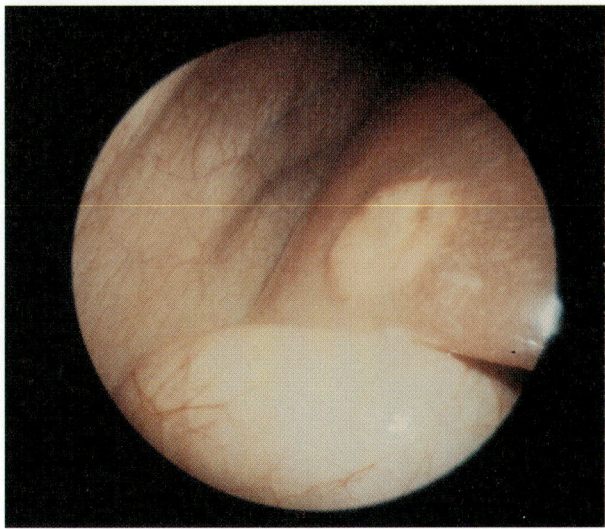

Figure 5.11 Liver metastases. Multiple nodules with neovascularity are present in the right hepatic lobe. Biopsy confirmed adenocarcinoma (courtesy of the Society of American Gastrointestinal Endoscopic Surgeons).

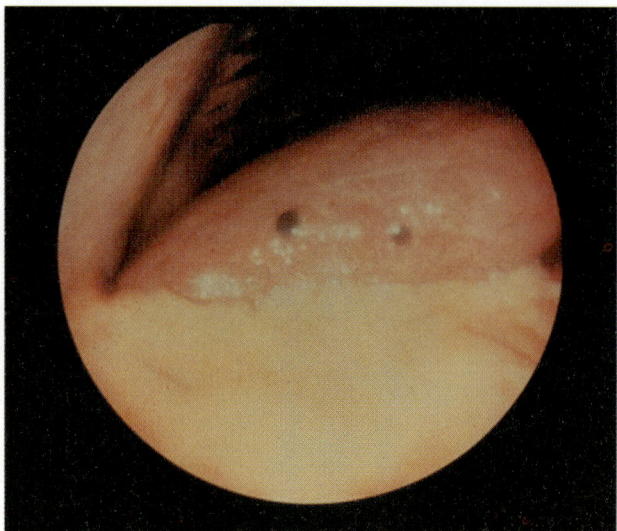

Figure 5.12 Biopsy of two darkly pigmented hepatic lesions revealed malignant spread of melanoma (courtesy of the Society of American Gastrointestinal Endoscopic Surgeons).

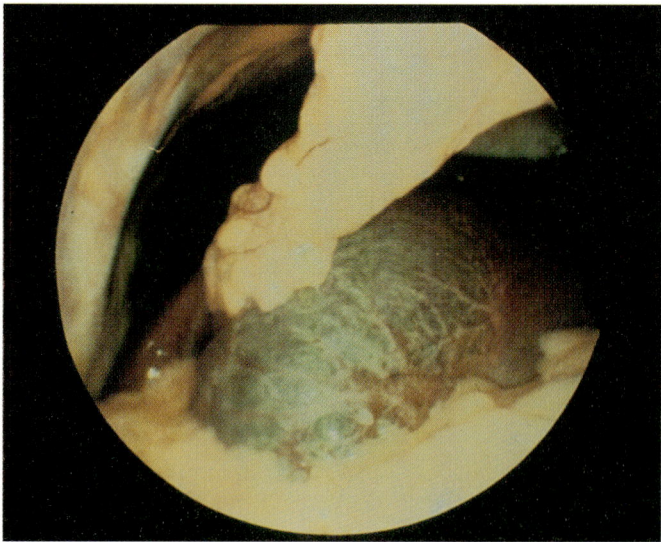

Figure 5.13 Hepatic cyst in the left hepatic lobe. This benign cyst has grown to displace surrounding subcapsular blood vessels, bile duct, round and falciform ligaments (courtesy of the Society of American Gastrointestinal Endoscopic Surgeons).

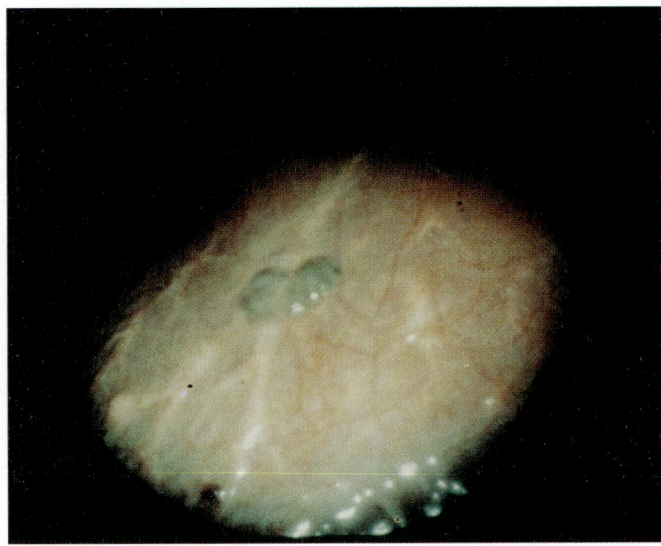

Figure 5.14 Hemangioma. Two nodular, dark blue subcapsular hemangiomas are located in the right hepatic lobe. If mistakenly biopsied, hemangiomas tend to bleed profusely (courtesy of the Society of American Gastrointestinal Endoscopic Surgeons).

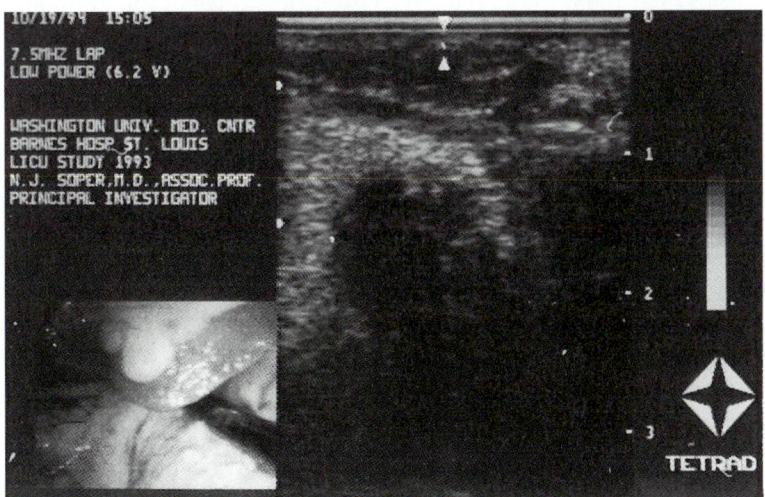

Figure 5.15 Cancer of the pancreas. Laparoscopic ultrasonography reveals a 3 cm mass invading the portal vein. This patient was deemed unresectable for a curative resection and was spared a laparotomy (courtesy of N.J. Soper M D).

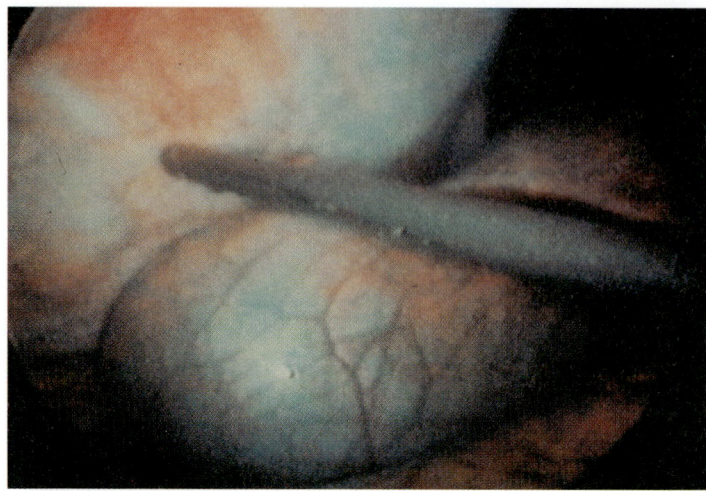

Figure 5.16   Courvoisier's gallbladder. Distal extrahepatic bile duct obstruction may cause massive distension of the gallbladder. This finding is associated with carcinoma of the pancreas and other lesions that obstruct the common bile duct (courtesy of the Society of American Gastrointestinal Endoscopic Surgeons).

hepatic obstruction may cause a dilated Courvoisier's gallbladder (Fig. 5.16). Transcholecystic cholangiography or laparoscopic ultrasonography (Yamamoto et al 1993) may be used to exclude stones in the gallbladder or bile ducts (Fig. 5.17). A pale or opaque gallbladder may represent chronic cholecystitis or tumor (Fig. 5.18).

Left upper quadrant

The normal spleen is usually not seen in the left upper quadrant; when visible, splenomegaly is often apparent. Further inspection of the spleen is best achieved by rotating the patient to the right in the head-up position. Although splenic biopsy has been performed, risks of severe hemorrhage usually warrant caution. The left hemidiaphragm can be inspected for hiatal hernia and esophageal varices. If the diaphragm bows inward, a pneumothorax should be suspected.

INDICATIONS FOR DIAGNOSTIC LAPAROSCOPY

Diagnostic laparoscopy may be used to optimize the work-up of abdominal pain and masses, triage trauma and stage malignancy. The current indications for diagnostic laparoscopy are listed in Table 5.2.

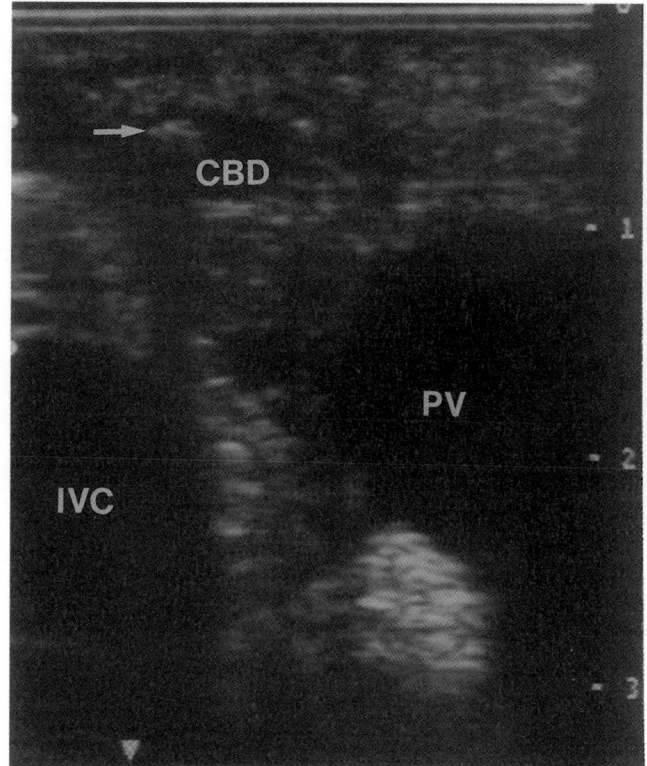

Figure 5.17   Common bile duct stone detected by laparoscopic ultrasonography during laparoscopic cholecystectomy CBD = common bile duct, IVC = inferior vena cava, PV = portal vein (reproduced with permission from Jones & Soper 1995).

Evaluation of abdominal pain

Acute pain

Acute right lower quadrant pain that may be due to acute appendicitis is ideally evaluated by laparoscopy. Traditionally, appendicitis was a clinical diagnosis, for which a 20% error rate with a normal appendix was considered acceptable because of the morbidity and mortality caused by appendiceal perforation from a delay in operation. With the use of laparoscopy, several studies have shown a markedly decreased rate of negative laparotomy for questionable appendicitis (Leape & Ramenofsky 1979).

Especially in young women, who experience gynecological problems which may mimic appendicitis, diagnostic laparoscopy has reduced the unnecessary laparotomy rate by one-third (Cox et al 1993, Deutsch et al 1982, Jadallah et al 1994, Olsen et al 1993). In a prospective randomized

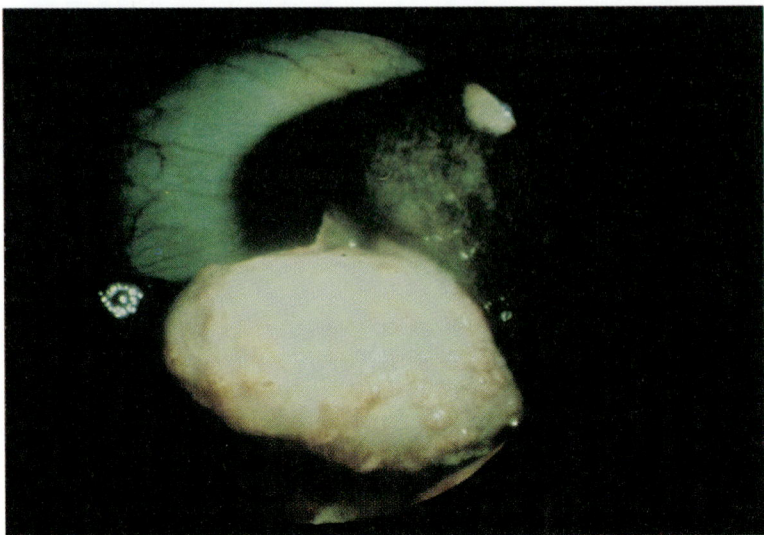

Figure 5.18 Gallbladder cancer. Multiple nodules are scattered over the gallbladder wall. A single metastatic nodule is seen in the right hepatic lobe. The liver appears greenish-black because of severe cholestasis. Biopsy confirmed adenocarcinoma (courtesy of the Society of American Gastrointestinal Endoscopic Surgeons).

trial of 100 patients with the clinical diagnosis of appendicitis, 50 underwent open laparotomy and 50 underwent diagnostic laparoscopy. In the latter group, 19 patients (38%) did not require appendectomy; moreover, there were no complications from laparoscopy (Jadallah et al 1994). If appendicitis is present, the appendix may be resected laparoscopically and its stump closed with a loop ligature or a stapler. If the appendix is perforated, laparoscopy allows thorough irrigation of the abdominal cavity. Two randomized prospective studies showed that laparoscopic appendectomy decreased postoperative pain and expedited return to full activity compared to conventional appendectomy (Attwood et al 1992, Frazee et al 1994).

Other causes of right lower quadrant pain may also be better evaluated via a laparoscope. Laparoscopic treatment of tubal pregnancy, for example, is as safe as treatment with laparotomy and has the benefit to the patient of decreased length of hospital stay, lower cost and earlier return to full activity (Brzezinski & Schenker 1994, Ou 1993). Laparoscopy was the definitive diagnostic modality in 176 patients with suspected pelvic inflammatory disease (Morcos et al 1993). In this study, laparoscopy was found to be 87% sensitive and 46% specific, with a positive predictive value of 84%.

Children, newborn to age 15 years, with ill-defined abdominal pain have been evaluated by laparoscopy and found to have problems ranging from appendicitis, adhesions, cysts, Meckel's diverticula or unappreciated hernias (Schier & Waldschmidt 1994). Most of these patients can be treated laparoscopically.

In the intensive care unit setting, diagnostic laparoscopy has been used to assess the patient with a suspected abdominal catastrophe. In a study of 25 such patients, 13 (52%) laparoscopies were negative and non-therapeutic operations were avoided (Brandt et al 1993).

Chronic pain

The cause of chronic abdominal pain may be confusing even after extensive preoperative diagnostic evaluation. Laparoscopy has been used to evaluate chronic abdominal pain and Easter et al (1992) found laparoscopy to yield positive findings in 47% of the cases. Laparoscopy has the advantage of adding therapeutic possibilities to its diagnostic value and when adhesions were detected, for example, laparoscopic adhesiolysis relieved the patients' symptoms.

Trauma

Laparoscopy may have a role in the evaluation of blunt and penetrating abdominal trauma. Following trauma, a surgical dictum has been to explore all penetrating wounds of the abdomen. This practice results in many negative laparotomies when operation is based on clinical impression alone. Hemodynamically stable patients with significant abdominal trauma are traditionally evaluated by peritoneal lavage or CT scan. With a 5 mm laparoscope inserted under local anesthesia in the emergency room, Berci et al (1991) showed in 150 blunt abdominal trauma cases that diagnostic laparoscopy was able to predict or exclude the need for laparotomy in >90% of patients. Sosa et al (1992) used laparoscopy in six patients with tangential gunshot wounds to the abdomen to exclude fascial penetration and avoid laparotomy. Diagnostic laparoscopy is also efficacious as an adjunct in patient selection after CT scan has demonstrated solid organ injury and in 15 patients with splenic and liver lacerations, Townsend et al (1993) managed eight (53%) conservatively without laparotomy. Fernando et al (1994) reported 33 stable patients with penetrating trauma (11 stab wounds, 22 gunshot wounds) and no clinical evidence of intraperitoneal injury. In these patients, diagnostic laparoscopy identified peritoneal penetration in ten patients, of whom nine had intraperitoneal injury at laparotomy, but 23 patients were spared a negative exploratory laparotomy. Fabian et al (1993) reported a larger prospective study of 182 hemodynamically stable patients following abdominal trauma in whom laparotomy was avoided in 44% after penetrating and in 47% after blunt trauma.

Diagnostic laparoscopy for trauma remains controversial despite its potential to avoid negative laparotomy because retroperitoneal wounds and hollow organ perforations may not be recognized and go untreated. Salvino et al (1993) found diagnostic laparoscopy to be better than peritoneal lavage in predicting the need for laparotomy for stab wounds but not following blunt trauma in a prospective study of 75 patients. Following penetrating abdominal trauma in a series of 100 patients, diagnostic laparoscopy was accurate in assessing for hemoperitoneum, solid organ injuries, diaphragmatic lacerations and retroperitoneal hematomas. For injuries to the hollow viscera, laparoscopy was 100% specific, but only 18% sensitive. Injuries to the flank and epigastric region were frequently missed, thereby limiting its usefulness (Ivatury et al 1993). Rossi et al (1993) performed laparoscopy prior to laparotomy in 32 patients. Laparoscopic findings correlated (97%) with the need for laparotomy, but several injuries to the liver, pancreas, stomach, duodenum, small bowel, intestinal mesentery, ureter and urinary bladder were missed by laparoscopy. In the future, perhaps a combined approach using laparoscopy to examine the peritoneum and spiral CT to image the retroperitoneum may increase diagnostic accuracy following abdominal trauma.

Liver and ascites

Inspection of the liver is probably the most common reason for performing diagnostic laparoscopy. Blind percutaneous biopsy of the liver may cause inapparent injury and will miss focal disease such as small metastases, while laparoscopy improves the accuracy of biopsy (Nord 1982). In addition, laparoscopic criteria may be predictive of outcome. In cirrhosis, although the interpretation of laparoscopic findings is largely subjective, the size and pattern of regenerating nodules, formation of lymphatic vesicles and presence of an enlarged spleen all predict a poor prognosis (Tameda et al 1990).

Laparoscopy is indicated in the evaluation of ascites after transabdominal ultrasonography, CT scan and paracentesis fail to determine its etiology (Brady et al 1991). Due to the 12–15-fold magnification and excellent ability to view the entire peritoneal surface, laparoscopy is particularly sensitive for small peritoneal implants. Pancreas, ovary, breast and colonic malignancy frequently spread to the peritoneum, while benign implants may include tuberculosis, listeria or liver fluke. In general, if the size of the miliary nodules is uniform, the nodules are more likely to be benign. Malignant nodules usually are of varying sizes (Geake et al 1981). Biopsy for histologic confirmation is essential to the diagnosis and ascitic fluid should be sent routinely for cytology and microbiology. In a study of 129 patients with ascites of unknown origin, Chu et al (1994) found that laparoscopy in combination with biopsy established the etiology of ascites in 111 (86%) patients.

Staging of malignancy

When performing laparoscopy to stage abdominal malignancy, pre-operative consideration should be given to the accessibility of specific viscera, tissue samples required for adequate staging and range of palliative interventions possible endoscopically and laparoscopically if the lesion proves unsuitable for curative operation. Following initial port placement and primary visual survey of the abdomen, accessory ports are placed under direct vision in appropriate locations. In this manner, the patient is best managed while preserving the goal of minimal invasion. Of 25 patients referred for evaluation, Easter et al (1992) found laparoscopy to be 100% accurate in the diagnosis or exclusion of various intraabdominal malignant neoplasms.

Liver cancer

Of patients thought to have resectable disease by preoperative trans-abdominal ultrasonography and/or CT scan, 40–70% with primary or metastatic hepatic malignancy are found to have unresectable disease at operation (Babineau et al 1994). Therefore, diagnostic laparoscopy prior to laparotomy is recommended to evaluate the extent of cancer and degree of cirrhosis.

Laparoscopy accurately diagnoses metastatic tumors to the liver. Lightdale et al (1979), in a study of 65 metastatic lesions, obtained tissue samples in 60. Histology was 92% sensitive and 100% specific. However, 40–50% of hepatomas <3 cm in diameter are not visible on the surface of the liver (Goletti et al 1994). For these small tumors, laparoscopic ultrasonography improves the sensitivity to 88%, while for tumors >3 cm the sensitivity by laparoscopic ultrasonography is 100% (Goletti et al 1994). Small hepatic cysts may be confused with metastases by surface imaging, while cysts usually appear as round, echo-free lesions with posterior enhancement by laparoscopic ultrasonography.

Ovarian cancer

Diagnostic laparoscopy has been used extensively to evaluate gyne-cological malignancy (Canis et al 1994, Gelman 1988). Canis et al (1994) evaluated 819 adnexal masses and found laparoscopy to have a sensitivity for the detection of malignancy of 100%, specificity of 97% and negative predictive value of 100%. However, the positive predictive value was only 41% because 27 tumors were incorrectly thought to be malignant. Ovarian cancer metastatic to the diaphragm is best identified by laparoscopy (Bagley et al 1973, Rosenhoff et al 1975) and in one study Bagley et al (1973) reported 11 of 14 patients to be upstaged by diagnostic laparoscopy.

Gastric cancer

With cancer of the stomach, laparoscopic examination can prevent 40–50% of unnecessary laparotomies (Kriplani & Kapur 1991, Kriplani et al 1992). Laparoscopy determines serosal infiltration, tumor fixation and metastases to the liver and peritoneum. Performing laparoscopy in 40 patients with gastric carcinoma, Kriplani & Kapur (1991) detected distant metastases in five cases and locally advanced unresectable cancer in 11 patients (27%). The overall diagnostic accuracy was 92%. Similarly, Possik et al (1986), who evaluated 360 patients with gastric cancer, found laparoscopy 89% accurate in detecting peritoneal spread and 97% accurate in identifying liver metastases. Intraoperative ultrasonography is complementary to the laparoscopic examination. Ultrasonography identifies small lymph nodes, gastric wall involvement and deep hepatic metastases (Goletti et al 1994).

Gallbladder cancer

Advanced gallbladder cancer has a dismal prognosis. If malignancy is suspected, diagnostic laparoscopy can confirm local and distant spread precluding resection in 85% of patients (Dagnini et al 1984, Kriplani et al 1992). Using laparoscopy, Bhargava et al (1983) correctly identified over 80% of patients with advanced malignancy, for whom laparotomy could be avoided. Fortunately, gallbladder cancer is rare. In the senior author's series of over 900 laparoscopic cholecystectomies, only three patients were diagnosed with cancer of the gallbladder, none of whom were resectable for cure.

Cancer of the pancreas

Diagnostic laparoscopy was recognized as early as 1911 by Berheim (1911) as a valuable procedure to exclude pancreatic cancer metastases. However, Meyer-Burg (1972) reported the first series using diagnostic laparoscopy for the staging of cancer of the pancreas. Since then, several different approaches to this retroperitoneal organ have been proposed. Cuschieri et al (1978) examined the pancreas through an infragastric opening into the lesser sac and were able to see the entire gland in 60% of patients. Ishida (1983), using a supragastric approach, visualized only 32% of tumors in the head of the pancreas but accurately identified 85% of cancers in the body of the pancreas.

Diagnostic laparoscopy is particularly helpful in those patients who have no evidence of metastasis on CT scan and transabdominal ultra-sonography. Laparoscopy identified metastases in over 40% of these patients (Warshaw et al 1986, 1990). More recently, intraoperative laparo-scopic ultrasonography has enhanced the ability to stage cancer of the pancreas laparoscopically. Murugiah et al (1993) reported that of 12 patients with suspected carcinoma of the head of the pancreas considered preoperatively to have resectable disease, four were found at laparoscopy to have advanced disease. Intraoperative laparoscopic ultrasonography clearly demonstrated another two patients with unresectable cancer. In addition to hepatic metastases, ultrasonography reveals lymphadeno-pathy, local infiltration, portal vein displacement or invasion and anomalous anatomy.

At our institution, intraoperative laparoscopic ultrasonography is routinely used to stage cancer of the pancreas prior to laparotomy. Patients unresectable at laparoscopy are considered for laparoscopic biliary bypass or gastrojejunostomy, maintaining the goal of minimal invasion. Patients without evidence of metastases or vascular invasion by tumor are converted to a laparotomy for curative resection.

Lymphoma

Laparoscopy completely stages lymphoma by liver biopsy, nodal sampling and full abdominal visualization (Greene & Cooler 1994). During diagnostic laparoscopy, Salky (1993) obtained adequate tissue samples in 12 of 12 patients (100%) after percutaneous biopsy was unsuccessful. Childers & Surwit (1992) have reported laparoscopic paraaortic lymph node biopsy for non-Hodgkin's lymphoma. Whether laparoscopic splenectomy is necessary for full staging remains contro-versial.

Esophageal cancer

Diagnostic laparoscopy has been advocated for staging esophageal cancer in those patients considered suitable for resection by CT scan. Dagnini et al (1986) reported that laparoscopy prior to laparotomy identified 14% of patients with metastases to the liver, peritoneum, omentum and lymph nodes precluding resection.

'Second look' procedure

After initial treatment of abdominal malignancy, second look may be better done laparoscopically rather than via a laparotomy. If early tumor recurrence is suggested by history, physical examination or rising tumor markers, but imaging studies (CT, MRI, ultrasound or PET scan) are negative, laparoscopy may be indicated. Imaging studies may be equivocal because of scar formation, altered anatomy from previous operation or possible reactive lymphadenopathy. Though abdominal exploration by laparoscopy may also be limited by adhesions, the finding of histologically confirmed distant metastases and/or peritoneal carcinomatosis may obviate further evaluation. In the future, radionuclide probes that detect tumors may improve the accuracy of diagnostic laparoscopy as a 'second look' procedure.

CONCLUSIONS

Diagnostic laparoscopy is being embraced rapidly in the United States and throughout the world. With minimal morbidity, lesions too small to be seen by CT scan, MRI and abdominal ultrasonography can be accurately described and biopsied via a laparoscope. Malignancy can be staged and vague abdominal complaints elucidated. Certainly, many unnecessary and morbid laparotomies can be avoided. For these reasons, diagnostic laparoscopy is being incorporated into modern diagnostic and management algorithms for more and more disease processes.

Occasionally, anatomic or physiologic considerations will preclude the laparoscopic approach and conversion to an open operation reflects sound surgical judgement and should not be considered a complication. The exact role for diagnostic laparoscopy in the elective and emergency situation is still evolving as laparoscopists become more adept technically and as technology improves.

Acknowledgement

The authors gratefully acknowledge the Washington University Institute for Minimally Invasive Surgery as funded by an educational grant from Ethicon-Endosurgery Inc.

REFERENCES

Albala D M, Clayman R V 1994 Postoperative care. In: Soper N J, Odem R R, Clayman R V, McDougall E M (eds) Essentials of laparoscopy. Quality Medical Publishing, St. Louis, pp 210–212
Anderson E T 1937 Peritoneoscopy. American Journal of Surgery 35: 136–139
Attwood S E A, Hill A D K, Murphy P G, Thorton J, Stephens R B 1992 A prospective randomized trial of laparoscopic versus open appendectomy. Surgery 112: 497–501
Babineau T J, Lewis W D, Jenkins R L, Bleday R, Steele G D, Forse R A 1994 Role of staging laparoscopy in the treatment of hepatic malignancy. American Journal of Surgery 167: 151–154

Bagley C M, Young R C, Schein P S et al 1973 Ovarian cancer metastatic to the diaphragm – frequently undiagnosed at laparotomy. American Journal of Obstetrics and Gynecology 116: 397–400

Banting S, Shimi S, Velpen G V, Cuschieri A 1993 Abdominal wall lift: low pressure pneumoperitoneum laparoscopic surgery. Surgical Endoscopy 7: 57–59.

Beck D H, McQuillan P J 1994 Fatal carbon dioxide embolism and severe hemorrhage during laparoscopic salpingectomy. British Journal of Anaesthesia 72: 243–245

Berci G, Dunkelman D, Michele S L, Sanders G, Wahlstrom E, Morgenstern L 1983 Emergency mini-laparoscopy in abdominal trauma. An update. American Journal of Surgery 146: 261–265

Berci G, Sackier J M, Paz-Partlow M 1991 Emergency laparoscopy. American Journal of Surgery 161: 332–335

Bernheim B M 1911 Organoscopy. Cystoscopy of the abdominal cavity. Annals of Surgery 53: 764–767

Bhargava D K, Sarin S, Verma K, Kapur B M L 1983 Laparoscopy in carcinoma of the gallbladder. Gastrointestinal Endoscopy 29: 21–22

Bleau B L, Ahlquist D A, Gostout J H, Donohue J H 1994 Laparoscopically-assisted panenteroscopy: a feasibility study in pigs. (Proceedings of World Congresses of Gastroenterology). Academy Professional Information Services, New York Abstract 3087

Brady P G, Peebles M, Goldschmid S 1991 Role of laparoscopy in the evaluation of patients with suspected hepatic or peritoneal malignancy. Gastrointestinal Endoscopy 37: 27–30

Brandt C P, Priebe P P, Eckhauser M L 1993 Diagnostic laparoscopy in the intensive care patient. Avoiding the nontherapeutic laparotomy. Surgical Endoscopy 7: 168–172

Brzezinski A, Schenker J G 1994 Current status of endoscopic surgical management of tubal pregnancy. European Journal of Obstetrics, Gynecology and Reproductive Biology 54: 43–53

Canis M, Mage G, Pouly J L, Wattiez A, Manhes H, Bruhat M A 1994 Laparoscopic diagnosis of adnexal cystic masses: a 12-year experience with long-term follow-up. Obstetrics and Gynecology 83: 707–712

Childers J M, Surwit E A 1992 Laparoscopic para-aortic lymph node biopsy for diagnosis of a non-Hodgkin's lymphoma. Surgical Laparoscopy and Endoscopy 2: 139–142

Chu C M, Lin S M, Peng S M, Wu C S 1994 The role of laparoscopy in the evaluation of ascites of unknown origin. Gastrointestinal Endoscopy 40: 285–289

Cox M R, McCall J L, Wilson T G, Padbury R T, Jeans P L, Toouli J 1993 Laparoscopic appendicectomy: a prospective analysis. Australian and New Zealand Journal of Surgery 63: 840–847

Cuschieri A, Hall A W, Clark J 1978 Value of laparoscopy in the diagnosis and management of pancreatic cancer. Gut 19: 672–677

Cuschieri A, Hennessy T P J, Stephens R B, Berci G 1988 Diagnosis of significant abdominal trauma after road traffic accidents: preliminary results of a multicenter clinical trial comparing minilaparoscopy with peritoneal lavage. Annals of the Royal College of Surgeons of England 70: 153–155

Dagnini G, Marin G, Patella M et al 1984 Laparoscopy in the diagnosis of primary carcinoma of the gallbladder. A study of 98 cases. Gastrointestinal Endoscopy 30: 289–291

Dagnini G, Caldironi M W, Marin G 1986 Laparoscopy in abdominal staging of esophageal carcinoma. Report of 369 cases. Gastrointestinal Endoscopy 32: 400–402

Deutsch A A, Zelikovsky A, Reiss R 1982 Laparoscopy in the prevention of unnecessary appendicectomies: a prospective study. British Journal of Surgery 69: 333–337

Easter D W, Cuschieri A, Nathanson L K, Lavelle-Jones M 1992 The utility of diagnostic laparoscopy for abdominal disorders. Archives of Surgery 127: 379–383

Fabian T C, Croce M A, Stewart R M, Pritchard F E, Minard G, Kudsk K A 1993 A prospective analysis of diagnostic laparoscopy in trauma. Annals of Surgery 217: 557–564

Fernando H C, Alle K M, Chen J, Davis I, Klein S R 1994 Triage by laparoscopy in patients with penetrating abdominal trauma. British Journal of Surgery 81: 384–385

Fitzgerald S D, Andrus C H, Baudendistel L J, Dahms T E, Kaminiski D L 1992 Hypercarbia during carbon dioxide pneumoperitoneum. American Journal of Surgery 163: 186–190

Frazee R C, Roberts J W, Symmonds R E et al 1994 A prospective randomized trial comparing open versus laparoscopic appendectomy. Annals of Surgery 219: 725–731

Geake T M S, Spitaels J M, Moshal M G, Simjee A E 1981 Peritoneoscopy in the diagnosis of tuberculous peritonitis. Gastrointestinal Endoscopy 27: 66–68

Gelman E P 1988 The role of laparoscopy in cancer management. Updates. Cancer Principles and Practices 2: 1–11

Golletti O, Buccianti P, Cavina E 1994 Laparoscopic sonography. Editoriale Grasso, Bologna

Graff T D, Arbgast N R, Phillips O C et al 1959 Gas embolism. A comparative study of air and carbon dioxide as embolic agents in the systemic venous system. American Journal of Obstetrics and Gynecology 78: 259–265

Gravenstein J S, Paulus P A, Hayes T J 1989 Carbon dioxide and monitoring. In: Gravenstein J S, Paulus P A, Hayes T J (eds) Capnography in clinical practice. Butterworth Publishers, Boston, pp 3–10

Greene F L, Cooler A W 1994 Laparoscopic evaluation of lymphoma. Seminars in Laparoscopic Surgery 1: 13–17

Gunatilake D E 1978 Case report. Fatal intraperitoneal explosion during electrocoagulation via laparoscopy. International Journal of Gynaecology and Obstetrics 15: 353–357

Ishida H 1983 Peritoneoscopy and pancreas biopsy in the diagnosis of pancreatic disease. Gastrointestinal Endoscopy 29: 211–218

Ivatury R R, Simon R J, Staht W M 1993 A critical evaluation of laparoscopy in penetrating abdominal trauma. Journal of Trauma 34: 822–828

Jadallah F A, Abdul-Ghani A A, Tibblin S 1994 Diagnostic laparoscopy reduces unnecessary appendicectomy in fertile women. European Journal of Surgery 160: 41–45

Jones D B, Soper N J 1994 Laparoscopic general surgery: current status and future potential. American Journal of Roentgenology 163: 1295–1301

Jones D B, Callery M P, Soper N J 1995 Strangulated incisional hernia after laparoscopy. Surgical Laparoscopy and Endoscopy (in press)

Kalk H 1929 Erfahrungen mit der laparoskopie. Zeitschrift fur Klinische Medizin 111: 303–348

Kelling G 1901 Ueber oesophagoskopie gastroskopie und koelioskopie. Muenchener Medicinische Wochenschrift 49: 21–24

Kriplani A K, Kapur B M L 1991 Laparoscopy for preoperative staging and assessment of operability in gastric carcinoma. Gastrointestinal Endoscopy 37: 441–443

Kriplani A K, Jayant S, Kapur B M L 1992 Laparoscopy in primary carcinoma of the gallbladder. Gastrointestinal Endoscopy 38: 326–329

Leape L L, Ramenofsky M L 1979 Laparosopy for questionable appendicitis. Can it reduce the negative appendectomy rate? Annals of Surgery 191: 410–413

Lightdale C J, Winawer S J, Kurtz R S, Knapper W H 1979 Laparoscopic diagnosis of suspected liver neoplasms. Value of prior liver scan. Digestive Diseases and Sciences 24: 588–593

Meyer-Burg J 1972 The inspection, palpation and biopsy of the pancreas by peritoneoscopy. Endoscopy 4: 99–101

Monk T G, Weldon B C 1994 Anesthetic considerations for laparoscopic surgery. In: Soper N J, Odem R R, Clayman R V, McDougall E M (eds) Essentials of laparoscopy. Quality Medical Publishing, St Louis, pp 24–33

Morcos R, Frost N, Hnat M, Petrunak A, Caldito G 1993 Laparoscopic versus clinical diagnosis of acute pelvic inflammatory disease. Journal of Reproductive Medicine 38: 53–56

Murugiah M, Paterson-Brown S, Windsor J A, Miles W F, Garden O J 1993 Early experience of laparoscopic ultrasonography in the management of pancreatic carcinoma. Surgical Endoscopy 7: 177–181

Nord H J 1982 Biopsy diagnosis of cirrhosis: blind percutaneous versus guided direct vision techniques – a review. Gastrointestinal Endoscopy 28: 102–104

Nord H J, Boyd W P 1994 Diagnostic laparoscopy. Endoscopy 26: 126–133

Olsen J B, Myren C J, Haahr P E 1993 Randomized study of the value of laparoscopy before appendicectomy. British Journal of Surgery 80: 922–923

Ou C S 1993 Laparoscopic management of ectopic pregnancy. Journal of Reproductive Medicine 38: 849–852

Possik R A, Franco E L, Pires D R, Wohnrath D R, Ferreira E B 1986 Sensitivity, specificity and predictive value of laparoscopy for the staging of gastric cancer and the detection of liver metastases. Cancer 58: 1–6

Rosenhoff S H, Young R C, Anderson T et al 1975 Peritoneoscopy: a valuable staging tool in ovarian cancer. Annals of Internal Medicine 83: 37–41

Rossi P, Mullins D, Thal E 1993 Role of laparoscopy in the evaluation of abdominal trauma. American Journal of Surgery 166: 707–710

Ruddock J C 1937 Peritoneoscopy. Surgery, Gynecology and Obstetrics 65: 623–639

Sackier J M, Wang Y 1994 Robotically assisted laparoscopic surgery. Surgical Endoscopy 8: 63–66

Salky B 1993 Diagnostic laparoscopy. Surgical Laparoscopy and Endoscopy 3: 132–134

Salvino C K, Esposito T J, Marshall W J, Dries D J, Morris R C, Gamelli R L 1993 The role of diagnostic laparoscopy in the management of trauma patients: a preliminary assessment. Journal of Trauma 34: 506–513

Schier F, Waldschmidt J 1994 Laparoscopy in children with ill-defined abdominal pain. Surgical Endoscopy 8: 97–99

See W A, Soper N J 1994 Selection and preparation of the patient for laparoscopic surgery. In: Soper N J, Odem R R, Clayman R V, McDougall E M (eds) Essentials of laparoscopy. Quality Medical Publishing, St Louis, pp 6–7

Smith R S, Fry W R, Tsoi E K et al 1993 Gasless laparoscopy and conventional instruments. The next phase of minimally invasive surgery. Archives of Surgery 128: 1102–1107

Smith R S, Eubanks S, Swanstrom L L, Wolfe B M 1994 Gasless laparoscopy: the next phase of laparoscopic surgery? Contemporary Surgery 45: 171–184

Soper N J, Hunter J, Petrie R H 1992a Laparoscopic cholecystectomy in pregnancy. Surgical Endoscopy 6: 115–117

Soper N J, Stockman P T, Dunnegan D L, Ashley S W 1992b Laparoscopic cholecystectomy: the new 'gold standard'? Archives of Surgery 127: 917–923

Soper N J, Brunt M L, Kerbl K 1994 Laparoscopic general surgery. New England Journal of Medicine 330: 409–419

Sosa J L, Sims D, Martin L, Zeppa R 1992 Laparoscopic evaluation of tangential abdominal gunshot wounds. Archives of Surgery 127: 109–110.

Sosa J L, Markley M, Sleeman D, Puente I, Carrillo E 1993 Laparoscopy in abdominal gunshot wounds. Surgical Laparoscopy and Endoscopy 3: 417–419

Spinelli P, Difelice G 1991 Laparoscopy and abdominal malignancies. Problems in General Surgery 8: 329–347

Stellato T A 1992 History of laparoscopic surgery. Surgical Clinics of North America 72: 997–1002

Tameda Y, Yoshiza N, Takase K, Nakano T, Kosaka Y 1990 Prognostic value of peritoneoscopic findings in cirrhosis of the liver. Gastrointestinal Endoscopy 36: 34–38

Townsend M C, Flancbaus L, Choban P S, Cloutier C T 1993 Diagnostic laparoscopy as an adjunct to selective conservative management of solid organ injuries after blunt abdominal trauma. Journal of Trauma 35: 647–651

Tverskoy M, Cozacor C, Ayache M, Bradley E L 1992 Postoperative pain after inguinal herniorrhaphy with different types of anesthesia. Anesthesia and Analgesia 74: 495–498

Yamamoto M, Stiegmann G V, Durham J et al 1993 Laparoscopy-guided intracorporeal ultrasound accurately delineates hepatobiliary anatomy. Surgical Endoscopy 7: 325–330

Warshaw A L, Tepper J E, Shipley W A 1986 Laparoscopy in the staging and planning of therapy for pancreatic cancer. American Journal of Surgery 151: 76–80

Warshaw A L, Gu Z, Wittenberg J, Waltman A C 1990 Preoperative staging and assessment of resectability of pancreatic cancer. Archives of Surgery 125: 230–233

6

Manometry
D. L. Wingate

INTRODUCTION

The digestive tract is a hollow tube composed of two layers of smooth muscle whose fibres are oriented at right angles. The longitudinal muscle enables the tube to lengthen or shorten, while the circular muscle alters the cross-sectional area. Complex programs of contractile events utilize the properties of these layers to propel the luminal content in a caudal direction or to provide a reservoir in which luminal contents can be retained for storage and processing. It is these structural and dynamic properties that enable the gut to accept material, move it at an appropriate velocity while it is undergoing physicochemical trans-formation and finally expel the residue; these processes are regulated so as to accommodate the biological requirements of different regions of the gut and to respond to the social regulation of ingestion and excretion.

The propulsive property of the gut is commonly referred to as 'motility', but this is an imprecise term because it is used to denote both the movements of the smooth muscle walls and the movement of material within the lumen. Disordered motility is common – reflux and consti-pation are examples – but is often inferred, either from the patient's history or through imaging of abnormal luminal transit, rather than defined. Motility refers to dynamic events; abnormal motility often occurs without detectable tissue lesions and therefore the description of both normal and abnormal motility depends upon the detection of movement of the gut wall and of luminal content. In theory, imaging techniques are ideally suited to this purpose, but in practice they are limited because they are two-dimensional, often imprecise and ill-suited either to prolonged continuous observation of activity or observation of the response to physiological events such as the ingestion of food. Appropriate treatment of motility disorders, however, often requires identification of the specific pathophysiology and manometry – the measurement of pressure within the gut lumen – is evolving into a powerful diagnostic technique. The appropriate use of manometry and the ability to interpret manometric data require some understanding of the technology of manometry and how it may be used to define the motor physiology of the different regions of the gut.

PRINCIPLES OF MANOMETRY

The measurement of atmospheric pressure by the vertical displacement of a fluid column is commemorated by the nomenclature of units of pressure as centimeters of water or mercury and the same technology was used in the early days of physiology to measure pressures within the body. Whereas atmospheric pressure changes only slowly, physiological pressures – vascular, airways, bowel, bladder – undergo rapid phasic changes due to the action of muscle systems and a continuous record of pressure change is therefore needed. Originally this was provided by a stylus floating on top of a fluid column that would mark a smoked paper mounted on a moving drum, but this has been superseded by the development of transducers that, in effect, respond to changing pressure with a proportional change in electrical output. Transduction of pressure into an electrical change can be accomplished in various ways, for example by the mechanical displacement of the core of an induction coil. Transducers now in general use are constructed from materials that change their electrical conductivity when deformed; when used as one arm of a Wheatstone bridge circuit, the change in resistance proportional to the applied force can be tracked and continuously recorded. Such devices, known as strain gauges, used as the sensing elements in systems for pressure measurement in the human body, may be external to the body and connected to it by a mechanical fluid coupling or, miniaturized through the use of microcircuitry, they may be placed directly in the region where pressure is being measured, with an electrical linkage to a recording or radiotelemetering device.

It is important to bear in mind that the relation between patterns of

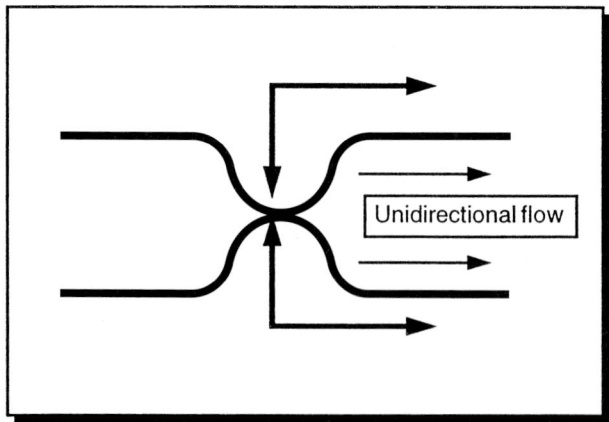

Figure 6.1 Schematic diagram of an occlusive contraction which is propagated by peristalsis, propelling the gut content in the same direction.

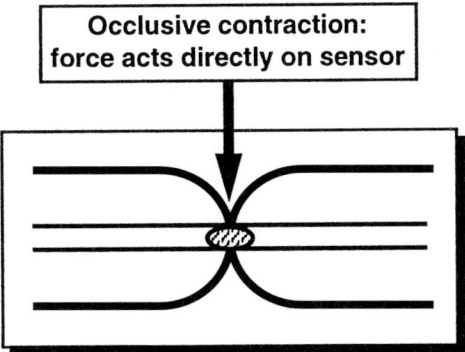

Figure 6.2 The passage of an occlusive contraction is accurately represented by an intraluminal sensor.

pressure change and the transit of material along the digestive tube depends upon whether contractions occlude the lumen. When this happens (Fig. 6.1), peristalsis will propel material in the direction of propagation and thus inferences about transit can be drawn from patterns of pressure activity (Fig. 6.2): the esophagus is a good example of this relationship. However, when contractions are not lumen-occlusive (Fig. 6.3), luminal content will move bidirectionally even though peristalsis is unidirectional and inferences about the direction and rate of flow of

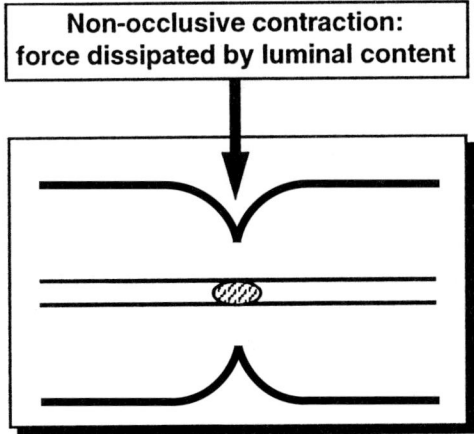

Figure 6.3 The force of a non-occlusive contraction is dissipated by luminal content, so that little or no pressure change is recorded by an intraluminal sensor.

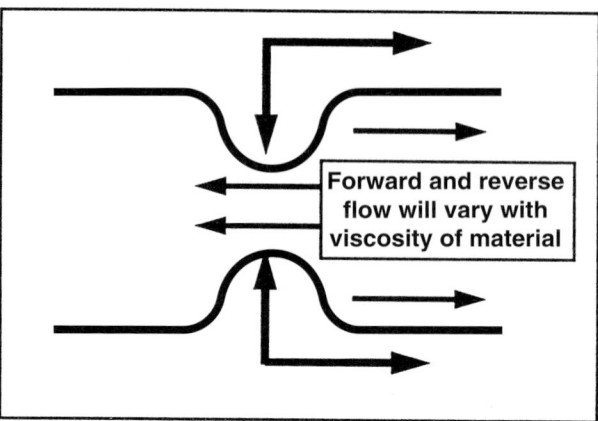

Forward and reverse flow will vary with viscosity of material

Figure 6.4 Propagated non-occlusive contractions produce backward as well as forward flow in the lumen.

material are not possible (Fig. 6.4); this applies to the stomach and colon. The mode of contact between the pressure sensor and the body cavity under study depends upon the geometry of the cavity. It is convenient to consider the systems used in gastroenterology, which can be located in the desired region of the digestive tract using appropriate techniques of intubation, as two types – *point* sensors and *volume* sensors.

Point sensors

Small volume sensors detect pressure change at a specific locus and are effective at detecting wall contraction in narrow tubes (esophagus, small bowel, bile duct, sphincters) where contractions occlude the lumen. The sensing device in common use in the gut is the continuously perfused open-tip tube. This usually takes the form of a fine-bore (<1 mm internal diameter) polyvinyl chloride (PVC) tube, attached to an external water reservoir and pump that delivers continuous flow through the tube. Occlusion of the outlet from the tube by the contraction of the smooth muscle that surrounds it raises the pressure in the fluid column and this pressure change is detected by an attached transducer. Several tubes can be bonded together to form a multilumen tube to detect pressure at a series of points along the gut; such tube assemblies are cheap and easy to build. The fluid load delivered by multiple perfused tube systems into the gut lumen can be minimized by the use of a pneumohydraulic pump – the 'Arndorfer pump' (Arndorfer et al 1977). In this system, compressed nitrogen is used to force water out of a reservoir through fine-bore steel capillary tubing; multiple identical capillaries can be matched to multiple perfused PVC tubes, giving uniform low flow in a low compliance system.

Transducers attached to the PVC tubes through T-junctions record pressure changes when the outflow from the open tips of the tubes is obstructed by contraction of the gut wall (Fig. 6.5).

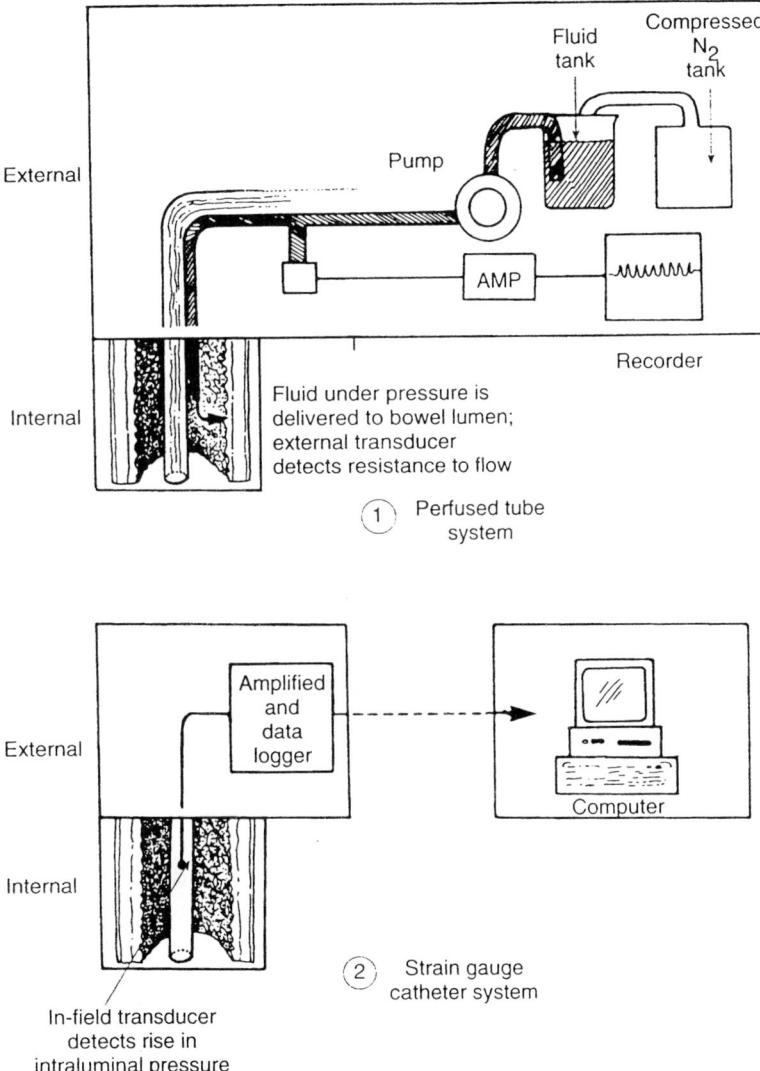

Figure 6.5 Perfused tube (above) and intraluminal strain gauge (below) systems perform identical functions, but with the perfused tube system, the subject must be continuously attached to the system elements contained in the upper rectangle, whereas in the intraluminal strain gauge system, the only required attachment to the patient is an electronic data-logger (reproduced from Schuster M M (ed) 1993 Atlas of gastrointestinal motility. Williams & Wilkins, Baltimore).

The perfused tube system is robust and reliable, but it has drawbacks for use over long periods of time. At an average flow rate of 0.2 mL/min, a 10-lumen tube will deliver 120 mL of water per hour and this may perturb normal physiology. During manometry, the patient must remain seated or recumbent, attached to bulky apparatus; this in turn requires the use of a clinical physiology facility. Because of the high pressure driving the fluid, continued supervision is required to make sure that the water reservoir does not run dry. These conditions pose problems that increase when continuous manometry is required for long periods of time and this is increasingly required for the investigation of antroduodenal and small bowel motor activity (Kellow et al 1990).

The solution to the problem of the fluid interface required to link the external strain gauge to the lumen of the bowel is to place the sensor directly within the lumen of the bowel (Gill et al 1990). This became possible when advances in electronic technology enabled strain gauges to be reduced in size. It is now possible to incorporate a number of strain gauges within a silicone rubber catheter less than 3 mm in diameter; the fine wire leads connecting the sensors to the external recording device run within the catheter, allowing it to retain the flexibility required to negotiate the curvatures of the nasopharynx and the digestive tract.

With the pump and reservoir made redundant, the remaining external elements of a manometric system can also be miniaturized, using solid-state components with low power requirements to provide the drive circuitry for the strain gauge resistors. These form the 'front end' of amplifying and recording systems powered by alkaline batteries that are small and light enough to be carried by the subject in a pouch or on a belt (Lindberg et al 1990).

It is generally assumed, for the sake of convenience, that point sensors located within the digestive tract have a precise anatomical location. Strictly speaking, this is untrue because it is not possible to fix sensors to the wall of the gut. Sensors are attached to inelastic tubes or catheters inserted into the proximal or distal end of an elastic tube that undergoes concertina-like elongation and shortening. Because of these movements, the sensors do not stay at anatomically fixed points. An example of this is the elongation of the stomach on feeding, which extends the distance between the mouth and the pylorus by about 3 cm, with the consequence that a sensor located just distal to the pylorus in a fasted subject will be retracted into the antrum when a meal is eaten. The reference points for the position of sensors are, therefore, either the points of entry (nose, mouth, anus) of the manometric system into the body or radiologically identifiable landmarks (cardia, ligament of Treitz, ileocecal valve).

Volume sensors

Volume sensors, in the form of air-filled or water-filled balloons connected to a pressure sensing device, were the first type of pressure sensor to be used in the digestive tract. A balloon connected to a water column requires no advanced technology. The height of the water column depended on the pressure within the balloon and a pointer mounted on a float on top of the water column could be arranged to make a mark on a moving sheet of paper previously coated with soot from a candle or gas flame. Such systems required only minimal technology and were well established in the nineteenth century.

Volume sensors have two disadvantages. The first is that they record the average pressure within a cavity but the locus of contraction in the wall of such a cavity is not identifiable and if the locus is moving, as for example with a peristaltic contraction, the volume sensor will record only a constant pressure elevation (Fig. 6.6). Since much of the information that is now sought from manometry is on the propagation or migration of localized contractions, this is clearly a disadvantage. The second problem is the use of elastic balloons made of rubber or similar materials; the elasticity of the wall contributes to the pressure recorded from the balloon. This problem has been overcome in recent years by the use of non-elastic plastic film, such as polythene, for the construction of volume sensors.

The problem of poor localization remains, but volume sensors still have their uses in large cavities of the digestive tract where contractions are not lumen-occlusive and are not detected by point sensors. In particular, their use in 'barostat' systems has been promising, although so far only in the research domain (Azpiroz & Malagelada 1987). In a barostat system, a non-elastic balloon attached to a catheter is filled with water by a

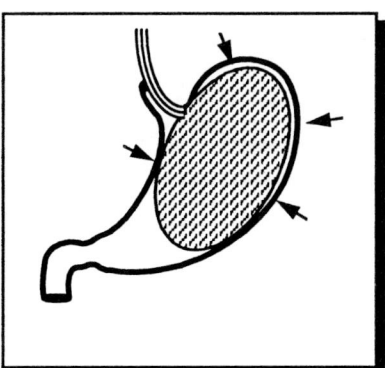

Figure 6.6 A volume sensor, such as an intragastric balloon, cannot discriminate between contractions arising at different points around its circumference and therefore has poor spatial resolution.

bidirectional pump. The system can be set so that either the volume in the balloon or the pressure recorded from the balloon remains constant; rapidly responsive pressure sensors in parallel in the fluid circuit are connected to computerized circuitry that controls the flow through the pump to achieve the desired effect. For *pressure* measurement, the system is set at a constant pressure; the volume in the balloon is then proportional to the pressure exerted by the viscus in which the balloon is confined. The set volume mode of operation is used to determine the response of the viscus to distension by a known volume.

Volume sensors are of value primarily in the stomach and colon, but standard study protocols for clinical diagnostic use have not been established, nor is there clear agreement on the dividing line between normal and abnormal motor activity detected by these systems.

The sphincter problem

Intraluminal recording from short sphincter segments poses particular problems because a sensor, attached to a catheter, which is initially stationed within a sphincter zone is easily dislodged by the natural elongation or shortening of the digestive tube between the sphincter and the pharynx (Fig. 6.7). 'Static' manometry, using a catheter in a constant position, is thus unreliable even for comparatively short periods of time. The traditional solution has been the 'pull-through' technique, in which the sensors are positioned on the aboral side of the sphincter. The catheter is then retracted, so that the sensors are drawn through the sphincter zone, with the reasonable assumption that at some point in the pull-through sequence (Fig. 6.8), they will be recording from the sphincter.

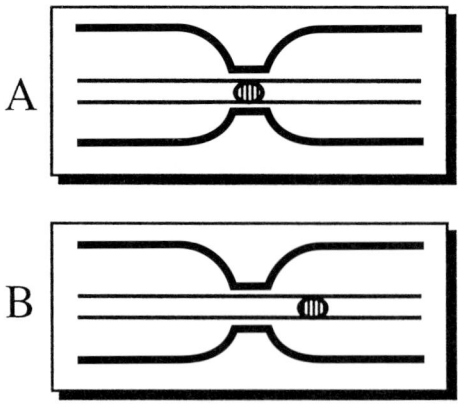

Figure 6.7 The sphincter problem. A sensor positioned initially within a sphincter zone will become dislodged from its position as recording proceeds.

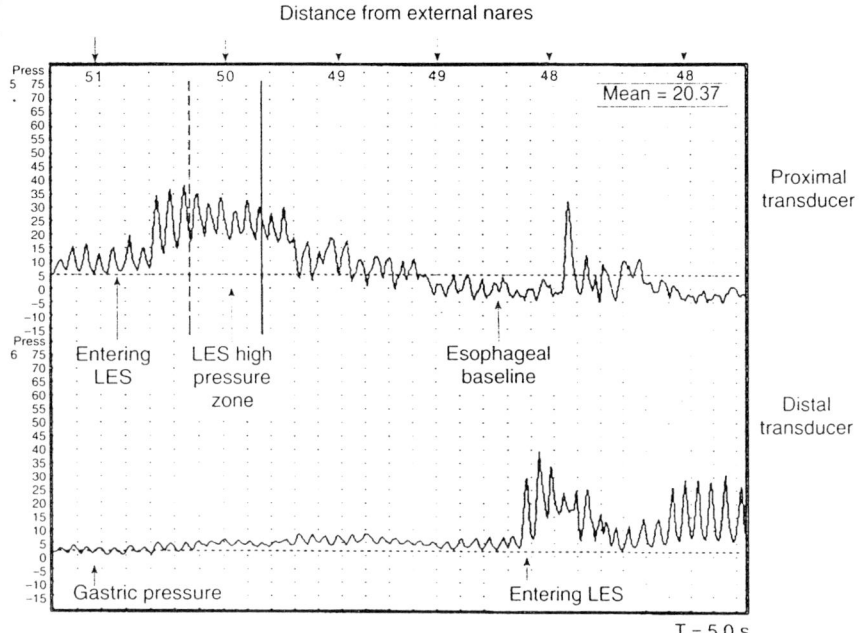

Figure 6.8 A 'pull-through' recording in the lower esophagus from two sensors. Initially, the catheter was passed into the stomach and then withdrawn. As it is withdrawn the high pressure zone of the lower sphincter is identified first in the proximal sensor and then in the distal sensor (reproduced from Schuster M M (ed) 1993 Atlas of gastrointestinal motility. Williams & Wilkins, Baltimore).

The pull-through technique is obviously inappropriate for prolonged recording activity and for this, the sleeve technique is required (Dent & Chir 1976). The sleeve consists of an elongated fluid-filled sac surrounding the catheter, which is in continuity with a sensor; the sleeve acts as an elongated sensor. If it is dislodged from its original position it will still remain within the sphincter (Fig. 6.9). The disadvantage of the sleeve is that the portions of the sleeve that are outside the sphincter zone are exposed to the pressure activity on either side of the sphincter and thus the pressure recorded from the sleeve is the integral of the pressure within the sphincter and the pressures on either side. This effect can be compensated for, at least to some extent, by adding additional sensors above and below the sleeve so that the perisphincteric pressures can be subtracted from the recorded sleeve pressure.

Data acquisition

For many decades, data acquisition in manometric recording consisted of no more than capturing the deflections of a pointer on a paper record.

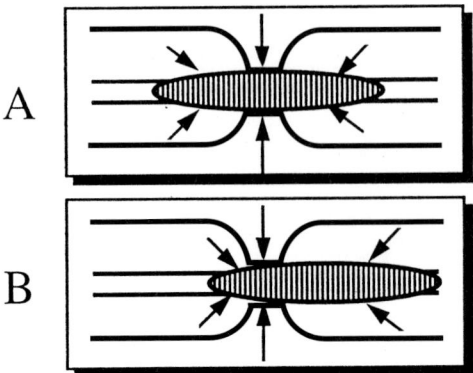

Figure 6.9 A sleeve sensor within a sphincter zone. Even if it is dislodged, part of the sleeve will remain within the sphincter zone because of its elongated shape (cf. Fig. 6.7). However, the sleeve is also subject to pressure changes from the segments on each side of the sphincter.

With the advent of electrical pressure transducers this process became more complicated, with an electrical signal transmitted from the sensors via electronic amplifiers to an ink or hot stylus pen pressed against a motor-driven paper record. It is important to remember that signals transferred to paper in this way cannot be quantified or processed; only the marks on the paper can be measured and related to the timing and amplitude of contractions. Before the advent of electronic signal processing, this did not appear to be a disadvantage since no alternative method of processing was available, but the 'visual analysis' or analysis by inspection and measurement of such pressure records is a laborious and inaccurate process compared with the use of computer methods.

The use of electronic media for data acquisition allows the signals to be reproduced in their original form when required and this development opened the door to the use of computer-based signal analysis techniques. Magnetic tape was the first such medium to be used. Magnetic tape has the advantage of a very high storage capacity and is especially useful for prolonged or simultaneous multichannel recording, but it has one major disadvantage for pressure recording. Only high frequency changes (for example, sound waves) can be stored directly on magnetic tape; low frequency (<1 Hz) changes, which are the frequency domain into which gut pressure activity falls, have to be converted, using frequency modulation (FM), into a high frequency signal in which frequency changes in a carrier signal are proportional to the frequency of the applied signal. The requirement for FM carrier recording increases the cost and complexity of recording systems.

Magnetic tape has now been replaced by digital storage, using computer diskettes, hard disks or solid-state digital memory. In digital systems, the pressure signal is sampled at a set frequency, usually 5 Hz, and each sampled signal is converted into a binary number which is then stored in memory. The stored signal is of high fidelity and there is no inherent 'noise' in the system, unlike magnetic tape where 'tape hiss' distorts low amplitude changes. Digital storage has the advantage of simplicity. In static laboratory-based systems, the same computer can be used for data acquisition and analysis; for mobile systems, small digital data-loggers (recorders) are available which can easily be carried by a subject and which have power requirements that are so low that a couple of small alkaline dry batteries are sufficient for 24 hours of recording. Once the recording is finished, the data are easily downloaded to a computer through a connecting lead.

Data analysis

The pressure within the gut lumen has two components – *tonic* and *phasic*. The tonic component is due to muscle tone, is not easily identified and is usually, for operational simplicity, ignored. Phasic pressure changes are due to circular muscle contractions at a specific locus and are easily identified as sinusoidal pressure changes. Phasic contractions are part of the sequence of peristalsis and such contractions normally travel in an aboral direction. The analysis of pressure data is a three-stage process consisting of (a) the identification of individual contractions, (b) the identification of propagation, and (c) the detection of specific physio-logical sequences of activity. An additional process, (d) the identification of movement 'artefacts', is sometimes required.

The identification of individual contractions

For simplicity, a phasic sinusoidal change can be treated as a triangle, since three points define the essential information. These are the times of deflection from the baseline, the pressure peak and the return to baseline (Fig. 6.10). The height of the triangle represents the maximal amplitude of the pressure change. This stage of the analysis is ideally suited to the computer (Benson et al 1993, Castell et al 1984) and simple algorithms for the detection of contraction are usually available in the software sold with modern electronic pressure measurement systems.

The identification of propagation

In the esophagus, stomach and small bowel, the velocity of migration of peristalsis in health is known and therefore when a series of point sensors

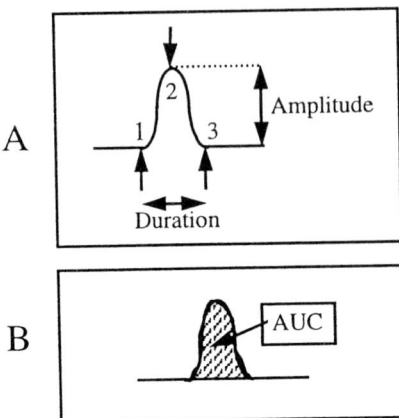

Figure 6.10 Characterization of gut contractions. Three points define the duration and amplitude of a single contraction (above). The area under the curve (AUC) can also be quantified by a computer (below) and the total AUC/unit time can be used as an index of motility. 'Motility indexes' have been popular as measures of average motility for many years, but their value is diminished since they do not indicate the number and timing of individual contractions required for the identification of patterns of motor activity.

is used, the times at which a peristaltic contraction will appear along the sequence of sensors can be estimated. It is therefore possible to distinguish between isolated contractions which proceed for a very short distance and those which travel further. This type of analysis is also suited to computer analysis; an algorithm is used to define a time window in which a contraction detected at a proximal sensor will be expected to appear at more distally placed sensors (Fig. 6.11). There is a caveat over the use of

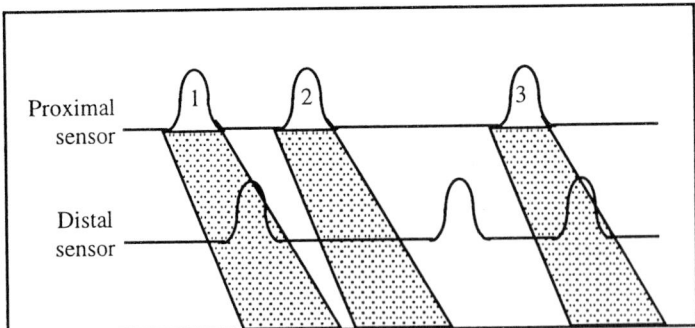

Figure 6.11 The use of a time window for the detection of propagation. The shaded areas represent 'windows' in which contractions detected by the proximal sensor would be expected to appear at the distal sensor according to the known velocity of the propagation of peristalsis. In this schematic example, contractions 1 and 3 are propagated, but contraction 2 is not.

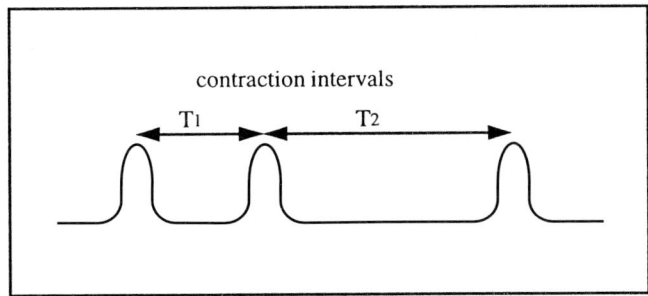

Figure 6.12 The interval between contractions often varies.

this type of analysis: the assumption that rates of propagation in disease will be identical with those in normal tissue may be invalid in disease of the smooth muscle or intrinsic innervation of the gut wall. In the esophagus at least, where peristalsis can be controlled by swallowing, it is possible to detect abnormal propagation because the time interval between swallows can be varied (Fig. 6.12) and the same time interval can be seen at successive sensors (Fig. 6.13).

The detection of specific physiological sequences of activity

Specific sequences of activity are less easily identified by computer, but more easily seen by inspection. Such sequences include swallowing (with peristalsis along the esophagus combined with lower sphincter relaxation), antroduodenal coordination and the identification of the three phases of the migrating motor complex (MMC). The two former patterns are brief temporal events, whereas the latter are prolonged activity

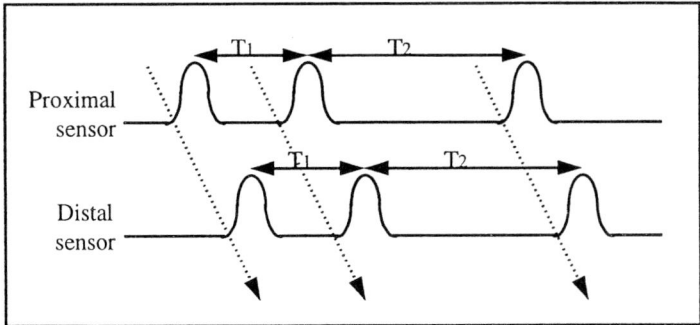

Figure 6.13 The variation in time interval can be used to detect propagation because the same sequence of time intervals can be predicted at successive sensors if the contractions are propagated.

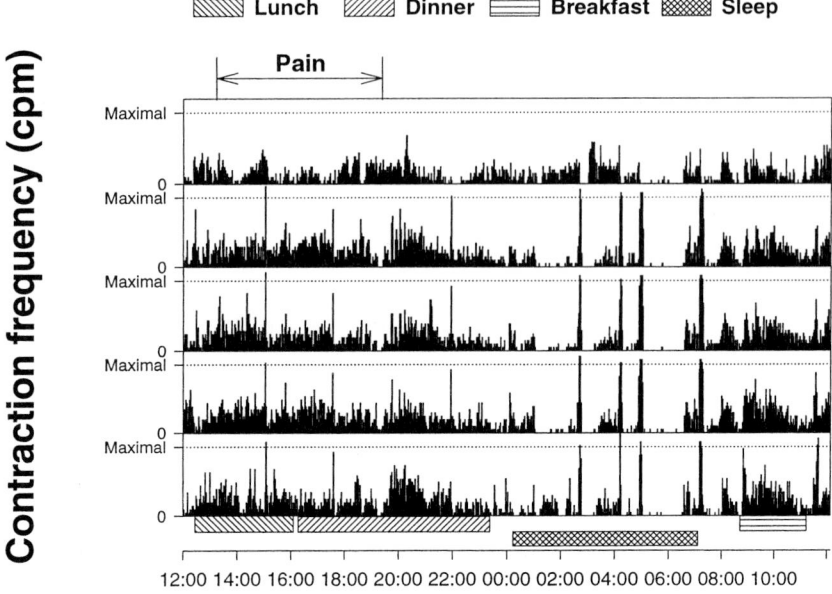

Figure 6.14 A computer-generated plot of small bowel manometry in an ambulant subject during 24 hours recorded from five sensors in the proximal small bowel. The computer has identified contractions, eliminated artefacts and provided an integrated record of contractions per minute (cpm) for each sensor. The maximal contractile frequency of ten contractions per minute is only achieved during phase III of the migrating motor complex (MMC). Four phase III episodes are clearly seen during the period of nocturnal sleep and can be identified as such by the computer program (courtesy of Dr F D Castillo).

patterns, in which phase III is most easily recognized by its characteristic burst of regularly recurring powerful contractions (Fig. 6.14).

The identification of movement 'artefacts'

One complicating factor in the analysis of motor activity from the intraabdominal portion of the digestive tube is the effect of changes in intraabdominal pressure due to the musculature of the abdominal wall. In recumbent subjects, activities such as coughing and sneezing cause large transient pressure changes and in ambulant subjects, such pressure changes are more frequent. These pressure changes are usually termed 'artefacts', not because they are artefactual, but because they are not generated by the contractile activity of gut smooth muscle. These pressure artefacts can usually be easily identified when recording is carried out from two or more intraabdominal sensors, because the pressure changes are simultaneous at all sensors. Compared with small bowel pressure changes, they are also usually of greater magnitude and the pressure changes are more abrupt. These differences can be used as the basis of algorithms for the detection and suppression of artefacts in computerized analysis. In esophageal manometry, artefacts are relatively unimportant, as intrathoracic pressures are less affected by such body movements.

REGIONAL MANOMETRY

While the principles of manometry do not change, their application in gastroenterology is governed by two major factors. First, a technology appropriate to the morphology of the area under study is required and this requirement has to take into account the problem of access to the region of interest. Secondly, the protocol of study has to be adapted to the specific nature of the physiological activity of the region of interest. In the esophagus, where the focus of interest is on peristaltic waves that traverse the organ in less than a minute, even a brief manometric study yields a good harvest of data. In contrast, in the stomach and small bowel, slow periodic biorhythms with an average periodicity of about 90 minutes require several hours of study in order to capture only a few cycles of activity.

In each of the sections that follow, the considerations appropriate to each major area of study are summarized, for easy reference, in an introductory tabulated overview; each summary is followed by an explanatory commentary. The format is intended to provide rapid guidance for clinicians; techniques that are still confined to the research laboratory are not reviewed so as not to confuse practical clinical techniques with those that are of only potential value.

The esophagus

The usual aim of esophageal manometry is to confirm the integrity of the swallowing process by the presence of normal swallow-associated peristalsis and the associated relaxation of the lower sphincter (Fig. 6.15). Manometry is essential for the detection and assessment of achalasia. While cases of advanced achalasia present with gross dilatation, less severe cases may be judged to be normal with endoscopy and radiology and misdiagnosis is not infrequent. Manometry is also useful for the assessment of sphincter integrity; although a low sphincter pressure is not synonymous with clinically significant acid reflux, the presence of a hypotonic sphincter may influence the choice of surgical repair rather than long-term acid suppression. While it is neither practicable nor necessary for all patients with gastroesophageal reflux disease to undergo manometry, it is important for it to be carried out, together with 24-hour pHmetry, before antireflux surgery.

Overview: Esophagus		
	Cavity	**Sphincters**
Motor physiology	Swallowing-induced and spontaneous peristalsis	Relaxation on arrival of peristaltic contraction
Pathophysiology	Abnormal peristalsis; simultaneous contraction	Failure of relaxation
Clinical aim	Detection of abnormal amplitude and progression of peristaltic wave *Achalasia*; '*nutcracker*'	Assessment of integrity of sphincter function *Incompetent sphincter achalasia*
Protocols	Brief recording of response to swallowing water	Brief 'pull-through' recording of response to swallowing water
Sensors	Point sensors (perfused tube or strain gauge)	Point sensors (perfused tube or strain gauge)
Special applications	Prolonged recording to detect sporadic symptom-associated abnormalities *Non-cardiac chest pain*	Prolonged recording via sleeve to detect inappropriate relaxation

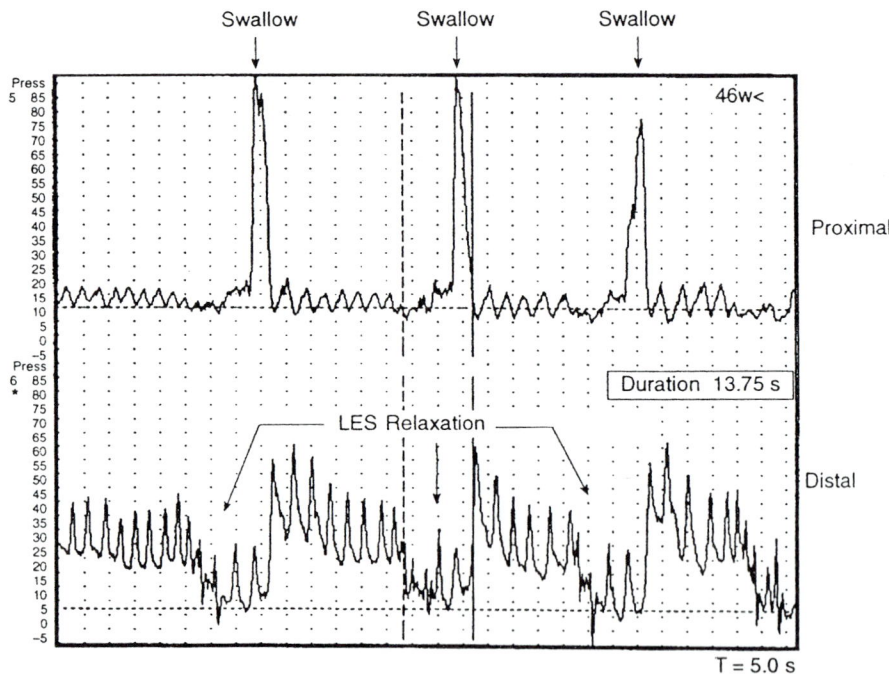

Figure 6.15 Swallow-induced peristalsis in the distal esophagus (upper trace) and the temporally associated relaxation of the lower sphincter (lower trace) in a normal subject (reproduced from Schuster M M (ed) 1993 Atlas of gastrointestinal motility. Williams & Wilkins, Baltimore).

At the time of writing, esophageal manometry is usually performed as a relatively brief procedure using the 'pull-through' technique, because this is appropriate for assessment of the lower sphincter. Prolonged manometry is reserved for diagnostic use in patients with unexplained chest pain, where the ability to record continuously for long periods that may include transient symptoms can be useful.

Esophageal manometry may be regarded as a secondary investigation; it is used when the conventional techniques of endoscopy and barium radiology have failed to provide an unequivocal diagnosis. This only occurs in a small proportion of patients with esophageal disorders but, because of the prevalence of reflux disease, it constitutes a significant and important clinical load.

The stomach

Because of the problems of recording the pressure activity of the stomach, gastric manometry has not evolved into a standard diagnostic method. Information on gastric motor function is normally obtained by imaging, either by radiology or scintigraphy with a gamma camera. Antroduodenal manometry is thus a secondary investigation, but it is the diagnostic method of choice in the investigation of gastroparesis (non-obstructive delayed gastric emptying) in diabetes mellitus and in pseudoobstruction

Overview: Stomach		
	Cavity	Sphincters
Motor physiology	Periodic fasting motor activity and sustained response to a meal (Fig. 6.16)	
Pathophysiology	Absent motor response to a meal, associated with gastric stasis	
Clinical aim	Detection of diminished amplitude and frequency of postprandial contractions *Gastroparesis*	
Protocols	5–6 hour recording of fasting and postprandial activity	
Sensors	Multiple antral point sensors (perfused tube or strain gauge)	
Special applications	'Barostat' recording of tonic and phasic response to distension *Visceral hypersensitivity*	'Sleeve' recording to detect appropriate pyloric relaxation *Pylorospasm*

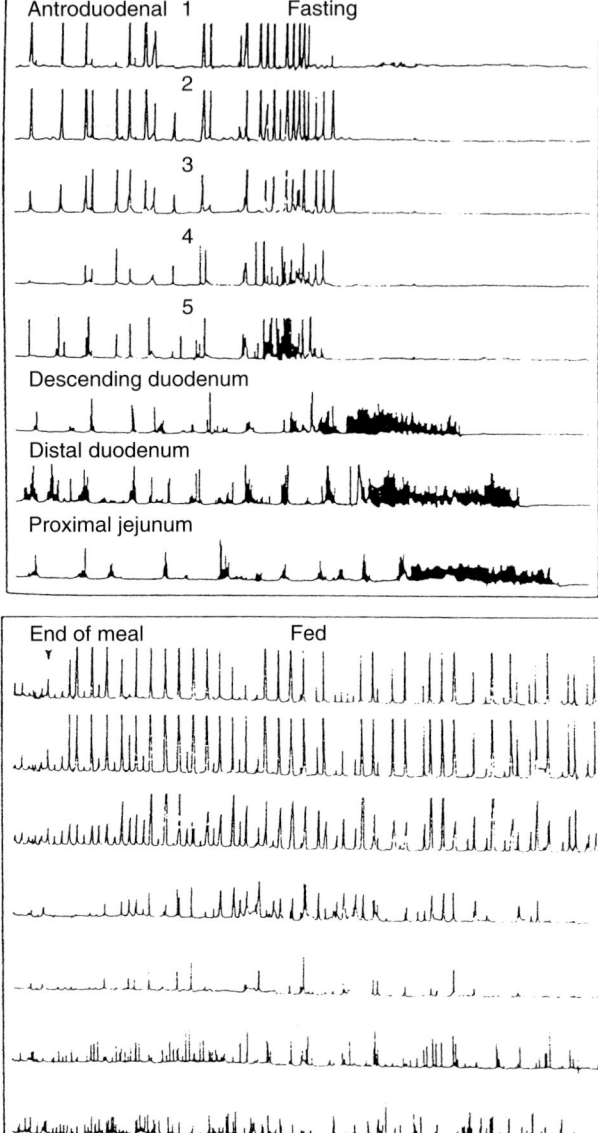

Figure 6.16 Normal antroduodenal manometric patterns of fasting (upper panel) and postprandial (lower panel) motor activity obtained by multilumen perfused tube manometry in a healthy subject. Phase III of the MMC followed by the quiescence of phase I and preceded by the irregular activity of phase II is clearly seen in the fasting record (adapted from Malagelada J R, Camilleri M, Stanghellini V 1986 Manometric diagnosis of gastrointestinal motility disorders. Thieme Inc, New York).

Overview: Biliary Tract	
Motor physiology	**Sphincter zone** Rhythmic contraction of sphincter of Oddi
Pathophysiology	Abnormal frequency of phasic and tonic contraction, possibly associated with pain
Clinical aim	Detection of dysrhythmias and/or hypertonicity 'Tachyoddia'
Protocol	Manometry via modified ERCP catheter
Sensors	Point sensors (perfused tube or strain gauge)

syndromes (Rees et al 1980). Manometry is the only way of distinguishing between an abnormal incidence of contractions and contractile inertia.

The use of the barostat for the assessment of gastric hypersensitivity is, at present, a research technique, but it may well be extended into clinical practice in the near future in the investigation of non-ulcer dyspepsia.

The biliary tract

Biliary manometry or – more accurately – manometry of the sphincter of Oddi, for clinical purposes is at present confined to a few specialist centers. Because it can only be done during endoscopic retrograde choledochography (ERCP), it requires the unusual conjunction of endo-scopic and manometric skills together with the supporting technology. Advocates of the technique (i.e. the few who can do it) assert that it is useful in the detection of motor abnormalities such as spasm that cause pain and are relieved by sphincterotomy; sceptics (i.e. the majority who don't do it) remain to be convinced. Thus the question of whether this is a useful technique depends upon your skill and inclinations but it is, at best, a secondary investigation.

The small intestine

Because, in contrast to the esophagus and stomach, there are no useful alternative technologies for the assessment of the motor function of the small bowel, small bowel manometry is a potential primary investigation. It is certainly a primary investigation for the diagnosis of intestinal pseudoobstruction. It has shown some promise for the diagnosis of the irritable bowel syndrome but in this respect it remains controversial.

The two characteristic motor activities of the organ are the periodic biorhythm of the migrating motor complex, best seen during sleep, and the motor response to a meal. There is general – but not universal –

Overview: Small intestine	
Motor physiology	**Cavity** Nocturnal periodic fasting (MMC) activity and sustained response to a normal mixed meal
Pathophysiology	Abnormal periodic activity due to intrinsic neuropathy; attenuated fed response due to intrinsic or extrinsic neuropathy; low amplitudes in myopathy
Clinical aim	Detection of abnormalities of phases 2 and 3 of the MMC and attenuated fed response *Chronic intestinal pseudoobstruction*
Protocols	Prolonged recording of proximal bowel motility to include response to a meal and overnight sleep
Sensors	Point sensors (strain gauge) incorporated in a nasojejunal catheter
Special applications	Prolonged recording to detect sporadic symptom-associated abnormalities *'Functional disorders'*

agreement that small bowel manometry should therefore consist of a prolonged recording that includes both the response to a normal mixed meal and also normal nocturnal sleep (see Fig. 6.14). This is an evolving field; manometry is a promising technique whose value remains to be defined with precision.

The colon

As is clear from the overview below, colonic manometry has not yet entered the clinical domain. The problems that remain to be overcome are the choice of appropriate sensors (volume sensors, including the barostat, may be more appropriate), their introduction into the colon without undue distortion of normal physiology (at present, sensing catheters are

Overview: Colon	
Motor physiology	**Cavity** Unknown
Pathophysiology	Unknown
Clinical aim	(Research only)
Protocols	No standard protocols
Sensors	Point sensors (strain gauge) incorporated in colonic catheter inserted at colonoscopy
Special applications	(Research only)

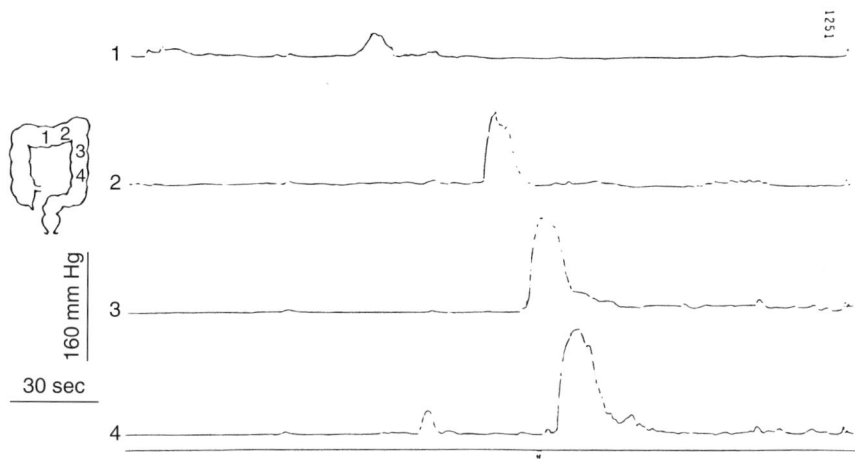

Figure 6.17 A high amplitude propagated contraction moving from the mid-transverse (1) to the mid-descending (4) colon in a healthy human subject during prolonged colonic manometry.

inserted using a colonoscope and guidewire into a previously cleansed colon) and the clear identification of normal physiological patterns of motor activity. The only physiological pressure events on which there is reasonable agreement are 'high amplitude propagating contractions' (HAPCs). These are pressure waves (Fig. 6.17) in excess of 90 mmHg that traverse the entire colon and may be temporally related to defecation. But, in health, only a few (2–5) HAPCs occur in 24 hours and therefore prolonged monitoring is required for their detection. Ambulatory monitoring has been attempted using peroral intubation, but it has not proved possible with this technique to place sensors with any degree of accuracy in desired locations because of the great variation in the length of the colon between different subjects (Soffer et al 1989).

The anorectum

Anorectal manometry is useful to assess the integrity of the internal and external anal sphincters and also the integrity of the rectoanal inhibitory reflex (RAIR), which is the reflex inhibition of the internal sphincter by rectal distension (Fig. 6.18). Absence of the RAIR is indicative of neurological damage. This is a specialist field of manometry that is useful in the management of fecal retention or incontinence. The use of rectal distension to test the sensory threshold is an emerging research activity, but there is controversy over the way in which distension should be carried out and also over the way in which findings should be interpreted.

Overview: Rectum	Cavity	Sphincters
Motor physiology	Rectal motor complexes	Rectoanal inhibitory reflex (RAIR)
Pathophysiology	Undefined	Absent RAIR due to denervation. Weak sphincter due to muscle or nerve damage
Clinical aim	Undefined	Absent RAIR; failure of sphincter relaxation *Neuropathy; anismus*
Protocols	No standard protocols	Brief recording of response to rectal distension
Sensors		Multiple point sensors in anal canal with rectal sensor and balloon
Special applications	Barostat recording to detect sensory and motor response to distension *Stiff or hypersensitive rectum*	Prolonged recording to detect sphincter relaxations *Incontinence*

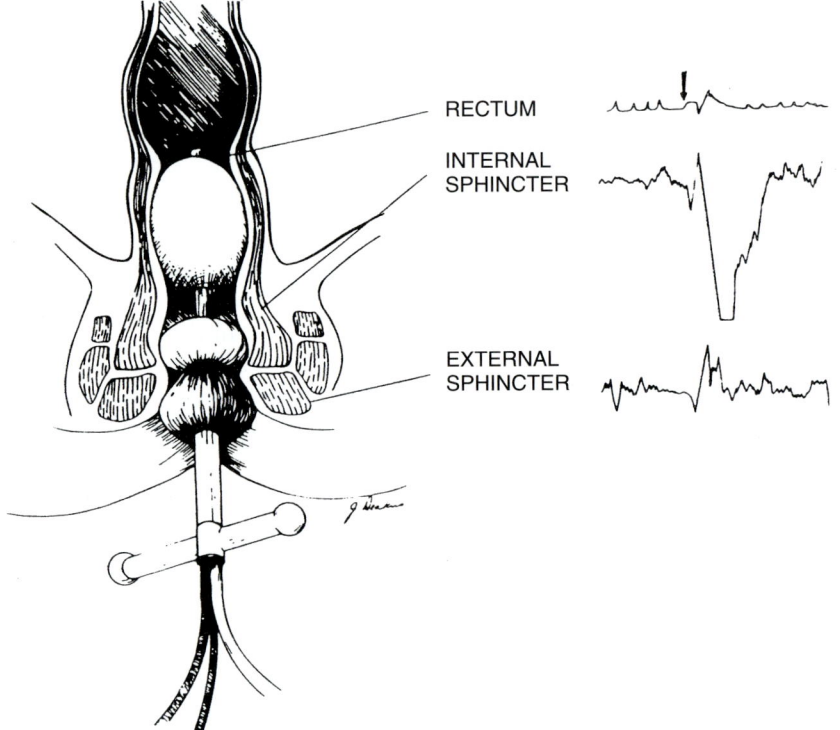

RECTUM

INTERNAL SPHINCTER

EXTERNAL SPHINCTER

Figure 6.18 The rectoanal inhibitory reflex (right) and the manometric assembly used in the recording. When the rectal balloon is inflated (arrow), the internal sphincter relaxes and the external sphincter contracts to maintain continence (reproduced from Schuster M M (ed) 1993 Atlas of gastrointestinal motility. Williams & Wilkins, Baltimore).

CONCLUSIONS

Manometry is a technique of clinical investigation in gastroenterology that was, for many years, considered to be of marginal value. The performance of manometry has been transformed by the advent of digital electronics, which has led to the design of user-friendly systems, often ambulant, in which computer technology controls the recording of pressure within the gut and is also used to analyze the data. Clinical advance is often driven by technology and the availability of safe, reliable and relatively inexpensive measurement systems is leading manometry into the repertoire of clinical skills. Esophageal manometry is now established as an important adjunct in the management of esophageal dysfunction and small bowel manometry is the definitive technique for the diagnosis of diffuse motor disorders of the bowel. The possibilities are intriguing; possible marriages of manometry with endoscopy, telemetry and ultra-sound will depend upon not only the ingenuity of clinical research workers but also investment decisions by industry. At least it is safe to conclude that this summary of the subject will be out of date in the not too distant future.

REFERENCES

Arndorfer R C, Stef J, Dodds W J, Linehan J H, Hogan W J 1977 Improved infusion system for intraluminal oesophageal manometry. Gastroenterology 72: 23–27
Azpiroz F, Malagelada J-R 1987 Gastric tone measured by an electronic barostat in health and postsurgical gastroparesis. Gastroenterology 92: 934–943
Benson M J, Castillo F D, Wingate D L, Demetrakopoulos J, Spyrou N M 1993 The computer as referee in the analysis of human small bowel motility. American Journal of Physiology 264: G645–654
Castell D O, Dubois A, Davis C R, Cordova C M, Norman D O 1984 Computer-aided analysis of human oesophageal peristalsis. Digestive Diseases and Sciences 29: 65–72
Dent J, Chir B 1976 A new technique for continuous sphincter pressure measurement. Gastroenterology 71: 263–267
Gill R C, Kellow J E, Browning C, Wingate D L 1990 The use of intraluminal strain gauges for recording ambulant small bowel motility. American Journal of Physiology 258: G610–G615
Kellow J E, Gill R C, Wingate D L 1990 Prolonged ambulant recordings of small bowel motility demonstrate abnormalities in the irritable bowel syndrome. Gastroenterology 98: 1208–1218
Lindberg G, Iwarzon M, Stal P, Seensalu R 1990 Digital ambulant monitoring of small bowel motility. Scandinavian Journal of Gastroenterology 25: 216–224
Rees W D W, Miller L J, Malagelada J-R 1980 Dyspepsia, antral motor dysfunction, and gastric stasis of solids. Gastroenterology 78: 360–365
Soffer E E, Scalabrini P, Wingate D L 1989 Prolonged ambulatory monitoring of human colonic motility. American Journal of Physiology 255: G601-G606

FURTHER READING

Schuster M M (ed) 1993 Atlas of gastrointestinal motility in health and disease. Williams & Wilkins, Baltimore
Wingate D L, Kumar D (eds) 1994 An illustrated guide to gastrointestinal motility, 2nd edn. Churchill Livingstone, London

pH Measurements
D. F. Evans

INTRODUCTION

pH measurements in the gastrointestinal tract have been of interest to physiologists and gastroenterologists since the discovery over 300 years ago that the stomach produced acid (Willis 1684). Early studies of gastric acid production involved either aspiration of gastric juice from the stomach by way of a tube passed either nasally or orally into the stomach or, in rare cases, by direct sampling from gastric fistulae (Beaumont 1833).

The development of pH–sensitive glass electrodes in the early twentieth century led to the eventual introduction of the intraluminal glass pH sensor (Rovelstad 1956) which allowed for continuous, uninterrupted measurement of hydrogen ion concentration in the stomach and small intestine. The development of novel sensors such as pH and pressure–sensitive telemetry capsules (Woolf 1961) enabled measurements to be made in otherwise inaccessible parts of the gut, for example the terminal ileum and cecum. The introduction of other types of sensors and the realization that pH measurements were useful in diagnosis, and a marker of treatment efficacy in acid–related diseases, have lead to the commercialization of pH recording equipment. In addition, the technological expansion over the past 10–20 years has led to the introduction of small, portable monitoring devices to enable long-term data collection under ambulatory conditions.

This chapter will describe the latest technology available for pH measurements in the human gut and general applications of the technique in medicine and research.

METHODOLOGY

Sensors

Active electrode

pH–sensitive electrodes have seen major advances in the last decade with size, comfort and unit cost very much in mind as the demand from the medical profession has grown. Miniature (<2 mm) glass and antimony electrodes are used as pH sensors with either combined or external reference electrodes (see below). Antimony electrodes may be of monocrystalline or polycrystalline construction but both types appear satisfactory in clinical practice. Electrodes may be disposable (single use), semidisposable (5–10 uses) or have an indefinite lifespan (usually glass). The cost of electrodes varies widely but currently the most inexpensive option is the semidisposable, single channel, antimony electrode with external reference at approximately £40. Glass electrodes with a combined reference are the most expensive, but are probably also the most accurate. A unit cost of up to £400 is offset by the potential of many uses.

Other sensing materials have been developed in an attempt to improve electrode efficiency and cost. Plastic (Rawlings & Lucas 1985) and ion-selective field effect transistors (ISFET) (Schepel et al 1984) have been developed as replacements for glass and antimony. However, none has made any real impact in the market place at present for various reasons. Sensor technology continues to explore new avenues. Electrode diameter is no longer a problem unless multiple channels and other parameters are to be measured (i.e. pressure). Recent developments using fiberoptic technology (Schneider et al 1990) and implanted telemetry capsules have great potential for the future (Kadirkamanathan et al 1993).

Reference electrode

All pH sensing devices require a stable reference electrode held at 0 volts. In a laboratory pH meter, the reference potential is usually a calomel or Ag–AgCl junction. In the case of in vivo devices, the reference electrode is either an Ag–AgCl skin electrode or a KCl or NaCl junction housed within the electrode casing, near to the active electrode. An internal reference is preferable but is more difficult to manufacture and makes for a larger diameter and more expensive catheter and patient contamination usually limits the electrode to single use only. External reference electrodes are satisfactory but there can be an offset potential set up between the skin and electrode which may affect the accuracy and stability of pH measurements. Another major problem is simply that of the reference electrode becoming detached from the body during the course of measurement.

Radiotelemetry capsules (RTC)

Radiotelemetry capsules have been available since the 1960s (Woolf 1961) and offer the potential for less invasive monitoring of intraluminal pH in comparison to catheter methods. RTCs are small (typically 28 × 8 mm), battery powered, pH–sensitive radio transmitters that are swallowed like any ordinary tablet (Colson et al 1981). The RTC may be free to transit the GI tract or tethered by some form of fine material such as silk or nylon thread. If untethered, the RTC moves through the GI tract unhindered, transmitting information with regard to intraluminal pH changes as it goes. If tethered, the RTC behaves in a similar way to a pH catheter. Untethered RTCs have been used mainly for pH measurements in the small and large intestine.

Signals from RTCs are detected by a body-borne aerial belt, decoded by a dedicated radio receiver and recorded on to pen recorders or ambulatory data-loggers (see below). New methods are being developed to implant RTCs in the gut lumen using endoscopically guided sewing machines (Swain et al 1992).

The advantage of the RTC is that it offers a very accurate means of pH detection. The large diameter glass electrode surface is stable and resistant to contamination by luminal content. This is particularly important in gastric pH measurements where contamination of smaller pH sensors (in particular antimony and micro glass) may be a problem. An inbuilt reference electrode ensures a stable non-polarizable zero voltage junction and when untethered or implanted, the RTC is totally undetectable by the patient. The disadvantages of RTCs are cost (currently £250 each) and the requirement for specialized receiver/ recorders (only one available worldwide in 1995). Some patients have difficulty swallowing the capsules, especially those attached to a long tethering thread.

Electrode calibration

All pH electrodes require calibration prior to use in solutions of known pH (buffers) to ensure accurate recordings. The selection of calibration values is determined by the measured pH range. As a general rule, the two calibration buffers should span the range to be measured. For example, if gastric pH is to be measured (average pH 1–5), then calibration buffers of pH 1 and 7 would be appropriate. If intestinal pH is to be measured (range pH 5–8), then buffers of pH 4 and 9 would be more suitable.

pH buffers

Generally, most standard laboratory buffers are suitable for glass electrodes, but in some cases electrode manufacturers will specifically recommend certain types. For antimony electrodes, non-phosphate buffers are recommended, as these do not affect electrode performance due to contamination. Buffers should be stored at 4°C to avoid bacterial contamination. It is also important not to contaminate buffers with themselves during calibration, especially acid (pH 1) into neutral (pH 7).

Calibration procedure

Temperature. Ideally, calibration should be performed at 37°C in a water bath. Practically, electrodes may be calibrated at room temperature, but pH electrodes and buffers are temperature sensitive, so in order to maintain accuracy in vivo, some form of electrical temperature compensation will be necessary.

In vitro calibration. Calibration is achieved by placing the active electrode and reference electrode in the buffer solution and cycling through the calibration procedure. This is possible only with electrodes with internal reference (including radiocapsules) and where external reference electrodes are the non-disposable type (Ag–AgCl). In this case there may be some offset potential and therefore inaccuracies in pH detection due to the presence of a small skin potential when the electrode is attached to the patient.

On-patient calibration – 'finger dip'. To overcome the possible skin potential offset problem, where an external reference electrode is used, the calibration procedure can be performed on the patient. The reference electrode is attached to the skin at a convenient place and the active electrode placed in the buffer solution. A finger is placed in the buffer to complete the circuit and the calibration cycle performed. In this way, there is no danger of offset problems as the skin reference potential is identical for both calibration and measurement.

Cleaning and sterilizing for reusable electrodes

Reusable and semidisposable electrodes require cleaning and disinfection between uses. Manufacturers almost universally recommend the following procedure.

1. Remove debris from electrode by rinsing in clean tap water.
2. Wash with diluted detergent (not Dettox as it reduces sensitivity).
3. Immerse in glutaraldehyde or equivalent for 10 minutes (overlong soaking may impair electrode performance).
4. Rinse with sterile water.
5. Store dry or in pH 7 buffer (see manufacturer's recommendation).

RECORDERS

Recorders may be static (i.e. mains driven and immovable) or portable. Data storage may be analog (stand-alone or portable, ambulatory tape recorders) or digital. Generally, portable, digital, solid-state recorders are now used. Recorders may be single or multichannel (up to four pH channels) or combined with other parameters, usually pressure (up to 14 channels).

Static recorders

Static recorders are rarely used for routine diagnostic pH studies. For research studies or where real-time on-line monitoring is desired, it is possible to connect ambulatory recorders with suitable patient electrical isolation to display computers with a real–time visual display of the pH signals. Analog chart recorders for on-line static monitoring have become virtually obsolete with the introduction of the portable, ambulatory devices.

Portable (ambulatory) recorders

pH recorders have seen much development. Most are digital, portable and solid-state (Evans 1987). In esophageal pH studies for GER disease, ambulatory outpatient recordings have been shown to be essential in order to express reflux in the real-life setting of the patient's home environment (Branicki et al 1982, Schlesinger et al 1985). Recorders incorporate event markers to record symptoms, meals and upright and supine periods, these being important factors in the accurate diagnosis of pathological GER. Symptom markers are particularly important where symptoms are atypical, for example in the diagnosis of non-cardiac chest pain. Even a negative test in this case may be helpful in diagnosis (Vantrappen et al 1987).

Commercial pH systems record for at least 24 hours, this period yielding the maximum information about circadian patterns of reflux. The most up-to-date recorders will store pH data for up to 96 hours on a single battery, although it is doubtful that such long-term measurements will be either tolerated by the patient or particularly useful in all but the most difficult diagnostic cases. Some recorders incorporate other features such as warning bleeps, informing patients to take medication, or automatic posture sensors to indicate body position.

There are currently at least ten manufacturers worldwide who now produce ambulatory pH equipment. Many specifically target the eso-phagus but the recorders can also be used for gastric measurements and other parts of the gut accessible to pH electrodes. Only one manufacturer markets a telemetry capsule capability, but this is virtually exclusively used for research. The choice of recorder will be mainly dictated by cost, availability and personal preference, but one important factor is after-sales back-up as, although modern recorders are very reliable, equipment faults and procedural problems can be rapidly resolved with a helpful, easily available company representative.

Multichannel capability

The majority of recorders now have the capability of recording two or more channels of pH. This is particularly useful in certain cases where a

---

Box 7.1 Multichannel recording

Esophageal – distal and proximal measurements

Adult	**Pediatric**
Regurgitation	Vomiting
Hoarseness	Cyanosis/Apnea
Wheeze/asthma	Near-miss cot death
Palatal tooth wear	Chest infection

Duodenogastric or gastroesophageal
Acid suppression treatment failures (on therapy)
Suspected duodenogastric or bile reflux

---

more accurate diagnosis might be made by the additional information from more than one channel. Box 7.1 illustrates some of the circumstances where multichannel recording may be helpful.

Analysis of recordings

Analog pH recordings have the disadvantage that data can only be analyzed manually, a long and laborious process. The main advantage therefore of digitally stored data is the ability to store, display and analyze data retrospectively by computer-generated programs using purpose-designed software, the whole process of data transfer, display and analysis taking only a few minutes with a fast PC, even for studies of 24–48 hours duration.

Most commercially available systems offer purpose-designed software for analysis of GER acid and alkaline reflux and gastric pH. As yet, analytical software for other parts of the GI tract is not widely available other than through individuals undertaking research studies (Evans et al 1988, Gilbert et al 1988). Detailed description of analyses will be discussed in the appropriate sections below.

APPLICATIONS OF pH MEASUREMENTS

Esophagus

Rationale for studies

Symptomatic (GER) and reflux esophagitis are common conditions affecting up to 60% of the adult population (Jones & Lydeard 1989). The accurate diagnosis of GER can be complicated by the absence of visible esophagitis in up to 40% of patients (Richter & Castell 1982) and in some cases, a poor correlation of GER with symptoms. Many tests have been developed to aid diagnosis, but intraesophageal pH measurement is the best discriminator between physiological and pathological reflux (DeMeester et al 1976) and is now regarded as the gold standard in the diagnosis of reflux disease.

Procedure

Single site. The pH sensor is introduced transnasally or orally and the tip positioned 5 cm proximal to the lower esophageal sphincter, this being determined by manometry, endoscopy, radiology or by a pH withdrawal technique, the first being the most accurate. When an external reference electrode is used, this is sited high on the chest over a bony area and secured with adhesive tape. The pH sensor lead is brought out of the nose, affixed to the cheek with waterproof adhesive tape and connected to the recorder by routing the cable underneath the clothing. This enables the patient to undress without disconnection and is also more cosmetically acceptable.

pH measurements should be performed for about 24 hours and must include at least one or two meals and the nocturnal period. This is to ensure that postprandial and nocturnal GER are assessed. Studies should be performed under near physiological conditions and patients should be encouraged to perform normal daily activities where possible. During diagnostic tests, free access to normal meals, smoking and alcohol should be allowed, but these events should be documented. Antireflux medication is usually withdrawn for up to 5 days prior to study (5 days proton pump inhibitors, 2 days H_2 receptor antagonists and prokinetics, 24 hours antacids and alginates) but in some circumstances may be continued, in which case the investigation may be useful in assessing the efficacy of treatment. This is particularly helpful when medication appears to be failing to control symptoms.

Multisite. With two or more sensors, the reference sensor is always the distal esophageal site (5 cm above LES) and the others may be positioned above or below at intervals set by the interelectrode distance (usually 5, 10, 15 or 20 cm). These studies are particularly useful in more detailed examinations of acid and alkaline levels around the gastroesophageal junction (Box 7.1).

Pediatric pH studies

Esophageal pH measurements are now widely used in pediatrics to investigate a variety of symptoms possibly associated with GER (Box 7.2). In general, the pH catheters and recording equipment are similar to those used in adults but there are some differences in the procedure and analysis due to the patient group.

Electrodes and positioning. In all but the smallest infants, pH electrodes are the same as used for adults, excluding the larger (>3 mm) combined

---

Box 7.2   Indications for 24 h esophageal pH monitoring

Adult
Angina-like (non-cardiac) chest pain
Dysphagia with normal motility
Nocturnal asthma or wheeze
Negative endoscopic esophagitis
Globus hystericus
Other symptoms suspicious of GER

Pediatric
Vomiting
Failure to thrive
Hematemesis
Near miss SID
Anemia
Apnea/cyanosis
Chest infection/wheeze

Symptoms unresponsive to therapy or frequent relapse
Patients being considered for surgery

---

glass and antimony types. In neonates, it may be preferable to use a smaller than standard electrode (<2 mm).

pH electrode positioning is rarely gauged by prior manometry as this is often not available and is also more difficult and distressing to perform in children. Nomograms have been devised (Strobhel et al 1979) to calculate esophageal length in children, but the two most widely used methods are radiological positioning (DeMeester et al 1980) and the pH withdrawal technique (Dehn & Kettlewell 1987). Radiological positioning involves radiation and relies on the identification of the diaphragm to pinpoint the GE junction. Without barium, the presence of a hiatus hernia may give rise to errors. In the pH withdrawal technique, the presence of GER at the time of positioning, or a hiatus hernia, may lead to errors in accurate sitting of the electrode.

Recording protocols. In infants and small children, feeds are frequent and sleep is not only restricted to the nocturnal period. In addition, the LES and esophageal motility may not be fully developed until some months after birth (Boix-Ochoa & Canals 1976). Consequently, the recording protocol will vary according to the age of the child and the analysis of the recordings will be adjusted accordingly.

Combined recordings

With recent advances in computer technology, the last few years have seen the introduction of data-loggers with high capacity solid-state memory and multichannel recording facilities. This type of equipment is useful in investigations of unexplained, non-cardiac chest pain (NCCP). Prior to this, combined, ambulatory esophageal pressure and pH recordings could only be achieved using a tape-based system (Janssens et al 1986).

The objective of such recordings is the simultaneous monitoring of esophageal motility, LES function and pH. This enables a comparison of abnormalities of motility and GER and any correlation with symptoms. Technically, the recordings can be achieved easily, using solid-state multichannel microtransducers, either combined with one or two pH channels or, as is more common, separate from the pH electrode. The investigation is more demanding for the patient due to the presence of a larger single catheter or two catheters and for the investigator because of the more complex analysis and interpretation of the recording.

Recent publications (Barham et al 1992) have suggested that the major use of combined recordings is the investigation of NCCP caused by diffuse esophageal spasm. It is also useful for exclusion of esophageal pain as a cause of NCCP as, sometimes, patients with microvascular angina can be missed on initial investigation. At present, in our practice, combined recordings are limited to patients who have no esophagitis, normal pH and stationary manometry but who remain symptomatic.

Analysis and interpretation

Since 1976, when Johnson & DeMeester published their analysis of 24-hour pH recordings and introduced the DeMeester scoring system (DeMeester et al 1976), there has been considerable debate as to the correct analytical methods in the interpretation of GER. Initially, such analyses were performed manually but now, with computer regeneration of data, analysis of GER is totally automated. Recordings are replayed using laser or other digital printer facilities, either compressed or as detailed hour-by-hour plots of esophageal pH. Figure 7.1 shows three pH traces taken from actual recordings and illustrates different types of GER.

GER analysis – adult. Records are normally analyzed for total time and also divided into epochs of upright, supine and also postprandial periods. This enables separation between nocturnal (supine) and daytime (erect) GER. A further subdivision of inter- and postprandial periods allows inclusion or exclusion of meal-related reflux and a correlation analysis between meals and GER.

Summary analyses can calculate numerous variables which have been suggested as useful discriminants between physiological and pathological GER. Box 7.3 illustrates the multitude of data that can be derived from the pH recordings.

Box 7.3 Data from pH recordings

Basic data	**Derived scores**
Frequency (episodes/h)	DeMeester scores
Duration (min/h)	Frequency – duration index
Longest episode (min)	Kaye score (postprandial)
No episodes >5 min	Cumulative pH plots
% time <pH 4	Reflux index
Total symptom score	Meal reflux index
Postprandial GER time	

Figure 7.1

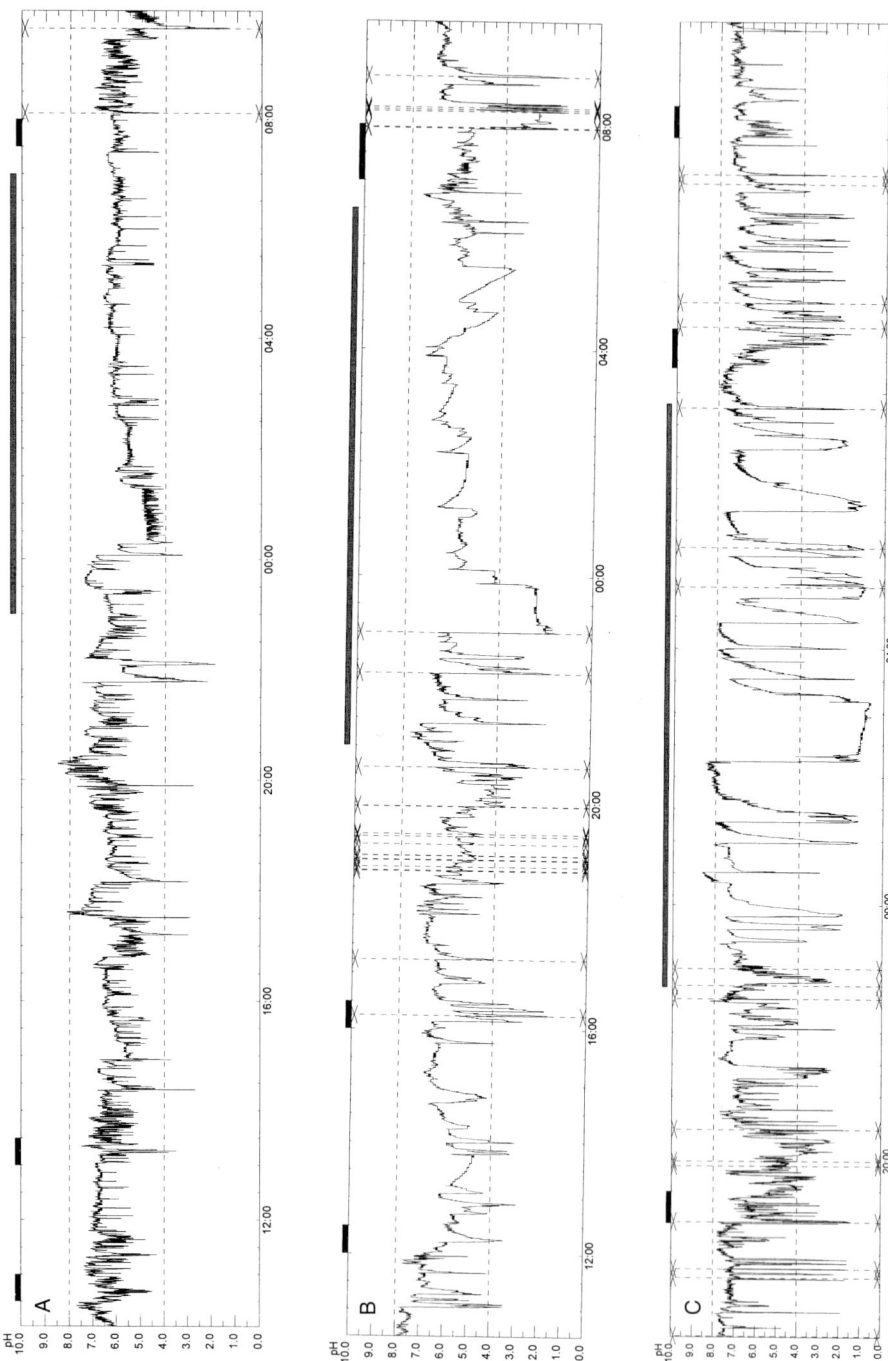

Ironically, the percentage time below pH 4 was initially advocated by DeMeester & Johnson as the best discriminant between physiological and pathological GER and this single figure remains the most widely recommended parameter in reflux assessment (Emde et al 1987). Most commercially available equipment has facilities to calculate all GER parameters, direct and derived, and reflux totals can also be compared with previously published upper physiological limits taken from asymptomatic controls. Most systems will produce a full analytical summary in a few minutes.

pH analysis – pediatrics. In pediatrics, basic analysis is performed as in adult studies although some differences exist. Normal ranges for physiological GER vary according to development. The LES and esophageal motility are not fully developed until at least 100 days after birth and in premature babies maybe even longer (Boix-Ochoa & Canals 1976). Upper physiological limits have been calculated in children and stratified by age (Vandenplas 1992) to achieve a better discriminant analysis taking development into account.

The influence of postprandial and nocturnal GER is also more difficult in pediatrics due to the nature and timing of feeds and the frequent interfood sleep cycles. In addition, the greater supine periodicity may also affect the normal calculation based on adult values.

Indications for investigation

Esophageal pH monitoring is most useful in patients with atypical symptoms or poor response to treatment. Thus patients with a good history and typical symptoms of GER, with visible esophagitis on upper GI endoscopy, will not require pH studies unless treatment fails. This is not a hard and fast dictum but avoids the temptation to 'overinvestigate' that is often the case when new technology becomes available in a particular center. Box 7.2 outlines the common indications for pH investigations for both adults and children.

Figure 7.1   Twenty four hour compressed single-channel pH traces from three GER patients. (A) This trace is essentially normal. Only physiological reflux is evident. The patient has pressed the event marker (vertical -----) on only two occasions. One event correlates with a brief reflux episode. GER is shortlived and acid clearance is good. There is little GER at night<pH 4. (B) This trace shows moderate day and severe nighttime reflux of greater severity and longer duration than (A). Symptoms correlate well with reflux episodes. (C) This trace is taken from a patient with a large hiatus hernia and shows severe reflux symptoms unresponsive to medication. One nocturnal reflux episode is undetected as the patient sleeps and continues for over 1 hour in the complete recording. Acid clearance increases on waking. Acid exposure <pH 4 is >30% in this recording. This type of reflux is often the most difficult to treat conservatively.

Gastric pH

Rationale for studies

pH can also be measured in the stomach. In the past, when peptic ulcer posed a serious problem, it was common to measure gastric acid output by aspiration of gastric content prior to and often after acid-reducing surgery. In recent years, the requirement for peptic ulcer surgery has reduced and acid secretion is mainly of interest to the pharmaceutical industry in the development of new acid-reducing drugs. It is now accepted that prolonged gastric pH measurements give a more representative picture of acid status and the methodology developed for the esophageal market has been adapted for gastric measurements (Rohmel et al 1990, Walt et al 1985).

Equipment

The majority of equipment suitable for esophageal studies is also used for gastric measurements. The major difference is in the choice of pH sensors and analysis of data.

pH sensors

One major problem with gastric pH measurements is the high acid levels that are present in the stomach and also the particulate nature of gastric chyme. Small changes in pH at acid levels (1–3) mean large changes in hydrogen ion concentration and therefore any electrical drift in the pH sensor at these levels will give rise to large errors in derived H^+ ion concentration. Small changes in reference electrode potential will have a similar effect and therefore an internal reference is also desirable. The particulate nature of stomach content means that a non-homogeneous environment surrounding the electrode tip may also lead to errors. This is most likely in the case of electrodes with a small sensor surface area.

The ideal gastric pH electrode is therefore a glass sensor with internal reference. The tethered pH-sensitive radiopill is therefore particularly suited to this type of study (Reynolds et al 1987) but, as with the other glass sensors with combined reference, these are expensive and often not as acceptable to subjects as the smaller antimony catheters.

pH sensors may be single or multisite. The advantage of multisite measurements is the ability to monitor pH at different levels in the stomach (fundus, body, antrum). This has been shown to be important as considerable pH differences can exist between the proximal and distal stomach (Mattioli et al 1992).

Sensor position is normally referenced to the gastroesophageal junction, i.e. a distance related to the distal margin of the LES. Generally, in adults, a single electrode is normally placed 10 cm from the GE junction to give an optimum pH assessment of gastric content. Sensor position can also be checked fluoroscopically for greater confidence of position.

Procedures

Investigations can be broadly divided into clinical and research studies. For clinical studies, protocols will depend on the rationale for the recording. For example, in patients failing to respond to acid suppression therapy, a pH study performed while the patient continues to take therapy will yield useful information regarding acid suppression levels. In research, study protocols will depend on the basic research objective but the following points may be relevant.

The major influence on gastric pH levels is food intake. Because gastric pH is a measure of hydrogen ion concentration and not gastric acid volume output, unless volume secretion is very low, the pH will predominantly also be at a low level, i.e. pH 1–3. The presence of ingested food, especially if this is alkaline in nature, will therefore buffer the pH to a higher level (up to pH 6 or 7) for a finite time (perhaps 1–2 hours) after a meal. The return to acid levels will depend on the acid secretion response as well as the rate of gastric emptying of the meal. In studies with a rigid protocol, it may therefore be necessary to standardize food intake and composition. This is particularly important in comparative crossover studies of drug efficacy, where meals may be the only additional influence on gastric pH profiles. Figure 7.2 is an example of a 24-hour gastric pH study on a patient taking acid suppression therapy. The intake of two meals and oral dosing has a marked influence on gastric pH.

Analysis and interpretation

The analysis of gastric pH recordings is determined by the specific information requirements. pH sampling rate is usually similar to esophageal pH recordings, i.e. 0.15 – 0.25 Hz. This rate allows pH changes of less than a minute time period to be accurately recorded. pH trends can be estimated by taking median pH levels of any number of samples, i.e. 0.5 minutes, 1 minute or even 30 or 60 minutes. pH data can also be expressed in other

---

Box 7.4 Analysis of gastric pH recordings

Direct data	**Derived parameters**
Mean or median pH	Hydrogen ion concentration
% time above or below threshold levels	Cumulative % pH graphs
Median pH trends	pH distribution tables

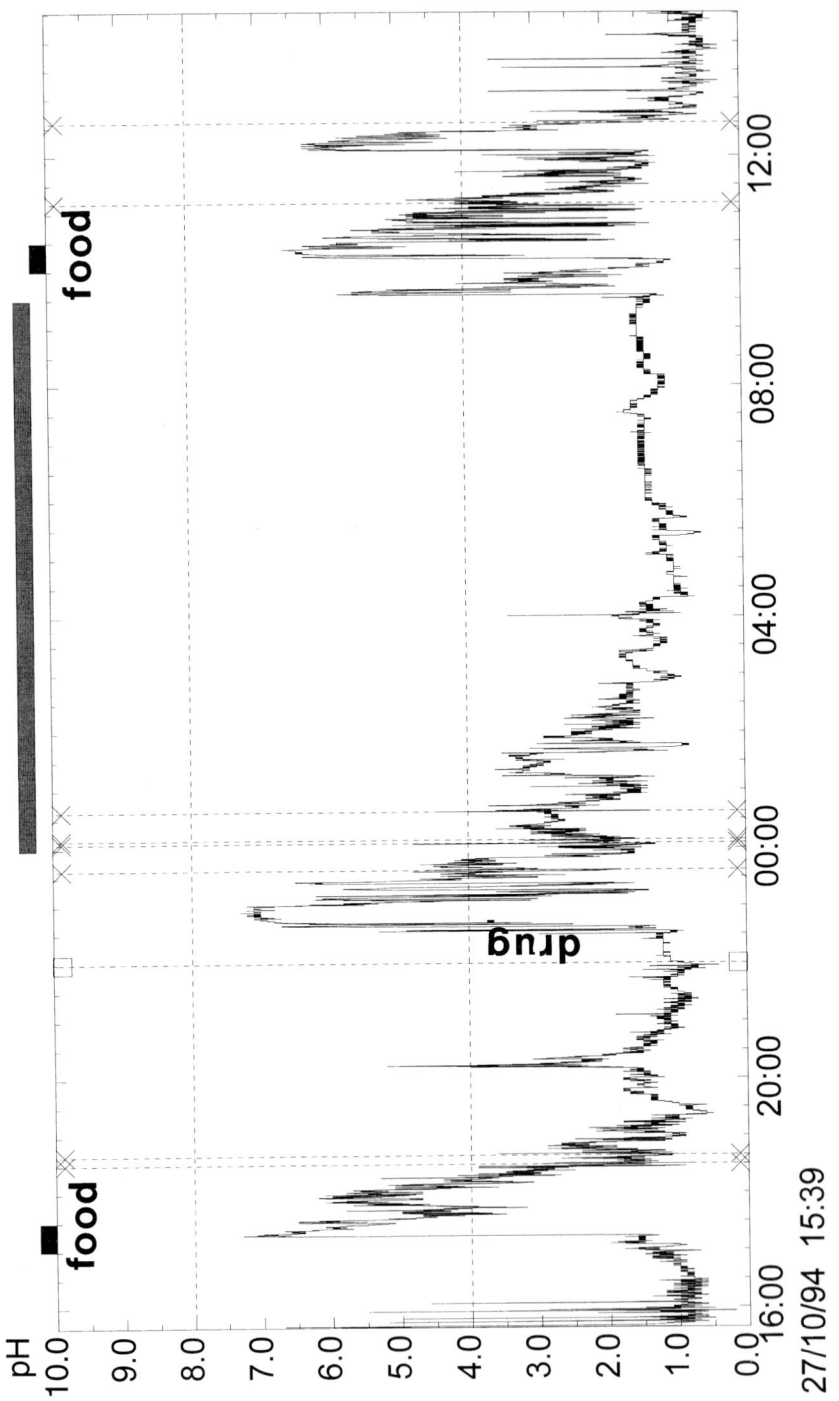

Figure 7.2   Gastric pH trace in a patient unresponsive to H_2 receptor antagonist therapy. The buffering effect of two meals and the brief elevation in gastric pH after evening dosing are clearly seen.

ways, for example as hydrogen ion concentration by direct arithmetic conversion of the pH scale. Box 7.4 illustrates a number of different parameters that can be used in the analysis of gastric pH recordings.

Small and large bowel and anorectum

Rationale for studies

The pH in the small and large intestine has not drawn much attention from medical researchers and clinicians, partly due to difficulties in measurement and partly due to a lack of need in terms of a relationship to pathophysiology or treatment. Where intestinal and anorectal studies have been carried out, there has always been a question to answer in relation to luminal pH and the causation or treatment of a particular illness. For example, pediatricians involved in the treatment of cystic fibrosis may wish to know the pH profile in the proximal jejunum in order to titrate doses of acid-blocking drugs to assist in jejunal neutralization and pancrease supplementation (Gilbert et al 1988). The pharmaceutical industry has also shown some interest in pH profiles through the gut due to the desire to specifically target drugs to the gut (Dew et al 1985), e.g. 5-ASA to the ileum and cecum in inflammatory bowel disease.

The methodology for intestinal pH measurements is somewhat different to the upper GI tract due to the difficulties in intubation of wire-connected pH sensors to distant parts of the gut such as the cecum. Although it is possible to intubate as far as the cecum, this practice has not been adopted for pH studies. The majority of studies have therefore been conducted using a free-moving pH RTC. Early studies were restricted to the laboratory environment (Bown et al 1974, Watson & Paton 1965) but recent studies have utilized portable, ambulatory systems (Evans et al 1988, Pye et al 1990).

Procedures

A calibrated pH-sensitive RTC is swallowed and allowed to pass through the GI tract under normal motility. Recordings are made using a body-borne aerial and a dedicated, combined, portable receiver-recorder (Flexilog 1010, Oakfield Instruments, Oxon). Gastric stasis of the RTC is likely if the subject has recently eaten prior to swallowing the capsule. This is due to the fact that large single indigestible objects are retained in the stomach until the passage of an interdigestive migrating motor complex.

Normal transit of the radiocapsule through the GI tract is around 24 hours although there may be wide variation (range 5 – >100 hours). The position of the capsule can be monitored by the pH recorded or, more accurately, by a unidirectional aerial attached to a portable receiver emitting a continuous tone when close to the RTC (Evans et al 1988).

Retrieval of RTCs is normally by fecal collection in specially designed devices which fit into a standard toilet. The passage of the capsule is determined by radiotransmission within the feces indicating the presence of the capsule.

Analysis and interpretation of data

Recorded data are downloaded to computer and pH profiles may be displayed on standard software packages designed for the RTC recorders. A normal whole gut profile is illustrated in Figure 7.3. Analysis of data is normally by site and by pH level. In the literature, analysis has mainly focused on establishment of pH values in health and disease. Very detailed analysis has not yet been undertaken.

Indications for measurement

This type of pH monitoring has mainly been used for research and the published literature has concentrated on establishing pH profiles at various sites along the gut in normal subjects and in specific diseases. The method has been used in cystic fibrosis (Gilbert et al 1988), colorectal cancel (Pye et al 1990) and inflammatory bowel disease (Raimundo et al 1992). The interest by the pharmaceutical industry in drug targeting is also arousing new interests in researchers involved in gastroenterology therapeutics (Ashford et al 1993).

SUMMARY

Ambulatory pH monitoring is now widely available and easily performed by medical technologists and research nurses in GI function laboratories. Clinically these investigations are mainly used in the diagnosis of gastroesophageal reflux disease and are best used in patients whose symptoms are atypical, where endoscopy findings show no esophagitis or in patients who are unresponsive to treatment. Studies are normally reserved as second-line investigations after endoscopy but may be used in place of endoscopy when this is not available or contraindicated.

In other parts of the GI tract, pH studies continue to be a research tool. As more knowledge regarding disease states is accrued, pH studies in the rest of the gut may help in the diagnosis of certain disorders and also in the determination of efficacy of targeted drug therapy.

At present, pH equipment costs under £5000 per unit, less than half the price of a gastroscope. The technique is therefore extremely cost effective in the diagnosis of GER disease and may become useful in other areas if indicated by current and future research.

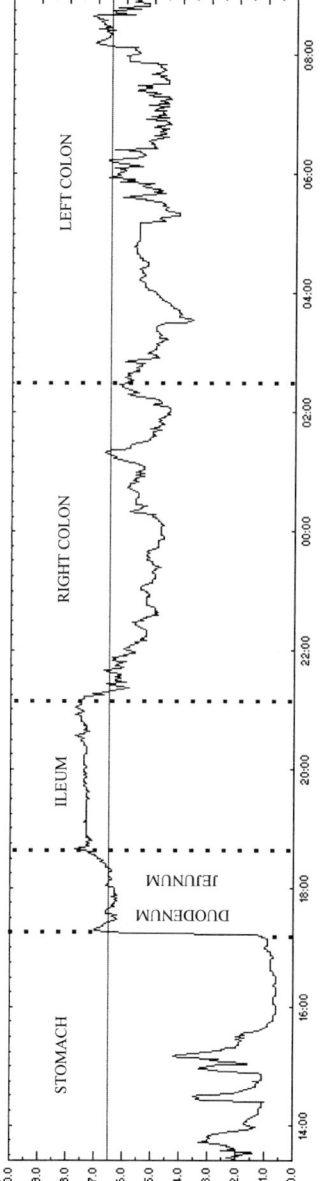

Figure 7.3 A total gut pH profile from a normal subject.

REFERENCES

Ashford M, Fell J T, Attwood P J, Woodhead P J 1993 An in-vitro investigation into the suitability of pH dependent polymers for colonic targeting. International Journal of Pharmaceutics 91: 241–245

Barham C P, Gotley D C, Miller R, Mills A, Alderson D 1992 Ambulatory measurement of oesophageal function: clinical use of a new pH and motility recording system. British Journal of Surgery 79: 1056

Beaumont W 1833 Experiments and observations on the gastric juice and the physiology of digestion. F P Allen, Plattsburgh, USA

Boix-Ochoa J, Canals J 1976 Maturation of the lower oesophageal sphincter. Journal of Pediatric Surgery 11: 749–756

Bown R L, Gibson J A, Sladen G E, Hicks B, Dawson A M 1974 Effects of lactulose and other laxatives on ileal and colonic pH as measured by a radiotelemetry device. Gut 15: 999–1004

Branicki F J, Evans D F, Hardcastle J D, Ogilvie A L, Atkinson M 1982 Ambulatory monitoring of oesophageal pH in reflux oesophagitis using a portable radiotelemetry system. Gut 23: 992–998

Colson R H, Watson B W, Fairclough P D et al 1981 An accurate long-term pH sensitive radiopill for insertion or implantation. Biotelemetry Patient Monitoring 8: 213–227

Dehn T C B, Kettlewell M 1987 24-hr monitoring of oesophageal pH in outpatients. Lancet i: 625–626

DeMeester T R, Johnson L R, Joseph G J, Toscano M S, Hall A W, Skinner D B 1976 Patterns of gastroesophageal reflux in health and disease. Annals of Surgery 184: 459–469

DeMeester T R, Wang C I, Wernley J A et al 1980 Technique, indications and clinical use of 24-hour oesophageal pH monitoring. American Journal of Gastroenterology 88: 629–632

Dew M J, Ryder R E, Evans N 1985 Colonic release of 5ASA from an oral preparation in active ulcerative colitis. British Journal of Pharmacology 28S: 1012–1014

Emde C, Garner A, Blum A 1987 Technical aspects of pH-metry in man: current status and recommendations. Gut 22: 1177–1188

Evans D G 1987 Twenty-four hour pH monitoring: an update. British Journal of Surgery 74: 157–161

Evans D F, Pye G, Bramley R, Clark A G, Dyson T J, Hardcastle J D 1988 Measurement of gastrointestinal pH in normal ambulant human subjects. Gut 29: 1035–1041

Gilbert J, Kelleher J, Littlewood J, Evans D F 1988 Ileal pH in cystic fibrosis. Scandinavian Journal of Gastroenterology 23(supp): 132–134

Janssens J, Vantrappen G, Ghillebert G 1986 24-hr recording of esophageal pressure and pH in patients with non-cardiac chest pain. Gastroenterology 90: 1978–1984

Jones R, Lydeard S 1989 Prevalence of dyspepsia in the community. British Medical Journal 298: 30–32

Kadirkamanathan S S, Swain C P, Gong F, Yazaki E, Evans D F, Williams N S 1993 Development of less invasive operations for gastro-oesophageal reflux. British Journal of Surgery 80: 1460

Mattioli S, Felice V, Pilotti V, Banchi M L, Pastina M, Gozzeti G 1992 Indications for 24 hr intragastric pH monitoring with single and multichannel probes in clinical research and practice. Digestive Diseases and Sciences 37: 1793–1801

Pye G, Evans D F, Ledingham S J, Hardcastle J D 1990 Gastrointestinal intraluminal pH in normal subjects and those with colorectal adenoma or carcinoma. Gut 31: 1355–1358

Raimundo A H, Evans D F, Rogers J, Jameson J, Silk D B A 1992 Intestinal pH in ulcerative colitis: acute (untreated) and in remission on 5ASA. Gut 33(supp): S63

Rawlings J M, Lucas M L 1985 Plastic pH electrodes for the measurement of gastrointestinal pH. Gut 26: 203–207

Reynolds J R, Walt R P, Clarke A, Hardcastle J D, Langman M 1987 Intragastric pH monitoring in acute upper GI bleeding and the effects of intravenous cimetidine and ranitidine. Alimentary Pharmacology and Therapy 1: 23–30

Richter J E, Castell D O 1982 Gastroesophageal reflux. Pathogenesis, diagnosis and therapy. Annals of Internal Medicine 97: 93–103

Rohmel O, Merki H S, Wilder-Smith C H, Walt R P 1990 Analytical and statistical evaluation of intragastric pH recordings. Disestive Diseases and Sciences 8(supp): 87

Rovelstad A 1956 Continuously recorded in situ pH of gastric and duodenal contents in patients with and without duodenal ulcers. Gastroenterology 31: 530–537

Schepel S J, de Rooj N F, Koning G, Oeseburg B, Zijlstra W G 1984 In vivo experiments with ISFET electrodes. Medical and Biological Engineering and Computing 22: 6–11

Schlesinger P K, Donahue P E, Schmid B, Layden T J 1985 Limitations of 24hr intra-oesophageal pH monitoring in a hospital setting. Gastroenteroloty 89: 797–804

Schneider J, Modler H, Kist R, Wolfelschneider H, Becker H D 1990 The Fabry Perot sensor. A long term monometry sensor for quantitative intraluminal pressure measurement of the gastrointestinal tract. Clinical Physics and Physiological Measurements 11: 319–325

Strobhel C T, Byrne W J, Ament M E et al 1979 Correlation of oesophageal lengths in children with height: application of the Tuttle test without prior manometry. Journal of Paedatrics 94: 81–86

Swain C P, Evans D F, Glynn M, Brown G, Mills T 1992 Endoscopic sewing machine used to achieve continuous non-invasive monitoring of gastric pH for 3 months in man. Gastrointestinal Endoscopy 38: 278

Vandenplas I 1992 Oesophageal pH monitoring of GER in infants and children. John Wiley, Chichester

Vantrappen G, Janssens G, Ghillebert G 1987 The irritable oesophagus – a frequent cause of angina-like pain. Lancet i: 1232

Walt R P, Reynolds J R, Langman M J et al 1985 Intravenous omeprazole rapidly raises intragastric pH. Gut 26: 902

Watson W C, Paton E 1965 Studies on intestinal pH by radiotelemetry. Gut 6: 606–612

Willis T 1684 A medico-philosophical discourse of fermentation of the intestine motion of particles in every body (Trans. S Podage). H Clark, Oxford

Woolf H S 1961 The radio pill. New Scientist 261: 419–421

8

Pathology interpretation in gastrointestinal diseases

F. Mitros

INTRODUCTION

The examination of biopsy and resected specimens in the pathology laboratory has become increasingly important in the practice of gastroenterology. If done properly these procedures can significantly aid in establishing the differential diagnostic possibilities and in making diagnoses. Gastrointestinal biopsies can aid greatly in monitoring modern therapies, both in assessing the effectiveness of therapy and in avoiding significant complications. This is a joint venture between two physicians, the one caring for the patient who judiciously chooses and obtains the specimen to be analyzed, and the one interpreting the specimen. The areas where cooperation is particularly important fall into one of two main categories: communication and specimen handling. These areas will be discussed in general terms and then the principles put forth in this discussion will be illustrated by describing a number of practical problems in the various topographical areas of the gastrointestinal tract.

There will be no attempt to provide a comprehensive description of all the areas of gastrointestinal pathology; the interested reader is referred to a number of comprehensive texts (Lewin et al 1992, Ming & Goldman 1992, Morson et al 1990, Whitehead 1989) and atlases (Misiewicz et al 1987, Mitros 1988, Morson 1988) currently available for more in-depth information and illustration. The examples chosen are those that reflect the author's experience in a large university medical center with an active gastroenterology division. They reflect areas where the principles of communication and specimen handling are particularly important, areas in which there is frequent significant misunderstanding or areas in which relatively new insights from the pathology laboratory may prove particularly useful to the gastroenterologist.

COMMUNICATION

In the opening chapter of this text we are told that the information gained from interviewing and examining patients guides all subsequent aspects of the physician–patient interaction. This is quite true, both for the gastroenterologist and for the pathologist. The experienced pathologist also knows that the eye often does not see what the mind does not know.

It is rare, if it happens at all, that the histologic appearance alone allows a specimen to be confidently assigned to one narrow diagnostic category. It is closer to the truth to consider that biologic variability results in a biopsy appearance that might fall into one portion of the spectrum of a number of disease processes and that these spectra may overlap. The experienced pathologist factors in the clinical probabilities in reaching the best biopsy interpretation. These clinical probabilities may also sharpen the focus of the pathologic examination.

Since it is impractical for the pathologist to interview and examine the patient associated with each biopsy specimen interpreted, he must rely on the physician providing the specimen for the history and physical findings (the clinical context). Since it is impractical for the gastroenterologist to provide a complete history and findings of physical examination with each biopsy specimen obtained, the gastroenterologist must develop skills in providing a highly selected summary of information appropriate for the particular patient and specimen in question (the clinical context). The experienced gastroenterologist soon becomes quite adept at this skill while the experienced pathologist soon becomes quite adept at understanding the needs and concerns of the clinician caring for the patient. For example, consider a rectal biopsy accompanied by the following histories; which is likely to lead to the more complete and more accurate interchange?

- **History 1:** 'diarrhea'
- **History 2:** '36-year-old man with well-documented ulcerative colitis for 12 years. Endoscopy shows quiescent colitis; no other lesions. Surveillance for dysplasia'.

The chance that a correct and complete diagnosis would be reached is greater with the second history. The person providing the first history was probably inexperienced; one hopes that the pathologist receiving the specimen with that meager history had sufficient experience to overcome the handicap!

SPECIMEN HANDLING

Communication is critical in respect of specimen handling. If an unusual situation is suspected, a brief conversation between clinician and pathologist prior to the procedure may alter sampling and fixation procedures and enhance information from the procedure. A particularly complete guide to specimen handling is included in one recent text (Lewin et al 1992); it is of interest that the text is coauthored by a gastroenterologist and two pathologists. What follows is a brief outline of some principles of specimen handling.

The choice of biopsy technique is important. The most common instrument used is the endoscopic *pinch biopsy forceps*; specimens obtained with these forceps tend to be relatively small and shallow, although some muscularis mucosae is usually included. A distinct advantage is the ability to direct the forceps at a specific lesion. The *suction biopsy* provides a larger and often deeper specimen; this allows for better orientation and the increased sample size may help improve the diagnostic yield. The disadvantage is the inability to target a specific site, although such diffuse processes as reflux esophagitis or small intestinal mucosal diseases are quite amenable to this method. *Electrocautery* ('hot biopsy') may be convenient in the endoscopy suite, but it is anathema in the pathology laboratory. The main use is in eradication of diminutive colon polyps, but there remains some danger that cautery artefact may be so severe as to preclude recognizing a small adenoma. The cautery artefact may be useful in snare polypectomy specimens where it acts as an indicator of the line of resection but it may prevent unequivocal identification of tumor involvement of the margin in some cases. The *large-particle biopsy* is of some use in particular circumstances, the most notable being the evaluation of large gastric folds.

Once the biopsy is obtained, the next step, a crucial one, is *orientation*. This is best done by an experienced assistant in the endoscopy suite. The biopsy specimen is gently uncurled and placed submucosal surface down on a dry flat surface. After several seconds the oozing protein from the submucosa results in adherence. Millipore filter paper is preferred, despite its expense, because the specimen can be kept on it throughout processing; it does not destroy microtome blades as do other types of filter paper, cards, plastic mesh, etc.

The choice of *fixative* is important. The standard is 10% buffered formalin and this will suffice in most instances. Such fixatives as Bouin's provide more nuclear detail, but Paneth cells and eosinophil granules are not well preserved; also the tissue may become brittle if left in this fixative too long. If electron microscopy is being considered, glutaraldehyde should be used to fix a small portion of the biopsy specimen (one or more 1 mm cubes).

It is also quite important to know when not to use a fixative. This is particularly important when the diagnosis of lymphoma is being considered. The immunohistochemistry involved in assessing lymphomas is more difficult than that for assessing epithelial and neuroendocrine cells. *Frozen tissue* is essential in these cases. Likewise modern molecular pathology techniques may be necessary in particularly difficult cases; frozen tissue is also required. In order to accomplish the logistics of getting the appropriate portion of the biopsy specimen properly and expeditiously frozen, communication with the pathology laboratory prior to obtaining the specimen is necessary.

Frozen section techniques in operating room biopsies may help in deciding what portion of the specimen should be used for a lymphoma work-up. They are of particular use with regard to the evaluation of colonic motility problems, where acetylcholinesterase stains may prove useful. They are of no value in evaluating inflammatory conditions of the mucosa and should not be used to evaluate whether or not polyps contain a focus of carcinoma except in extraordinary circumstances (see below). In fact, in these latter circumstances, the irreversible artefacts introduced during the frozen section procedure may prove deleterious.

Cytologic examination of gastrointestinal specimens so far has been of limited use. It requires a good deal of expertise to interpret such specimens. The esophagus has been most amenable to this technique; cytology may aid in identifying dysplasia and carcinoma (squamous as well as glandular in esophageal epithelium).

SPECIFIC EXAMPLES

Esophagus

The evaluation of reflux esophagitis and its complications accounts for most esophageal biopsies. The presence of intraepithelial eosinophils or neutrophils allows one to diagnose esophagitis and can be recognized even in poorly oriented biopsies (Brown et al 1984). Frequently, however, the diagnosis will rest on alterations in the basal layer and papillary height (Ismail-Beigi et al 1970). In order to assess these properly it is imperative that the biopsy be well oriented. It has also been shown that the changes in papillary or basal layer height are of significance only if they are 2 cm or more proximal to the gastroesophageal junction (Weinstein et al 1975). Simply labeling a biopsy 'distal esophagus' may not give enough information to establish a diagnosis. The ideal biopsy for evaluating reflux esophagitis is a carefully oriented suction biopsy a least 2 cm above the junction.

The description of the endoscopic appearance is of some importance. The white patches of *Candida* esophagitis are often obvious to the endoscopist but can be subtle and not evident to the pathologist. If the clinical impression is of candidiasis, we will perform a silver stain for fungus in our laboratory; we use the GMS (Gomori methenamine silver). The cost in money and technician time precludes staining all esophageal biopsies in this fashion. The salmon-pink color indicative of Barrett's epithelium should be noted on the pathology sheet if present. More importantly, the location of this epithelium with respect to the gastroesophageal junction should be noted. This is particularly important when a hiatal hernia is present. There are three basic forms of columnar epithelium present in Barrett's epithelium (Paull et al 1976). One, the so-called specialized epithelium, is unique; it has a villiform architecture with a mixture of gastric foveolar cells and intestinal goblet cells at its surface. This epithelium is usually found just distal to the squamous epithelium and is the usual site in which dysplasia and carcinoma develop.

The recognition of specialized epithelium is based on recognition of architectural and cytologic features on standard H&E sections. The intestinal component may be confirmed by using mucin stains, but we do not recommend using mucin stains as a routine on all biopsies from the gastroesophageal area. The diagnosis of Barrett's epithelium should not be made based solely on small amounts of mucin seen only with a sensitive mucin stain. The other two forms of columnar epithelium found in Barrett's epithelium closely mimic gastric cardia or fundus. Location is key to their recognition as representing metaplasia. If present in distal esophagus they may merely represent a biopsy from the physiologic Z-line. If from well within the tubular esophagus (e.g. 35 cm) they allow one to diagnose Barrett's epithelium. The pathologist should identify the epithelial type or types present in the pathology report with special attention being paid to the presence of specialized epithelium since this is the epithelial type in which dysplasia is most likely to be found (Hamilton & Smith 1987).

When tumor is suspected pinch biopsies of the lesion should be performed. Multiple biopsies (3–7) from different aspects of the lesion will increase the diagnostic yield. With *squamous carcinoma* there is almost invariably an endoscopically evident exophytic lesion; the biopsy merely confirms the clinical impression. Dysplasia in the squamous epithelium is uncommonly encountered in the absence of nearby invasive neoplasm. One should be aware that a mistake made frequently by pathologists inexperienced in interpreting gastrointestinal biopsies is misinterpreting reactive atypia near erosions in reflux esophagitis as representing dysplasia.

Adenocarcinoma presents another set of problems. Dysplasia and even carcinoma may not be endoscopically apparent. The interpretation of dysplasia is difficult and subjective. Once Barrett's epithelium is identified, the biopsy should be characterized as having no dysplasia, as being indefinite for dysplasia or as having dysplasia (Hamilton & Smith 1987). If dysplasia is present, it is characterized as low grade or high grade; the latter includes carcinoma in situ. Biopsies indefinite for dysplasia or with low-grade dysplasia should shorten the interval to the next biopsy. High-grade dysplasia can be used to justify surgery; it should be confirmed by a second opinion or second biopsy or both before esophagogastrectomy is performed. Because of the acknowledged difficulties in recognizing and grading dysplasia, Barrett's epithelium has proven an area of active research in the areas of mucin histochemistry and flow cytometry. The latter in particular appears promising, although to date the interpretation of H&E sections remains the standard for making therapeutic decisions.

Stomach

In contrast to the esophagus, duodenum and colon where the endo-scopic and histologic appearances in inflammatory processes correlate closely with each other, the endoscopic and microscopic appearances in *gastritis* are often divergent. In spite of this, or perhaps because of it, there is all the more need to try to relate the two. One of the major positive aspects of the recently proposed Sydney system is the emphasis it places on this attempt (Price 1991). The need to biopsy and analyze different regions of the stomach has become obvious as knowledge about gastritis has expanded in recent years.

Pivotal to the increased knowledge about gastritis has been the recog-nition of the importance of *Helicobacter pylori* in the common form of gastritis. As the ability to recognize this organism and the reaction pattern to it has grown, the recognition of other patterns of injury has become easier and more certain. In particular, the recognition that *H. pylori* is a common pathogen producing a characteristic histopathology has opened the door to the recognition of the pattern of damage due to bile reflux and pharmaceutical agents (NSAIDs).

When the importance or *H. pylori* became clear (Marshall & Warren 1984) it was thought that recognition depended on performing arduous and capricious silver stains. As experience increased, the recognition of these organisms became easier. At this time, the organism is readily recognized by experienced observers on standard H&E-stained sections (Fig. 8.1). The organisms are always seen related to foveolar epithelium, which lines the surface of the stomach. The predilection for this epithe-lium is so great that *H. pylori* can be seen related to it even when it occurs outside the stomach, as in foveolar metaplasia in Barrett's epithelium, peptic duodenitis and even in Meckel's diverticulum. The mucin produced by foveolar epithelium appears to provide a microenvironment conducive to the growth of *H. pylori*. Denser adherent mucin and wisps of mucin form plumes at the surface. Often there are neutrophils in the lamina propria or between epithelial cells in such areas. The curvilinear rods are usually readily visible in such areas at 40× magnification. Rarely, oil immersion is necessary to confirm their presence. If a special stain is judged necessary, we have employed the simple and reliable Diff-quik method (Skipper & DeStephano 1989). Silver stains or immunoperoxidase techniques are probably not necessary for typical clinical specimens.

When *gastric neoplasia* is suspected the possibility of sampling error should be kept in mind. If there is a suspicious ulcerated lesion, both the raised edge and the base of the ulcer should be sampled, preferably at more than one site. Sampling is also important for the pathologist to keep in mind. Signet ring cells may be sparse and readily missed if step sections and mucin stains are not examined with the specific intent of finding such

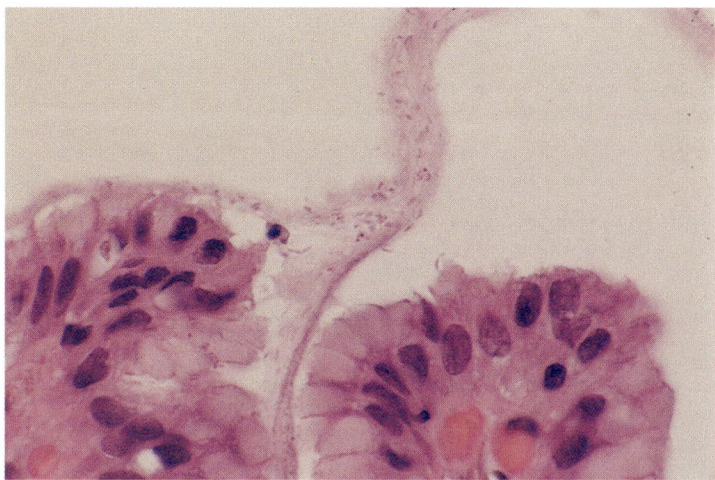

Figure 8.1 *Helicobacter pylori* are present in this dense plume of mucus emanating from inflamed gastric foveolar epithelium (×250, H&E).

cells. The stomach is also the most common site of extranodal lymphoma; lymphomas may be subtle endoscopically and histologically, requiring multiple biopsies, particularly with regard to MALT (mucosa-associated lymphoid tissue) lesions (Isaacson & Spencer 1987).

Another area of increasing interest in gastric biopsy pathology relates to *neuroendocrine proliferations* and tumors. Much of the information concerning the gastric neuroendocrine system comes from studies of patients with pernicious anemia (Solcia et al 1991). In these subjects there is a proliferation of gastrin-producing cells in the antrum, with consequent hyperplasia of the enterochromaffin-like cells (ECL) in the proximal stomach. Immunoperoxidase stains are particularly useful in showing such changes. General neuroendocrine markers such as chromogranin A and synaptophysin readily demonstrate the increased numbers of neuroendocrine cells. Gastrin antibodies can help to document the severity of hypergastrinemic states (Fig. 8.2). Unfortunately, to date there is no specific antibody to ECL cells. Sequential steps of hyperplasia of varying severity with progression to carcinoid tumors have been described (Solcia et al 1988). With the widespread use of H_2 blockers and proton pump inhibitors a pharmacologic hypergastrinemic state with neuroendocrine hyperplasia can be created (Lamberts et al 1993). These drugs alone have not been convincingly shown to produce carcinoid tumors in patients who do not have complicating disease processes such as Zollinger–Ellison syndrome. Close communication between gastroenterologist and pathologist greatly enhances the recognition and correct interpretation of these interacting proliferative processes.

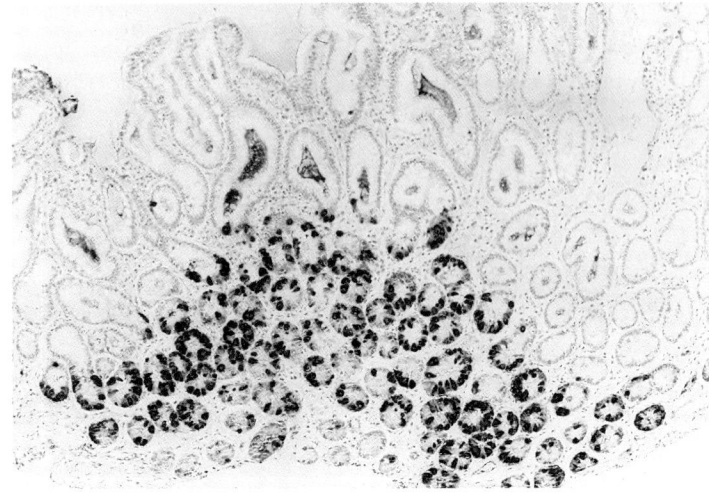

Figure 8.2 There is a striking increase in gastrin-producing cells, both linear and diffuse, in this antral biopsy from a patient with a hypergastrinemic state produced by chronic renal failure (×33, immunoperoxidase with antigastrin antibody).

The evaluation of large gastric folds is difficult. In this situation the large particle biopsy is useful. With such a biopsy specimen lymphoma and carcinoma can be confidently excluded as the cause of the large rugae. There may be positive evidence for Menetrier's disease (cystically dilated protein-filled spaces lined by foveolar epithelium) or for Zollinger–Ellison syndrome (striking parietal cell hyperplasia).

Small intestine

Small intestinal mucosal biopsies are important in the evaluation of patients with malabsorption. A normal biopsy in these patients may be as useful as an abnormal one in that it directs attention elsewhere (for example, to the colon). However, it is important to be sure that the biopsy is normal before excluding small intestinal disease.

Celiac disease has been underdiagnosed because the clinical diagnosis is not considered until a late stage. The patient may not present with the classic picture of wasting with steatorrhea and the biopsy may not show severe inflammation or be devoid of villi. Patients may present with symptoms such as isolated iron deficiency anemia and the biopsy may only show subtle attenuation of villous architecture. A very useful histologic finding in the more subtle presentation of celiac disease is the presence of distinctly increased numbers of intraepithelial lymphocytes in the surface epithelium (Marsh 1992). This is usually expressed as the number of lymphoid nuclei per 100 epithelial nuclei. A reasonable estimate can be made on a well-oriented, well-stained thin H&E section (Fig. 8.3). A continuous segment of several hundred (preferably 1000) surface epithelial cells is counted; the number of lymphoid cells in the same segment is then counted. If there are 40 or more lymphocytes per 100 epithelial nuclei the diagnosis of celiac disease must be considered. Confirmatory tests such as those for antiendomysial or antigliadin antibody may prove useful. The clinical response of the presenting symptom and the improvement in the histologic appearance after a gluten-free diet are often the most rewarding outcome of a perfect collaboration between the gastroenterologist and the pathologist.

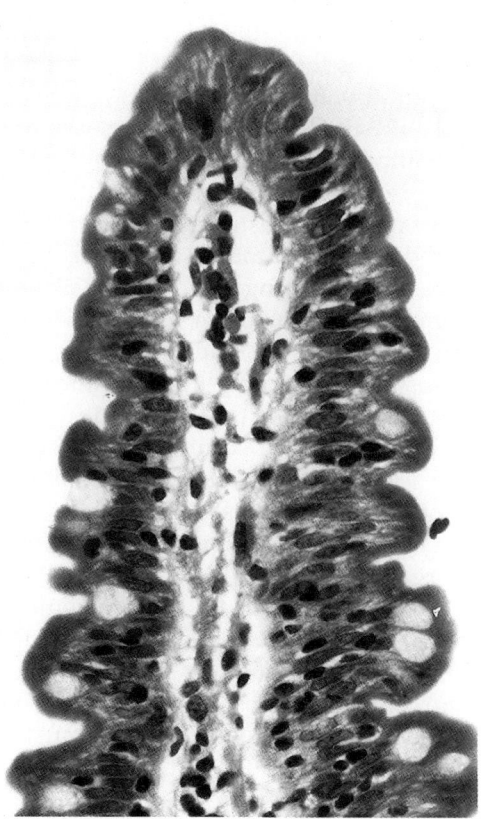

Figure 8.3 There is a striking increase in intraepithelial lymphocytes despite the preservation of villous architecture; this is a valuable clue to the presence of celiac disease (×120, H&E).

The most common inflammatory condition seen in the small intestine is *non-specific duodenitis*. It is seen in biopsies from the proximal duodenum usually in patients with peptic ulcer disease. Patchy foveolar metaplasia and neutrophils in the lamina propria near the surface are characteristic (Shousa et al 1983). This pattern differs from the lymphocytosis described in celiac disease. A gastric antral biopsy will frequently show an active *Helicobacter*-related gastritis. In fact, *H. pylori* may even be present on the patches of metaplastic foveolar epithelium. Brunner's glands may be prominent as a response to the excess secretion of gastric acid. This contributes to the nodularity commonly seen endoscopically in duodenitis. Such nodularity often needlessly arouses the clinical suspicion of lymphoma. Physiologic lymphoid aggregates are seen in ileal biopsies and are sometimes misinterpreted as representing inflammation.

Some small intestinal diseases present an entirely characteristic histologic appearance. Chief among these is Whipple's disease. The bulged villi, distorted by an infiltrate of foamy macrophages which are PAS positive as well as by the presence of lipid-filled lacteals, are quite characteristic. Electron microscopy confirms the presence of large numbers of rod-shaped bacteria, but it is unnecessary. It is also not necessary to perform PAS stains routinely on all small intestinal biopsies. If there are only scattered PAS-positive cells the significance is uncertain; many substances containing polysaccharides will cause PAS positivity in macrophages.

The identification of microorganisms may be difficult. *Giardia,* the most commonly encountered organism, can be recognized confidently on H&E sections. Examination of a 'hanging drop' of small intestinal fluid or a smear of this fluid stained by the Giemsa stain is useful, but the diagnosis may not be considered until it is too late to do these examinations. Other more specialized stains offer little help in recognition, although scanning electron microscopy may prove useful in difficult cases. Paraffin-embedded materials can be used for scanning electron microscopy. Foamy macrophages may be seen with *Mycobacterium avium intracellulare*, but the infiltrate is not so massive as that seen in Whipple's disease nor are dilated lacteals ordinarily present. A simple acid-fast stain will document the presence of this organism.

The patient with AIDS presents diagnostic problems for the pathologist as well as the gastroenterologist. There is a wide spectrum of organisms to be considered and the organisms may be sparse or otherwise difficult to identify. Special stains may prove useful and should be employed liberally in this setting. For this reason the pathologist must be alerted that the biopsy is to be scrutinized for opportunistic infections. Cytomegalovirus infection is ordinarily diagnosed by the presence of characteristic nuclear and cytoplasmic inclusions on H&E, but immunoperoxidase techniques are available to enhance identification. Cryptosporidia are usually numerous at the surface but must be distinguished from particles of mucin or epithelial debris. Acid-fast stains or scanning electron micro-scopy may help in this regard. The acid-fast stain is doubly useful in that cells with *Mycobacterium avium intracellulare* in low density may be revealed. Microsporidia may resist detection unless transmission electron microscopy is used. This may be necessary in patients with resistant diarrhea in the appropriate clinical setting.

Appendix

In addition to documenting classic appendicitis or identifying the un-common appendiceal tumors, the examination of the appendix may yield other clues to diagnosis. The unexpected finding of a granuloma may prove to be a clue to the presence of Crohn's disease, although not all granulomas in the appendix indicate Crohn's disease. The examination of the appendix does not identify the neural or muscular lesion in patients with a motility disorder with the possible exception of long segment Hirschsprung's disease.

Colon

The colon and rectum are the most commonly biopsied sites in the gastro-intestinal tract. Recognition of normal histology can be difficult. There is a general tendency to overinterpret normal lamina propria cellularity as indicating inflammation. Precise quantitative studies have been done (Lee et al 1988). A good general guideline suggests that about half the biopsy area should be epithelial and about half lamina propria. The lamina propria should be about half cellular and half connective tissue. Plasma cells are the normal predominant cellular component, followed by mature lymphocytes; evenly dispersed eosinophils are normal, even if they constitute up to 7% of the nuclei. The right side of the colon (near the ileocecal valve) has a greater lamina propria cellularity than the distal colon. Neutrophils in the lamina propria or between epithelial cells are abnormal. Crypts (when well oriented) should be straight and relatively parallel. Paneth cells at the base of crypts are normal in cecum and ascending colon in adults. They may be seen more distally in children. They are abnormal in the rectosigmoid and represent metaplasia which is a marker of chronic inflammation, as is irregular crypt branching.

The most common error in interpreting colorectal biopsies is over-interpretation of chronicity. The clinical history is the most important guideline. If diarrhea is of short duration (several days or weeks) that should be clearly stated. One should avoid making the diagnosis of ulcerative colitis or Crohn's disease when the duration of symptoms is less than several months. Infection and inflammatory bowel disease share many common histologic features, including crypt abscesses and cryptitis.

While some histologic features, such as Paneth metaplasia, distinct crypt branching and a plasma cell infiltrate in the deep (basal fifth) mucosa (Kumar et al 1982) are strong evidence of chronicity, it is best not to diagnose inflammatory bowel disease until both the clinical and histologic parameters of chronicity are certain. The diagnosis 'acute colitis, non-specific, severe' does not exclude inflammatory bowel disease.

The distinction of ulcerative colitis from Crohn's disease is not always possible from biopsy pathology. The gastroenterologist must communicate information about the presence of small intestinal involvement, strictures and fistulae that would make a definitive diagnosis of Crohn's disease. If the colon only is involved, both gastroenterologist and pathologist face a difficult task. For the pathologist evaluating chronic colitis the distribution within the colon (pancolitis, distal predominance, rectal sparing, 'skip' lesions) is one key factor. The other is the distribution of the inflammation within the wall of the colon in the involved area (superficial and diffuse versus transmural and aggregated). Biopsy pathology is of little use in evaluating the depth of inflammation, but it is helpful in mapping the distribution throughout the length of the colon. This requires multiple mapping biopsies taken endoscopically. Care should be taken in this process to biopsy 'normal' areas if these represent 'skip' areas or areas of distal sparing. What appears to be normal to the endoscopic observer may show atrophy, crypt distortion and mild inflammation to the pathologist. Good mapping requires review of prior biopsies. This may require requesting slides from outside hospitals; the pathologist should check his own files routinely for old material on any patient whose biopsy is being evaluated.

Another way of increasing sampling is by cutting additional sections from the block containing a mucosal biopsy. This may be done with serial sections or with step sections. A 3 mm rectal biopsy can be processed to produce hundreds of sections (serial 4–6 micron sections). While serially cutting a block ensures that a 40–60 micron granuloma will not be missed because of sampling, time and expense make this impractical in a busy clinical laboratory. A reasonable compromise is to examine step sections. In this process a ribbon of several 4–6 micron sections is cut and then some portion of the block (ordinarily about 50 microns) is cut away before the next ribbon of 4–6 micron sections is taken. Three to five such ribbons are ordinarily stained; the efficacy of such step sections nearly equals that of serial sections for finding focal lesions such as granulomas. Even with resected specimens it may not be possible to accurately separate ulcerative colitis from Crohn's disease. This is especially true when the colectomy was performed during the fulminant stage (Price 1978).

Colitis due to toxins such as that produced by C. *difficile* or E. *coli 0157* (*verotoxin*) is probably underrecognized. Not all such cases produce typical pseudomembranes endoscopically or histologically. At times there may be focal hemorrhage and coagulative necrosis, mimicking ischemia; this is particularly true with regard to verotoxin (Kelly et al 1987). On the other hand, very mild cases may produce subtle damage that can be missed completely. In these cases there may be focal damage to the intercryptal surface epithelium, producing a cluster of damaged vacuolated epithelial cells ('summit' lesion) (Price & Davies 1970). While not specific for toxin-related damage, the association is strong enough that toxin assays should be done; the pathologist who suspects toxin-related damage should call the gastroenterologist and suggest that toxin assays be ordered.

Hemorrhage and coagulation necrosis suggest *ischemic damage,* but such damage is not limited to the relatively low blood flow regions. As noted above, toxin damage may need to be considered. Other situations producing the appearance of ischemic damage on biopsy include such diverse conditions as radiation-related damage, vasculitis, cryoglobulinemia and solitary rectal ulcer syndrome.

Adenomas and carcinoma of the colon present a challenge for biopsy evaluation. Endoscopic polypectomy specimens are becoming more frequent; the endoscopist performing the polypectomy should record the site of the polyp as accurately as possible, since if invasive cancer is found in the polyp further surgery may be necessary. Both the gastroenterologist and the pathologist need to handle the specimen carefully to preserve as much of the polyp stalk as possible and to orient the specimen carefully so that the relationship of the polyp to the stalk and the line of resection can be evaluated. The diagnosis of invasive carcinoma is made if there is severely atypical epithelium beneath the muscularis mucosae or if there is a fibrous stromal response (desmoplastic reaction) to the atypical epithelium. Many pathologists avoid using carcinoma in situ as a diagnostic term, preferring such euphemisms as 'severe atypia'. The reason for this reluctance is the fact that carcinoma in situ in the colon has not been shown to have a potential for metastasis and the use of the term carcinoma in situ for biologically benign lesions frequently results in unnecessary surgery (Haggitt et al 1985). Even after invasive carcinoma is identified, great care is necessary in evaluating a polyp, in writing the pathology report and in advising further therapy.

Three criteria suggest that further surgery is necessary for a carcinoma identified in a colon polypectomy specimen (Cooper 1988). The most common and most important of these is involvement of the resection margin (Fig. 8.4); the other two are the presence of high-grade dysplasia and the presence of vascular invasion. Frozen sections make orientation difficult and may result in the inability to evaluate the above parameters. Frozen sections should be employed only in the intraoperative situation. Biopsy of a very large lesion may not give the pathologist enough tissue to identify invasion. A 'negative' biopsy does *not* exclude carcinoma in such circumstances.

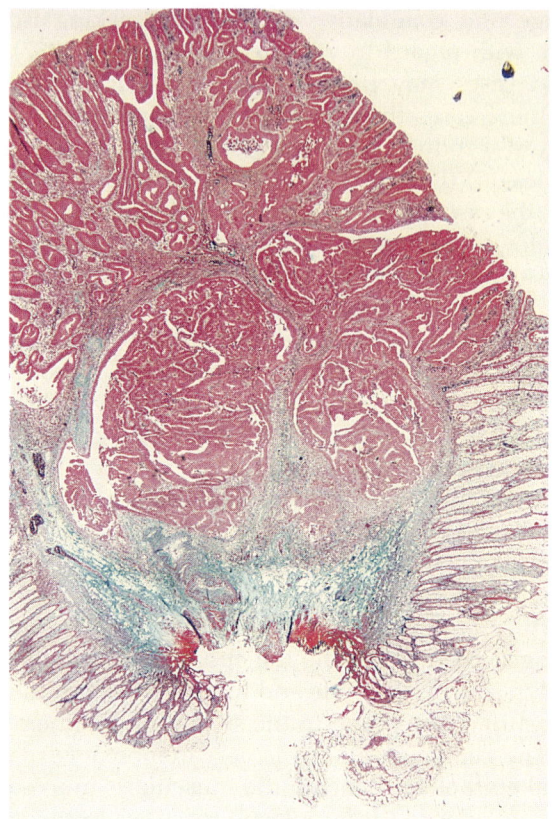

Figure 8.4 Moderately differentiated adenocarcinoma arising in an adenoma and invading the stalk in this polypectomy specimen. The margin of resection of the stalk (bottom of photograph) is free of tumor. No further surgery is necessary (×4, trichrome).

The most common indication for frozen section histology in the colon is the evaluation of possible lymphoma. Another indication is to determine the length of the Hirschsprung's disease segment using peroperative biopsies. Submucosal ganglion cells in the rectum are sparse enough that they may not be present in small samples; also, there is a zone of physiologic hypoganglionosis in the one or two centimeter zone proximal to the pectinate line. The acetylcholinesterase stain, which can only be done with frozen tissue, shows a positive finding in Hirschsprung's disease, namely a hyperplasia of the positive-staining parasympathetic fibers in the lamina propria between the crypts.

Liver

The history and supporting laboratory information are particularly important in evaluating liver biopsies. The spectrum of disease processes is wide but the patterns of histologic response are narrow.

The presence of risk factors (alcohol abuse, intravenous drug abuse, therapeutic drugs, obesity) and the pattern of the laboratory abnormalities (transaminase ratios, 'biliary' enzymes, etc.) will guide the pathologist in the evaluation of the biopsy. Similarly, serologic information (hepatitis A, B, C, delta; autoimmune markers; antimitochondrial antibody; antineutrophil cytoplasmic antibody) is also helpful. One should not rely on the immunoperoxidase demonstration of hepatitis B surface antigen when the serologic test is more sensitive, more reliable and less expensive.

It is particularly important to note a history of medication use, particularly if the drugs used have been associated with hepatic injury or were started shortly before hepatic disease was identified. Drug-induced damage can mimic virtually any of the hepatic diseases, including alcohol-related damage, chronic hepatitis and biliary tree damage.

The diagnosis of alcohol-related liver disease should not be made in the absence of confirmed history of significant alcohol intake. The possibility of non-alcoholic steatohepatitis (Ludwig et al 1980) must always be kept in mind, since it may mimic the histology of alcohol-related damage. Risk factors (particularly obesity, diabetes or amiodarone use) must be sought.

When viral hepatitis is being evaluated, the pathologist must know the duration of illness. Duration may express either the period of time since the onset of symptoms or the period of time during which transaminase elevation has been documented. One should not make a diagnosis of

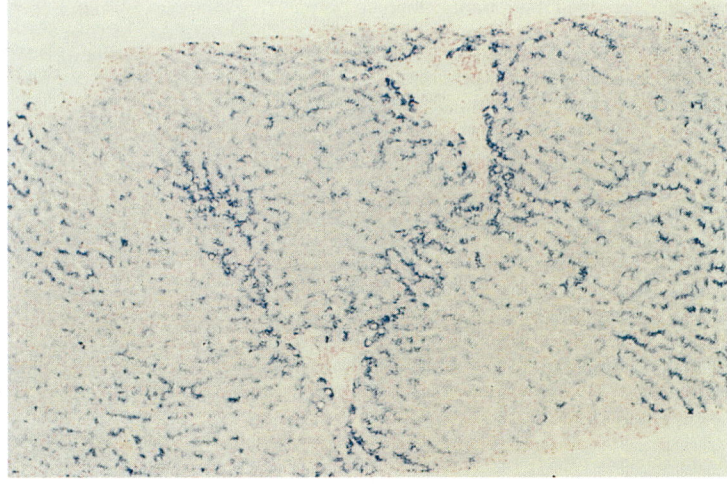

Figure 8.5 An iron stain revealing abundant hemosiderin in periportal hepatocytes. This much iron, or more, provides strong evidence for a diagnosis of hemochromatosis (×25, Perls' stain).

chronic hepatitis B or C with a symptom duration of less than 6 months. There is considerable overlap in the appearance of the liver in acute and chronic hepatitis for both types B and C. When reporting a biopsy showing features of chronic hepatitis, the pathologist should also make a statement regarding the degree of activity and the amount of fibrosis. This is preferable to the use of such terms as 'chronic persistent hepatitis' or 'chronic active hepatitis', terms which are now beginning to disappear (Ludwig 1993). The reason for this change in terminology was the realization that even innocuous-appearing chronic hepatitis C ('chronic persistent hepatitis') could unpredictably progress to more severe disease.

The pathologist must be diligent in searching for unexpected histologic clues. Polarization should be done routinely on all liver biopsies; the talc crystals so identified indicate intravenous drug use. An iron stain should be performed on all liver biopsies. A liver biopsy showing 3+ paren-chymal iron (Fig. 8.5) suggests hereditary hemochromatosis. Hemo-chromatosis is more common than generally believed (3–5 cases per 1000, Edwards et al 1988); the diagnosis is often missed in the early stages and the disease is amenable to readily available and inexpensive therapy (phlebotomy).

REFERENCES

Brown L F, Goldman H, Antonioli D A 1984 Intraepithelial eosinophils in endoscopic biopsies of adults with reflux esophagitis. American Journal of Surgical Pathology 8: 899–905

Cooper H S 1988 The role of the pathologist in the management of patients with endoscopically removed malignant colorectal polyps. In: Pathology annual. Rosen P P, Fecknes R E (eds). Appleton & Lange, New York, pp 25–43

Edwards C Q, Griffin L M, Goldgar D, Drummond C, Skolnick M H, Kushner J P 1988 Prevalence of hemochromatosis among 11,065 presumably healthy blood donors. New England Journal of Medicine 318: 1355–1362

Haggitt R C, Glotzbach R E, Soffer E E, Wruble L D 1985 Prognostic factors in colorectal carcinomas arising in adenomas: implications for lesions removed by endoscopic polypectomy. Gastroenterology 89: 328–336

Hamilton S R, Smith R R L 1987 The relationship between columnar epithelial dysplasia and invasive adenocarcinoma arising in Barrett's esophagus. American Journal of Clinical Pathology 87: 301–312

Isaacson P G, Spencer J 1987 Malignant lymphoma of mucosa-associated lymphoid tissue. Histopathology 11: 445–462

Ismail-Beigi F, Horton P F, Pope C E 1970 Histological consequences of gastroesophageal reflux in man. Gastroenterology 58: 163–174

Kelly J K, Pai C H, Jadusingh I H et al 1987 The histopathology of rectosigmoid biopsies from adults with bloody diarrhea due to verotoxin-producing *Escherichia coli*. American Journal of Clinical Pathology 88: 78–82

Kumar N B, Nostrant T T, Appelman H D 1982 The histopathologic spectrum of acute self-limited colitis (acute infectious-type colitis). American Journal of Surgical Pathology 6: 523–529

Lamberts R, Creutzfeldt W, Stüber H G, Brunner G, Solcia E 1993 Long-term omeprazole therapy in peptic ulcer disease: gastrin, endocrine cell growth, and gastritis. Gastroenterology 104: 1356–1370

Lee E, Schiller L R, Fordtran J S 1988 Quantification of colonic lamina propria cells by means of a morphometric point-counting method. Gastroenterology 94: 409–418

Lewin K J, Riddell R H, Weinstein W M 1992 Gastrointestinal pathology and its clinical implications, vol 1. Igaku-Shoin, New York

Ludwig J 1993 The nomenclature of chronic active hepatitis: an obituary. Gastroenterology 105: 274–278

Ludwig J, Viggiano T R, McGill D B, Ott B J 1980 Nonalcoholic steatohepatitis: Mayo clinic experiences with a hitherto unnamed disease. Mayo Clinic Procedures 55: 434–438

Marsh M N 1992 Gluten, major histocompatibility complex and the small intestine. Gastroenterology 102: 330–354

Marshall B J, Warren J R 1984 Unidentified curved bacilli in the stomach of patients with gastritis and peptic ulceration. Lancet i: 1311–1315

Ming S, Goldman H 1992 Pathology of the gastrointestinal tract. W B Saunders, Philadelphia

Misiewicz J J, Bartram C I, Cotton P B, Mee A S, Price A B, Thompson R P H 1987 Atlas of clinical gastroenterology. Gower Medical Publishing, London

Mitros F A 1988 Atlas of gastrointestinal pathology. Gower Medical Publishing, New York

Morson B C 1988 Color atlas of gastrointestinal pathology. H Miller, London, England

Morson B C, Dawson I M P, Day D W, Jass J R, Price A B, Williams G T 1990 Morson & Dawson's gastrointestinal pathology, 3rd edn. Blackwell Scientific Publications, Oxford

Paull A, Trier J S, Dalton M D, Camp R C, Loeb P, Goyal R K 1976 The histologic spectrum of Barrett's esophagus. New England Journal of Medicine 295: 476–480

Price A B 1978 Overlap in the spectrum of non-specific inflammatory bowel disease – 'colitis indeterminate'. Journal of Clinical Pathology 31: 567–577

Price A B 1991 The Sydney system: histologic divison. Journal of Gastroenterology and Hepatology 6: 209–222

Price AB, Davies D R 1970 Pseudomembranous colitis. Journal of Clinical Pathology 30: 1–12

Shousha S, Spiller R C, Parkins R A 1983 The endoscopically abnormal duodenum in patients with dyspepsia: biopsy findings in 6 cases. Histopathology 7: 23–34

Skipper R, DeStephano D B 1989 A rapid stain for *Campylobacter pylori* in gastrointestinal tissue sections using Diff-Quik. Journal of Histotechnology 12: 303–304

Solcia E, Bordi C, Creutzfeldt W et al 1988 Histopathological classification of nonantral gastric endocrine growths in man. Digestion 41: 185–200

Solcia E, Fiocca R, Villani L et al 1991 Morphology and pathogenesis of endocrine hyperplasias, precarcinoid lesions, and carcinoids arising in chronic atrophic gastritis. Scandinavian Journal of Gastroenterology 26: 146–159

Weinstein W M, Bagoch E R, Bowes K L 1975 The normal human esophageal mucosa: a histologic reappraisal. Gastroenterology 68: 40–44

Whitehead R 1989 Gastrointestinal and oesophageal pathology. Churchill Livingstone, Edinburgh

9

Psychological measurement
C. K. Burnett   W. E. Whitehead

INTRODUCTION

Gastrointestinal disorders and psychological disturbances have long been considered to be related. For example, between 46% and 100% of patients with irritable bowel syndrome exhibit a diagnosable psychological disorder (Whitehead 1994). The purposes of this chapter are to outline an approach to psychological screening and assessment for the practicing gastroenterologist and to provide some suggestions for using common psychological screening instruments.

Psychological assessment refers to a number of techniques for recording and quantifying the psychological differences between individuals. Individual differences of interest may include such characteristics as thoughts, beliefs, attitudes, values, knowledge, overt behavior, psychophysiological indices and exposure to stressful events. The fundamental questions underlying psychological assessment are: (1) what are the relevant psychological characteristics of a given person? and (2) how does an individual's psychological characteristics differ from those of other people? The psychological characteristics considered relevant depend on the context of the assessment. For the gastroenterologist, relevant psychological characteristics include the presence of psychiatric disorders (especially depression), personality features that may interfere with treatment compliance, cognitive functioning and exposure to stress. The assessment of the extent to which one person differs from another indicates the severity of the psychological distress. The ability to interpret differences largely depends on the reliability and validity of the assessment instrument.

THE PURPOSES OF PSYCHOLOGICAL ASSESSMENT

The screening approach

Most physicians will be interested in psychological assessment primarily to assist in identifying subjects for whom psychological factors may be affecting the expression of physical symptoms or in whom psychological issues may be interfering with treatment compliance or progress. This situation calls for a screening approach to psychological assessment. Screening for psychological disorders follows the logic of screening for any other condition; the goal is to rapidly identify those at risk of developing a condition or who currently suffer from a given condition. Examples of psychological disorders suitable for screening are depression, anxiety, excess life stress and cognitive deficit. Specific recommendations for instruments of psychological screening in gastroenterological practice are given later in this chapter.

Differential diagnosis

Another frequent use of psychological assessment is in differential diagnosis. A common diagnostic issue is how to differentiate between organic pathology and psychological factors as contributing causes in somatic complaints. Understanding the extent to which symptoms are exacerbated by psychological factors such as anxiety, stress or depression can be useful in interpreting the results of diagnostic tests and in estimating the likely yield from further invasive procedures.

Another issue in differential diagnosis is how to distinguish among various psychological diagnoses. Psychologically distressed patients often present with mixed symptoms that could fit several diagnostic categories such as anxiety, depression or personality disorders. Patients diagnosed with anxiety or depression can often be managed with medication, counseling or psychotherapy. However, patients with a suspected personality disorder such as the obsessive–compulsive, dependent or borderline personality disorders usually require referral to a psychologist or psychiatrist for diagnosis and management. Accurate diagnosis of psychological disturbances allows prioritization and selection of treatments such as antidepressant or anxiolytic medication or psychotherapy.

Documentation and treatment planning

Other uses of psychological assessment are in documenting diagnoses and for treatment planning. The results of psychological assessment can provide necessary documentation in support of functional diagnoses, for example. For treatment planning, documented diagnostic information can be used to justify and guide referral for psychological or psychiatric treatment.

Treatment progress and long-term follow-up

Monitoring changes in psychological status is useful to assess progress in treatment, to assess the need for psychotherapy and to provide the physician with information for medical decisions. For example, a patient who becomes non-compliant with medication and begins to miss appointments yet reports worsening physical symptoms without a change in physical findings could be significantly depressed.

In gastroenterological practice, then, psychological assessment may be thought of as serving three major functions. The first function is psychological screening to identify patients likely to be depressed, anxious, overly stressed or cognitively impaired. Second, more extensive psychological assessment can provide diagnostic information and treatment suggestions. Finally, psychological status can be tracked over time to assess progress and to assist in understanding compliance and responses to treatment.

USING AN INTERVIEW FOR PSYCHOLOGICAL ASSESSMENT

The most widely used psychological assessment method is the patient interview. An interview can be structured to achieve a number of goals such as screening for mood disorders, diagnosis or ongoing monitoring. The goal of any interview is to obtain information from the patient. The physician usually focuses on obtaining data from the patient about the symptoms of the presenting illness. This format, although time-efficient and directive, provides limited opportunity for the patient to reveal feelings and thoughts.

Increasing the time allowed to obtain psychological information from the patient is essential in conducting a psychological interview. Patients have a story to tell about their symptoms and about themselves. Despite careful questioning on the part of an interviewer, a great deal of the psychological information gleaned from an interview will come from the patient's story. Listening to what is said, how it is said and to what is *not* said can provide a great deal of insight into a patient's psychological status and motivation for seeking treatment. Exploring the basic dimensions of *what* is going on, *when* did it start and *why* the patient has come to the doctor at this particular time usually provides most of the structure needed to facilitate the telling of the story. Encouraging patients to fit their story into the available time and assisting them in focusing on information related to the presenting complaint will often provide the greatest challenge.

THE SCREENING INTERVIEW

For purposes of psychological screening, it is often helpful first to elicit a description of symptoms and presenting complaints, second, to explore the patient's reasons for seeking medical advice and third, to facilitate discussion of more psychologically-related issues. A few strategically-placed questions about mood, sleep, appetite, current stresses and quality of personal relationships usually suffice.

To assess affect, patients may be asked if they have been feeling 'sad', 'down' or 'blue' lately or if they have been feeling 'nervous' or 'jittery'. Patients will often be able to respond to these types of descriptors more readily than to potentially more threatening labels such as 'depression' or 'anxiety'. The former, more subtle approach can serve to *open* dialogue by providing the physician with an opening into the patient's own story about what is happening. The latter approach can serve to *close* dialogue by asking the patient to provide a 'yes or no' response to whether or not they fit into a diagnostic category. For example, if a patient answers 'no' when asked if he is depressed, the physician's options for the next question are limited. A power struggle may ensue with the interviewer asking an increasingly broader range of questions in an attempt to elicit depressive symptoms, while the patient retreats and resists being labeled as depressed. Conversely, if the patient answers 'yes' to the depression question, he may feel the need to justify the diagnosis by overly elaborating symptoms and level of distress. Either option pits physician and patient against each other in a struggle to discover 'the truth', rather than emphasizing a physician–patient partnership whose goal is to collaborate in understanding how the patient feels. The ability to encourage a patient to describe feelings while retaining the responsibility for making a diagnosis yourself are essential for a successful psychological interview.

THE DIAGNOSTIC INTERVIEW

When conducting a diagnostic interview, in contrast to a screening interview, the goal is to focus attention on the indepth exploration of a previously identified psychological issue. For example, during an initial screening interview, a patient might indicate feelings of sadness and listlessness. A later, longer appointment should be scheduled for a diagnostic interview to determine the extent of depression and formulate treatment and referral plans.

Usually, a diagnostic interview is more directive and requires more direct questioning than a screening interview. For diagnostic purposes, the question shifts from what is going on to how much difficulty the patient is experiencing due to the particular psychological distress that has been identified. An overall format, using the A-B-C algorithm, can help the patient identify A (what tends to occur before the symptom – Antecedents), B (exactly what the symptom entails – Behavior) and C (what happens as a result of the symptom – Consequences). If a suicidal tendency is a concern, direct questioning regarding the patient's intent, method and access to the method is preferable to indirect questioning.

As in a diagnostic interview, an interview to assess progress is focused and generally quite directive. This type of interview will usually assume the character of a problem solving session. Often a patient will indicate difficulty complying with medication, diet or other treatments. Framing the difficulty as a problem that can be solved by a collaborative discussion between physician and patient sets the stage for problem solving. For example, a problem with medication compliance may be related to misinformation, unresolved fears or other psychological features of the patient. Additional information gained from a follow-up interview can be helpful in targeting patient education, in altering treatment recommendations and in considering referral for psychological treatment.

DIARIES

An important method for collecting behavioral self-report data for psychological assessment in gastroenterology is the use of symptom diaries. Patients may be instructed to monitor symptoms such as stool frequency, pain level and stool form. Self-monitoring of stress and anxiety levels or behaviors such as exercise, participation in social activities or engaging in pleasant and distracting activities can also be recorded. Diary keeping is also useful for tracking thoughts, especially for identifying patterns of negative or maladaptive thinking that may be impeding therapeutic progress. A diary is useful for:

1. identifying possible cause–effect relationships (e.g. interactions with the boss lead to diarrhea);
2. assessing compliance with treatment (e.g. how many times sphincter exercises were performed);
3. evaluating progress (e.g. reduction in frequency or severity of abdominal pain).

Numerous formats for recording diary information are possible. Patients should not be asked to identify more than one or two events that they can reliably record. Expecting too much information from a diary often leads to frustration and unusable data. Patients need to understand the purpose of the diary and the specific symptoms or behaviors to record. Usually, 10 days to 2 weeks of data are sufficient to identify trends or patterns of symptoms or behavior. For straightforward or easily described symptoms, patients can be mailed a diary to collect baseline data prior to a first appointment. It is usually better to initiate diary recording of more complex data or symptoms after the data collection process has been explained in person.

A daily diary can be organized in columns corresponding to the categories of information to be recorded. For example, a simple diary should include columns for the date, number of bowel movements, average pain intensity and average stress rating. These latter ratings can be made on a scale of to 0 to 10, with 0 being no pain or stress and 10 being the worst pain or stress imaginable. This simple format will provide data on stool frequency and its relationship to daily pain and stress level. More detail can be obtained by asking for pain and stress ratings for each bowel movement. Stool form should also be obtained using a rating scale such as the Bristol stool form scale devised by O'Donnell & Heaton (1988). Additional data on diet, medication, exercise, mood or other behaviors of interest should also be included.

It is vital, however, to design the diary so that it provides maximum information but is simple and brief enough to be accurately completed. A blank diary form, consisting of four to six columns and seven to ten lines per page, can be easily produced and kept on hand. This diary form can then be customized for the specific information desired from each patient.

PSYCHOLOGICAL SCREENING QUESTIONNAIRES

The psychological conditions that the gastroenterologist is most interested in identifying are current state characteristics such as level of general psychological distress, depression, anxiety and quality of life. Of second-ary interest are the assessment of personality characteristics or traits that may not be directly amenable to treatment but that might affect com-pliance or outcome. Numerous questionnaires have been developed for use in screening for psychological symptoms. Although several of these have been extensively used in research with medical patients, few have been widely used in clinical practice.

To assist the practitioner in selecting psychological screening instru-ments, the selected questionnaires that are recommended for clinical use are described below. The major criteria employed for recommending instruments include adequate reliability (e.g. consistency of measurement across the questionnaire items and stability of measurement over time) and validity (e.g. relationships with other measures of the same concept). Other criteria include brevity, ease of administration, scoring, inter-pretation and clinical utility. The selected screening instruments assess generalized psychological distress, mood disorders, quality of life, personality and cognitive functioning.

Screening for general psychological distress

The Symptom Checklist 90, revised (SCL-90-R)

The most widely used questionnaire for screening for general psycho-logical distress is the SCL-90-R (Derogatis 1994). The SCL-90-R was derived from the Cornell Medical Index and the Hopkins Symptom Checklist. These earlier scales were primarily research instruments and the SCL-90-R includes both additional items and additional symptom scales for clinical use.

The SCL-90-R consists of 90 items describing a variety of psychological symptoms. The respondent is asked to indicate how distressing each symptom was during the past week on a scale of 0 'not at all' to 4 'extremely'. Scores on the SCL-90-R include a Global Symptom Index and nine symptom-specific dimension subscales: Somatization, Obsessive–Compulsive, Interpersonal Sensitivity, Depression, Anxiety, Hostility, Phobic Anxiety, Paranoid Ideation and Psychoticism. The SCL-90-R takes about 12–15 minutes for most people to complete. Internal consistency reliabilities for the SCL-90-R dimension subscales range from 0.77 to 0.90 and test-retest reliabilities range from 0.68 to 0.83 over a 10-week time period (Derogatis 1994). The validity of the SCL-90-R is supported by correlations ranging from 0.40 to 0.75 with the clinical and content scales of the Minnesota Multiphasic Personality Inventory (MMPI) (Hathaway & McKinley 1940). Dimension scales of the SCL-90-R also correlate from 0.48 to 0.74 with the dimensions of the Midddlesex Hospital Questionnaire (Derogatis 1994). These and other studies have established a broad base of evidence supporting the validity of the SCL-90-R with a variety of patient and non-patient groups.

A study comparing SCL-90-R scores with MMPI scores in a group of 38 consecutive patients with constipation also demonstrated the utility of the SCL-90-R for gastroenterological patients. Wald et al (1992) found substantial correlations between comparable SCL-90-R and MMPI scale scores, supporting the validity of the SCL-90-R. Patients with normal transit constipation scored consistently higher on both instruments than did those with slow transit constipation. However, the SCL-90-R provided greater discrimination between groups than did the MMPI, demonstrating that the SCL-90-R is more sensitive for detecting psychological distress in constipated patients than is the MMPI. Wald and colleagues (1992) thus recommended the use of the SCL-90-R for its apparently greater sensitivity and for its relative ease of use. The SCL-90-R is available from NCS Assessments Inc, Minneapolis, Minnesota, USA.

Stress

There are consistent relationships between stressful experiences and a variety of somatic symptoms. For example, stressful events precede the onset of irritable bowel syndrome (IBS) (Hislop 1971) and trigger exacerbations of IBS symptoms (Whitehead et al 1980). Stress management training appears to reduce IBS symptom severity (Neff & Blanchard 1987). Stress also affects colonic motility and transit time (Fukudo & Suzuki 1987, Welgan et al 1988).

Although the role of stress in physical illness has received a great deal of research attention, the clinical utility of assessing stress remains uncertain. For the gastroenterologist, measuring life events or patients' perception of stress can aid in estimating the possible contribution of environmental stresses to symptoms. For highly stressed patients, interventions can be targeted toward modifying life stresses if possible or increasing coping skills to reduce the negative impact of stress on health.

The magnitude of the relationship between stress level and bowel symptoms is unclear. There is a modest but significant correlation between irritable bowel symptoms and stress. Stress, assessed with a life events scale, is related to current and later bowel symptoms among IBS patients studied over a 1 year time period (Whitehead et al 1992).

The SCL-90-R Global Symptom Index and domain scales are sensitive to a number of both chronic and acute stressors (Derogatis & Coons 1993). The use of a general psychological distress measure allows assessment of the impact of stressors on psychological functioning, regardless of the nature of the specific stressors. Thus, the SCL-90-R can be recommended for use in evaluating the degree of psychological distress associated with stressful events.

The Social Readjustment Rating Scale (SRRS)

The SRRS was developed by Holmes & Rahe (1967) to assess exposure to both positive and negative life events perceived as stressful by most people (e.g. death of a spouse, change in employment, illness, financial problems). The SRRS allows quantification of the number of stressful events a patient has experienced in the preceding 6 months. The potential impact of these stressors can also be estimated by summing life change units or weights assigned to each of the 42 life events. The SRRS has since been revised to simplify the reading level of certain questions, to break complex questions into simpler sentences (Paykel et al 1971) and to assess positive as well as negative events (Sarason et al 1978).

The Hassles and Uplifts Scale (HUS)

The HUS was developed by DeLongis et al (1982) to assess the amount of subjective distress caused by commonplace events. The HUS emphasizes individual differences in reactivity to common events, in contrast to life events scales such as the SRRS that attempt to quantify exposure to less common and universally stressful life events. The HUS consists of 117 hassles (e.g. having too many responsibilities, problems at work, health problems) rated on a 3-point scale of severity. A parallel set of 135 uplift items assesses pleasure or support derived from daily events (e.g. relaxing, fulfillment from work, enjoying good health).

Three scores can be derived from the hassle items of the HUS:

1. a count of the number of hassles;
2. the sum of item severity ratings;

3. an intensity rating that is the severity rating divided by the number of hassles.

Hassles are more highly related to physical symptoms than are life events (Miller 1993). However, the HUS is correlated with measures of neuroticism and psychological distress.

Quality of life assessment

An increasingly common method for assessing the impact of illness on psychological as well as physical functioning is the use of a measure of quality of life. Health-related quality of life measures have been devised for assessing both general well-being (e.g. the Sickness Impact Profile, Bergner et al 1981; the SF-36, Stewart et al 1988) and for evaluating the impact of specific diseases on functional status, such as the Rating Form of Inflammatory Bowel Disease Patient Concerns Questionnaire (Drossman et al 1989). In general, these studies have found that quality of life assessments discriminate between patients and non-patients and are sensitive to changes in symptoms from pre- to posttreatment (Garret et al 1990, Ware 1993).

While disease-specific quality of life measures are available for some conditions, the practicing gastroenterologist would probably find a general quality of life scale most useful. A general scale has the advantage of applicability to patients with any condition, as well as allowing ready comparison among patients. Furthermore, patients may be less reluctant to complete these questionnaires than psychological tests such as the SCL-90-R because they are presented as measures of how physical disease has affected physical and psychological functioning. Nevertheless, quality of life scales provide a method of screening for psychological distress.

The MOS Short-form General Health Survey (SF-36)

The SF-36 was developed for use in the 1986 Medical Outcomes Study (Stewart at al 1988). The SF-36 consists of 36 items assessing two major domains of self-reported health status: (1) ability to function in physical activity, work and social domains of life; and (2) well-being in terms of mental health, perceived general health and level of bodily pain. The SF-36 is sensitive to deficits in functioning and well-being associated with a number of acute and chronic illnesses (Stewart et al 1989). Eight multi-item scales and one single-item scale of the SF-36 assess self-reported degrees of limitation, over the past year, on each of the following health concepts:

- physical functioning (e.g ability to ambulate);
- role-physical (e.g. ability to work);

- bodily pain;
- general health;
- vitality;
- social functioning;
- role-emotional;
- mental health;
- health transition (i.e. change in health relative to the previous year).

Median internal consistency and test-retest reliabilities for SF-36 scales range from 0.76 to 0.95 in published studies (Ware 1993).

A recent study using the SF-36 found significantly poorer quality of life among IBS patients than among asymptomatic controls (Whitehead et al 1994). Further, IBS patients who had consulted a physician about their bowel symptoms reported significantly poorer quality of life than IBS patients who had not consulted a physician. The difference between consulters and non-consulters persisted after statistical removal of the effects of psychological distress and neuroticism scores. This study suggests that quality of life assessment, using the SF-36, contributes useful information about patient functioning that is not entirely captured by measures of psychological distress or personality. Thus, the SF-36 could be useful in assessing functional status and sense of well-being in gastroenterological practice.

Mood disorders – depression

A primary concern when screening for psychological distress in medical patients is the ability to detect the condition of interest both sensitively and specifically. Screening for depression is a good example. If a patient's medical condition imposes a substantial somatic burden of deficits in appetite, sleep or energy, the patient may register as severely depressed on a screening instrument that is heavily loaded with somatic items. In such a case the patient may exhibit few cognitive symptoms of depression and yet appear to be depressed because of expected somatic symptoms. Thus, to avoid losses in specificity, the practitioner should use instruments with a greater number of cognitive items relative to somatic items when screening somatically ill patients.

The Beck Depression Inventory (BDI)

The BDI (Beck et al 1961) is the most widely used screening questionnaire for depression. The BDI consists of 21 items with five response choices for each item and assesses the severity of cognitive and somatic depressive symptoms. BDI items place a greater emphasis on cognitive aspects of depression such as hopelessness and sadness than on somatic aspects of depression such as decreased appetite and lethargy.

The BDI is self-administered and takes 5–10 minutes for most patients to complete. The total score on the BDI ranges from 0 to 63 and is the sum of the item intensity ratings which range from 0 to 3. The BDI has shown substantial internal consistency reliability, averaging 0.81 in non-psychiatric samples. Test-retest reliabilities range from 0.60 to 0.90 in non-psychiatric sample studies over intervals up to 3 weeks. The BDI has been validated against a number of other depression questionnaires and structured interviews with correlations exceeding 0.60 (Beck et al 1988).

The most commonly used cut-off scores on the BDI for a diagnosis of depression are 10–18 for mild to moderate depression, 19–29 for moderate to severe depression and 30–63 for severe depression (Beck et al 1988). Some investigators have suggested that higher cut-off scores, up to 17, should be used for medical patients to correct for the potential confounding effects of somatic illness on depression scores (Rodin & Voshart 1987).

The advantages of the BDI include its brevity, ease of administration and interpretation and emphasis on cognitive rather than somatic aspects of depression. The major disadvantage of the BDI is the ease with which patients are able to distort their responses so that they can appear more or less depressed. This potential bias can be best dealt with by establishing honest, open communication with patients about the purpose of screening and by projecting a non-judgemental attitude about psychological issues and assessment. The BDI is available from the Psychological Corporation, San Antonio, Texas, USA.

Mood disorders – anxiety

State-Trait Anxiety Inventory (STAI)

The STAI (Spielberger 1983) is the most widely used screening instrument for anxiety. The state anxiety items are constructed to assess current, transitory anxiety while the trait anxiety items are devised to assess stable anxiety-proneness. Each version of the scale, state anxiety and trait anxiety, is assessed with 20 items. The response options lie on a 4-point scale, from 'not at all' to 'very much so' for state anxiety and from 'almost never' to 'almost always' for trait items. Both subscales can be completed in about 10 minutes.

The median internal consistency reliabilities for the STAI across several normative groups were 0.93 for state anxiety and 0.90 for trait anxiety. Test-retest reliabilities have been reported as 0.77 for trait anxiety and 0.33 for state anxiety across 104 days (Spielberger 1983). These reliability data also support the difference between the constructs of state and trait anxiety, since state anxiety would be expected to be less stable over time than trait anxiety. The STAI has been used quite extensively in studies of gastrointestinal conditions, especially in studies of functional disorders. The STAI is available from Consulting Psychologists Press Inc, Palo Alto, California, USA.

Personality screening instruments

The assessment of personality traits typically requires more extensive evaluation than does screening for a patient's current state of psychological distress. Diagnosing personality traits or disorders such as obsessive–compulsive, dependent or borderline personality is best accomplished by psychological or psychiatric referral which usually includes formal personality testing. The length of most personality inventories and the complexity of scoring and interpretation make these instruments less desirable for use by gastroenterologists. Information from interviews and interactions with a patient may be all that is necessary for the physician to become aware that a referral is indicated. However, personality assessment can sometimes be useful to physicians in understanding and dealing with problems in treatment adherence.

Minnesota Multiphasic Personality Inventory (MMPI-2)

The MMPI-2 (Hathaway & McKinley 1994) provides extensive information on personality and psychopathology. The MMPI-2 consists of 567 items forming ten clinical subscales and three test validity subscales that assess domains of affective, personality and cognitive functioning. Numerous additional special scales for specific content areas are also available. Most patients require at least 1 hour to complete the MMPI-2.

The MMPI-2 can provide a great deal of diagnostic information. However, the length of the instrument, the complexity of the scoring and the specialized training required for interpreting test results make the MMPI-2 generally unsuitable for use by gastroenterologists. In situations where psychologists or other specially trained personnel are available, the MMPI-2 can become a valuable component of a comprehensive psychological assessment.

NEO Personality Inventory (NEO PI-R)

The NEO PI-R (Costa & McCrae 1992) assesses five major personality domains: neuroticism, extraversion, openness, agreeableness and conscientiousness. The neuroticism scale score, in particular, has been shown to differentiate patients with IBS from those without chronic bowel symptoms (Whitehead et al 1992).

Internal consistency reliabilities of the five NEO PI-R domain scale scores have been reported to range from 0.87 to 0.95. Validity of the domain scores and their component facet scores has been supported by numerous studies relating the NEO PI-R scores to other psychological measures (Costa & McCrae 1992). Most patients require 30–40 minutes to complete the NEO PI-R.

Screening for cognitive disorders

The need to assess cognitive functioning is sometimes apparent from a patient's behavior in the office or from reports about compliance problems from relatives or other caregivers. When a deficit in comprehension or memory is suspected, referral for appropriate neurological or psychiatric evaluation is usually appropriate. Initial screening for cognitive functioning is often useful, however, and can be accomplished with a brief mental status examination.

The Mini-Mental State Examination (MMS)

The MMS (Folstein et al 1975) is a standardized mental status screening instrument. The use of the MMS allows for tracking changes in function over time and for more valid comparison between patients than informal examination. The MMS takes about 5–10 minutes to administer and is easy to score and interpret. The total score ranges from 0 to 30. Conventional cut-off scores of 24–30 for no impairment, 18–23 for mild cognitive impairment and 0–17 for severe impairment have been established (Tombaugh & McIntyre 1992).

Internal consistency reliabilities for the MMS vary considerably due to the heterogeneity of the items included in the scale and the degree of cognitive deficit present in the populations studied. However, reliabilities for community samples range from 0.68 to 0.77 and a group of general medical patients demonstrated internal consistency reliability of 0.96 (Tombaugh & McIntyre 1992). Test-retest reliabilities generally range from 0.80 to 0.95 over a period of 2 months or less. Sensitivity and specificity also vary according to the diagnostic groups studied, but are generally adequate (Tombaugh & McIntyre 1992). Correlations with other cognitive and memory scales have been reported to range from about 0.70 to 0.90, indicating adequate construct validity. The MMS is reproduced in the publications by Folstein et al (1975) and Tombaugh & McIntyre (1992).

SUMMARY

Psychological assessment can add breadth and depth of understanding of patients in gastroenterological practice. The major function of assessment in gastroenterological practice is to identify patients with significant psychological distress or possible risk of suicide who need psychological help. Several brief yet reliable screening instruments are available that can provide useful information for treatment and referral. The major barriers to full utilization of psychological assessment are limitations in time and resources.

The gastroenterologist interested in psychological assessment should rely on the SCL-90-R as a first-line psychological screening instrument. The SCL-90-R has many advantages in psychological screening such as brevity, reliability, validity, ease of interpretation and substantial supporting research. Other more specialized instruments such as the Beck Depression Inventory (BDI), the State-Trait Anxiety Inventory (STAI), the SF-36 quality of life measure and the Mini-Mental State Examination (MMS) are recommended as first-line tools when interview or other findings suggest depression, anxiety, decrements in functioning or cognitive impairment, respectively. These tools may also be used to further investigate hypotheses about psychological problems suggested by the results of the SCL-90-R. The other instruments reviewed are available for the assessment of psychological functioning in other domains such as life events, stress or personality. However, these instruments are less likely to be of value to the gastroenterologist than the more generalized screening measures.

The primary screening instrument in gastroenterology remains the interview. No questionnaire can replace the insight into symptoms and life situations that can be gleaned from a skillful and sensitive interview. Even when a great deal of data are available from screening questionnaires, a patient interview is crucial to further explore and test hypotheses constructed from questionnaire findings. Much can also be gathered from symptom diaries to identify patterns in symptoms and behaviors that can direct treatment strategies. Such diaries can serve therapeutic purposes as well, helping patients to understand the relationship between behavior and symptoms.

Familiarity with all of the instruments described above will provide the physician with a collection of tools for assessing psychological status and screening for psychological distress, life stress, quality of life and affective, personality and cognitive disorders. These instruments can help to systematize and supplement clinical judgement, but do not replace it. Neither do these methods supplant the need for referral to qualified psychologists or psychiatric consultants. By employing some level of psychological assessment in the office, treatment strategies can be fine-tuned, referral questions can be sharpened and unnecessary referrals can be reduced.

REFERENCES

Beck A T, Ward C H, Mendelson M, Mock J, Erbaugh J 1961 An inventory for measuring depression. Archives of General Psychiatry 4: 561–571

Beck A T, Steer R A, Garbin M G 1988 Psychometric properties of the Beck Depression Inventory: twenty-five years of evaluation. Clinical Psychology Review 8: 77–100

Bergner M, Bobbit R, Carter W, Gibson B 1981 The Sickness Impact Profile: development and final revision of a health status measure. Medical Care 19: 787–805

Costa P T, McCrae R R 1992 Revised NEO Personality Inventory (NEO PI-R) and NEO Five-Factor Inventory (NEO-FFI) professional manual. Psychological Assessment Resources, Odessa, FL

DeLongis A, Coyne J C, Dakof G, Folkman S, Lazarus R A 1982 Relationship of daily hassles, uplifts, and major life events to health status. Health Psychology 1: 119–136

Derogatis L R 1994 SCL-90-R: administration, scoring and procedures manual. National Computer Systems, Minneapolis, MN

Derogatis L R, Coons H L 1993 Self report measures of stress. In: Goldberger L, Breznitz S (eds) Handbook of stress: theoretical and clinical aspects. The Free Press, New York, p 200

Drossman D A, Patrick D L, Mitchell C M, Zagami E A, Applebaum M I 1989 Health related quality of life in inflammatory bowel disease: functional status and patient worries and concerns. Digestive Diseases and Sciences 34: 1379–1386

Folstein M F, Folstein S E, McHugh P R 1975 'Mini-mental state': a practical method for grading the cognitive state of patients for the clinician. Journal of Psychiatric Research 12: 189–198

Fukudo S, Suzuki J 1987 Colonic motility, autonomic function, and gastrointestinal hormones under psychological stress on irritable bowel syndrome. Tohoku Journal of Experimental Medicine 151: 373–385

Garrett J W, Drossman D A, Patrick D L 1990 Inflammatory bowel disease. In: Spilker B (ed) Quality of life assessments in clinical trials. Raven, New York, p 367

Hathaway S R, McKinley J C 1940 A multiphasic personality schedule (Minnesota): I. Construction of the schedule. Journal of Psychology 10: 249–254

Hathaway S R, McKinley J C 1994 MMPI-2, Minnesota Multiphasic Personality Inventory-2: manual for administration and scoring. National Computer Systems, Minneapolis, MN

Hislop I G 1971 Psychological significance of the irritable colon syndrome. Gut 12: 452–457

Holmes T H, Rahe R H 1967 The social readjustment rating scale. Journal of Psychosomatic Research 11: 213–218

Miller T W 1993 The assessment of stressful life events. In: Goldberger L, Breznitz S (eds) Handbook of stress: theoretical and clinical aspects. The Free Press, New York, p 161

Neff D F, Blanchard E B 1987 A multicomponent treatment for irritable bowel syndrome. Behavior Therapy 18: 70–83

O'Donnell L J D, Heaton K W 1988 Pseudo-diarrhea in the irritable bowel syndrome: patients' records of stool form reflect transit time while stool frequency does not. Gut 29: A1455

Paykel E S, Prusoff B A, Uhlenhuth E H 1971 Scaling of life events. Archives of General Psychiatry 25: 340–347

Rodin G, Voshart K 1987 Depressive symptoms and functional impairment in the medically ill. General Hospital Psychiatry 9: 251–258

Sarason I G, Johnson J H, Siegel J M 1978 Assessing the impact of life changes: development of the life experiences survey. Journal of Consulting and Clinical Psychology 46: 932–946

Spielberger C D 1983 Manual for the state-trait anxiety inventory. Consulting Psychologists Press, Palo Alto, CA

Stewart A L, Hays R D, Ware J E 1988 The MOS short-form general health survey: reliability and validity in a patient population. Medical Care 26: 724–735

Stewart A L, Greenfield S, Hays R D et al 1989 Functional status and well-being of patients with chronic conditions: results from the Medical Outcomes Study. Journal of the American Medical Association 262: 907–913

Tombaugh T N, McIntyre N J 1992 The Mini-Mental State Examination: a comprehensive review. Journal of the American Geriatrics Society 40: 922–935

Wald A, Burgio K, Holeva K, Locher J 1992 Psychological evaluation of patients with severe idiopathic constipation: which instrument to use. American Journal of Gastroenterology 87: 977–980

Ware J E 1993 SF-36 health survey: manual and interpretation guide. The Health Institute, Boston

Welgan P, Meshkinpour H, Beeler M 1988 Effect of anger on colon motor and myoelectric activity in irritable bowel syndrome. Gastroenterology 94: 1150–1156

Whitehead W E 1994 The disturbed psyche and the irritable gut. European Journal of Gastroenterology and Hepatology 6: 483–488

Whitehead W E, Engel B T, Schuster M M 1980 Irritable bowel syndrome: physiological and psychological differences between diarrhea-predominant and constipation-predominant patients. Digestive Diseases and Sciences 25: 404–413

Whitehead W E, Crowell M D , Robinson J C, Heller B R, Schuster M M 1992 Effects of stressful life events on bowel symptoms: subjects with irritable bowel syndrome compared with subjects without bowel dysfunction. Gut 33: 825–830

Whitehead W E, Burnett C K, Cook E B, Taub E W 1994 Health-related quality of life in IBS patients compared to IBS non-consulters and asymptomatic individuals. American Journal of Gastroenterology 89: A340

Objective assessment of common clinical symptoms

10

Evaluation of dysphagia, heartburn and non-cardiac chest pain

J. L. Conklin

INTRODUCTION

The organs involved in swallowing – the pharynx and esophagus – serve three primary functions: to transport swallowed material from the oropharynx to the stomach, to prevent the reflux of gastric contents into the esophagus, pharynx and respiratory tract, and to clear refluxed gastric contents from the esophagus. Peristaltic contractions of the muscular walls of the pharynx and esophagus propel swallowed materials from the mouth to the stomach. The failure or discoordination of peristaltic contractions may disrupt the propulsion of swallowed material along the conduit. This leads to the symptoms of *dysphagia* (difficult swallowing) or *odynophagia* (painful swallowing). The reflux of gastric contents into the esophagus and pharynx is prevented primarily by specialized, tonically-contracted sphincter muscles that impede the retrograde movement of gastric contents. Their failure to do so may lead to reflux esophagitis and *heartburn* (a substernal and epigastric burning sensation). Noxious gastric contents that are refluxed into the esophagus are normally cleared by peristaltic contractions that sweep them back into the stomach. Therefore, derangement in esophageal peristalsis may exacerbate reflux esophagitis.

STRUCTURE AND FUNCTION OF THE SWALLOWING ORGANS

The pharynx and esophagus form a tubular conduit made up of distinct neuromuscular elements that are functionally integrated to perform the task of swallowing. The pharynx is a tapered hollow cylinder that connects the mouth and nasopharyngeal cavity to the esophagus and trachea. The muscular wall of the pharynx is composed of three over-lapping sheets of striated muscle, the pharyngeal constrictors (Donner et al 1985). The most caudal of these muscles, the inferior pharyngeal constrictor, thickens to give rise to a distinct band of striated muscle, the cricopharyngeus. The cricopharyngeus is positioned at the inlet of the esophagus where it functions as the upper esophageal sphincter.

Below the pharyngoesophageal junction, the esophagus forms a continuous tube to the stomach. The esophageal musculature consists of an outer longitudinal and an inner circular layer that are named according to the axial orientation of their constituent muscle cells. Both layers of the esophageal musculature are striated down to about the level of the aortic arch (22–24 cm from the incisor teeth). There is a transition zone of several centimeters at about the level of the tracheal bifurcation over which the striated muscle mixes with and is replaced by smooth (visceral) muscle. Smooth muscle makes up the distal esophagus. The circular muscle layer thickens a little at the esophagogastric junction to form a muscular ring called the lower esophageal sphincter.

At rest, the pharyngeal musculature generates a weak tonic contraction that stiffens the pharyngeal wall without occluding the lumen. The upper esophageal sphincter (cricopharyngeus) generates a powerful, tonic contraction at rest which occludes the lumen at the junction between the pharynx and esophagus (Code & Schlegel 1968, Conklin & Christensen 1994, Donner et al 1985). Similarly, the tonic contraction of the lower esophageal sphincter completely occludes the lumen at the gastroesophageal junction. The striated and smooth muscle portions of the esophagus between the two sphincters form a flaccid tube without tone at rest.

Swallowing starts as a phase of preparation including mastication of the food and the formation of the bolus to be swallowed. The tongue assumes a cup shape to hold the bolus in the oral cavity. As the swallow is initiated, the tongue elevates against the palate in a sequential manner from anterior to posterior to squeeze the bolus into the pharynx. As the bolus is propelled into the pharynx, the soft palate elevates to make contact with the posterior pharyngeal wall. This seals the oropharynx from the nasopharynx so that nasopharyngeal reflux does not occur. At about the same time the larynx is elevated and the arytenoids are displaced anterior to make contact with the epiglottis, thereby closing the laryngeal opening.

Two types of pharyngeal contraction facilitate the movement of the bolus towards the esophagus. Early in the swallow the pharynx shortens in its long axis, decreasing the distance the bolus must travel in transit through the pharynx. Pharyngeal shortening also obliterates the laryngeal vestibule and the pyriform sinuses so that none of the bolus is caught in these recesses. A peristaltic contraction of the pharyngeal musculature behind the bolus occludes the pharyngeal lumen as it sweeps caudad to force what has been swallowed towards the esophagus. The tonically contracted upper esophageal sphincter relaxes as the pharyngeal peristaltic contraction advances towards the esophagus and is actively pulled open as the larynx is elevated. The upper esophageal sphincter contracts powerfully as the pharyngeal peristaltic sequence passes and then rapidly reestablishes its basal tone. This facilitates the transfer of the bolus from the oropharynx to the esophagus. The peristaltic contraction sweeps without interruption from the upper esophageal sphincter along the esophageal body to the stomach. The tonically contracted lower esophageal sphincter relaxes long before the peristaltic contraction reaches the gastroesophageal junction. It remains relaxed until the peristaltic contraction arrives to strip the bolus into the gastric cavity. Arrival of the peristaltic contraction at the lower esophageal sphincter closes the sphincter with a transient, forceful contraction which soon subsides to the tonic contraction of the resting state.

NEUROMUSCULAR CONTROL OF SWALLOWING

The contractile behavior of the swallowing organs composed of striated muscle – the pharynx, upper esophageal sphincter and proximal eso-phageal body – is controlled by somatic nerves that originate in the nuclei of the glossopharyngeal (IX) and vagus (X) nerves (Bieger & Hopkins 1987, Holstege et al 1983). Axons from nerve cell bodies in these nuclei project through cranial nerves without synaptic interruption to end in motor endplates on the striated muscle cells. The continuous discharge of these nerves is responsible for the maintenance of tone in the striated muscle of the oropharynx and upper esophageal sphincter (Doty 1968). Relaxation of these muscles results from the inhibition of this tonic somatic neural discharge. The peristaltic contraction that sweeps along these organs represents a vigorous discharge of their somatic innervation. The contraction is peristaltic because the motor units, single motor neurons and striated muscle cells that they supply, are activated in a fixed craniocaudal sequence.

The neuromuscular control of the smooth muscle esophagus is quite different from that of the striated muscle organs. The central innervation of the smooth muscle portion of the esophagus arises from nerve cell bodies in the dorsal motor nucleus of the vagus (Doty 1968). Axons from these preganglionic parasympathetic neurons travel with the vagus nerve to synapse with neurons in the myenteric plexus. The terminal motor innervation of the smooth muscle of the esophagus, the postganglionic neurons, comes from these nerve cell bodies in the myenteric plexus.

The neural systems seem to be inactive at rest in the smooth muscle segment of the esophagus. The resting contraction of the lower esophageal sphincter reflects, mainly, the myogenic tone of the sphincter muscle rather than a strong tonic discharge of nerves; however, some fluctuations in baseline tone may represent neural activity (Christensen et al 1973, Goyal & Rattan 1976). The first swallow-induced event in the smooth muscle esophagus is relaxation of the lower esophageal sphincter. This relaxation results from the vagal activation of inhibitory myenteric nerves that release nitric oxide (Murray et al 1991).

The progressive nature of the peristaltic contraction in the smooth muscle esophageal segment, unlike peristalsis in the striated muscle part of the esophagus, is not programmed in the brainstem. Instead, it is controlled by neuromuscular mechanisms that are intrinsic to the esophagus. Nitric oxide-releasing myenteric nerves supply the circular muscle of the smooth muscle esophagus. Swallowing activates these inhibitory nerves simultaneously throughout the esophageal body, to cause a nearly simultaneous inhibition along the length of the smooth muscle esophagus (Du et al 1991, Serio & Daniel 1988). The duration of the inhibition is progressively longer at the more distal sites in the smooth muscle esophagus. Excitation that follows the period of inhibition is responsible for the progressive nature of the peristaltic contraction (Rattan et al 1983, Sugarbaker et al 1984).

DYSPHAGIA – DIFFICULTY SWALLOWING

Dysphagia is the perception of difficulty in swallowing. Normally, people are aware only of the oral and most of the pharyngeal phases of swallowing; that is, chewing, the formation of a bolus in the mouth and the initiation of a peristaltic sequence in the oropharynx. The symptom of dysphagia may be only a nondescript feeling that something is amiss after the pharyngeal portion of the swallow, it may be sensed as an evanescent slowing of the food bolus or it may be the sensation of a bolus getting stuck. These symptoms result when the transport of a swallowed bolus along the pharyngoesophageal conduit is impaired by either a mechanical obstruction of the lumen or neuromuscular failure causing disordered peristalsis.

   Dysphagia is usually classified as either oropharyngeal or esophageal. This distinction is more than anatomical because the neuromuscular mechanisms controlling these regions are dissimilar (see above) and the pathological processes that underlie disordered swallowing in the two regions differ (Box 10.1). Oropharyngeal dysphagia most commonly results from either neuromuscular disorders or structural abnormalities such as oropharyngeal tumors.

Evaluation of the patient with dysphagia

Historical features

Taking a detailed medical history regarding the characteristics of dysphagia and the symptoms associated with it is critical. The patient will often indicate *where* he senses the dysphagia. The perception of sticking anterior in the throat above the suprasternal notch reliably predicts that the dysphagia is oropharyngeal in origin. Esophageal dysphagia is sensed at the suprasternal notch, substernally or on the anterior chest wall. The location of the sensation does not predict the level of the lesion. In most

---

Box 10.1 Causes of dysphagia

Dysphagia from the oropharynx and striated muscle esophagus
- **Neuromuscular diseases**
  Diseases of the central nervous system
  Cerebral vascular accident
  Multiple sclerosis
  Amyotrophic lateral sclerosis
  Parkinson's disease
  Tumors of the brainstem
  Diseases of the peripheral nervous system
  Poliomyelitis
  Myasthenia gravis
  Peripheral neuropathies (diabetes mellitus)
  Myopathic diseases
  Muscular dystrophies
  Polymyositis, dermatomyositis
  Metabolic myopathic processes (myxedema, thyrotoxicosis, steroid-induced myopathy)
- **Structural abnormalities**
  Neoplasms (squamous cell carcinoma, lymphoid tumors)
  Infectious processes
  Compression from external lesions (enlarged thyroid, lymph nodes, cervical vertebral osteophytes)
  Esophageal rings or webs (Plummer–Vinson syndrome, congenital webs)

Esophageal dysphagia
- **Mechanical obstruction**
  Esophageal neoplasms (mucosal or intramural tumors)
  Peptic stricture
  Foreign bodies
  Paraesophageal hernia
  Mediastinal tumors
- **Esophagitis**
- **Myopathic diseases** as above
- **Peripheral neuropathies** (diabetes)
- **Primary motor abnormalities**
  Achalasia
  Diffuse esophageal spasm

---

cases, the sensation is cephalic to the lesion. Dysphagia is seldom perceived in the middle of the back or epigastrium.

Exacerbating and relieving factors

Asking the patient what triggers the dysphagia or makes it better or worse often provides valuable clues to the origins of the problem. Patients with oropharyngeal dysphagia often have more difficulty swallowing liquids than solids. They frequently learn that cautious eating and swallowing or getting the head into certain positions brings some relief. Patients with esophageal dysphagia arising from mechanical lesions obstructing the lumen of the esophagus complain that their dysphagia is worse with solids than with liquids. The most troublesome foods are those that are not chewed well: meats, breads and peanut butter. Patients with mechanical lesions may gain relief by 'washing it down' with liquids. Dysphagia for both solids and liquids suggests either a nearly complete obstruction of the esophagus or disordered esophageal motor function. Dysphagia brought on or worsened by drinking very cold liquids or by eating ice cream is suggestive of esophageal spasm.

Chronology of symptoms

Patients with esophageal dysphagia often note that their symptoms started as mild, intermittent dysphagia and progressed over time. Dysphagia that remains intermittent and is not progressive, or only slowly progressive over a long period of time, suggests a benign cause like a stable stricture or a motor abnormality. Long asymptomatic periods punctuated by brief episodes of relatively severe dysphagia suggest the presence of an esophageal mucosal ring (Schatzki's ring). Dysphagia for solids that worsens over time to dysphagia for both solids and liquids suggests an esophageal neoplasm. The sudden onset of dysphagia is uncommon and should make the physician think of such things as a lodged foreign body or an infection.

Associated symptoms or illnesses

Questioning the patient about other symptoms associated with dysphagia or intercurrent illnesses often helps to determine the etiology of the dysphagia. People with oropharyngeal dysphagia complain of difficulties initiating the swallowing process, nasopharyngeal reflux of swallowed liquids and choking or coughing with swallowing. These patients may also present with other symptoms of the neuromuscular disease that underlies the swallowing problem (see Box 10.1).

Heartburn associated with dysphagia suggests that an inflammatory process, usually chronic gastroesophageal reflux disease (GERD), is responsible for the dysphagia. Chronic esophagitis may lead to the formation of an esophageal stricture or precipitate an abnormality of esophageal motor function that interferes with esophageal transit. The symptom of odynophagia (painful swallowing) associated with dysphagia suggests a more severe inflammatory process like esophageal ulcers resulting from GERD, a tablet lodged in the esophagus or infections (cytomegalovirus, *Herpes* or *Candida*).

Immunocompromised patients, such as those being treated with chemotherapeutic or immunosuppressive agents and those suffering from AIDS, may have dysphagia arising from infections. The most common agents identified in biopsies of esophageal ulcers are cytomegalovirus, *Herpes* or *Candida*. Kaposi's sarcoma involving the esophagus can also produce dysphagia in patients with AIDS. Dysphagia may also be a manifestation of systemic diseases such as collagen vascular diseases (especially scleroderma), diabetes mellitus and hypothyroidism.

Radiographic evaluation of the patient with dysphagia

Customarily, the first diagnostic test to be performed in patients with dysphagia is a barium X-ray during swallowing.

Videofluoroscopy is essential for evaluating oropharyngeal dysphagia. This examination involves the videotaping of fluoroscopic images of the patient swallowing boluses of barium. The video images can then be reviewed in slow motion or frame by frame to analyze the complex muscular movements of the oropharynx during swallowing. Uncoordinated movements of the tongue impair the formation of the bolus and its propulsion through the pharynx. Dysfunction of the soft palate leads to regurgitation of the bolus into the nasopharynx. Impaired closure of the larynx leads to aspiration. Weak or uncoordinated contraction of the pharyngeal musculature is manifest as residue left in the valleculae or pyriform sinuses after the swallow. Videofluoroscopy can also identify the cricopharyngeal bar, a thickened cricopharyngeus muscle, and/or a Zenker's (pharyngoesophageal) diverticulum, both indicating failure of opening of the upper esophageal sphincter.

The barium swallow and cine esophagram are also useful in identifying the etiology of dysphagia arising from the esophagus. Many endoscopists hold the view that endoscopy is superior to barium studies in the evaluation of dysphagia arising from the esophagus because endoscopy will be required to determine if a lesion is malignant and to treat obstructing lesions. In fact, the barium swallow is a very effective way to rule out neoplasms of the esophagus or strictures as the cause of dysphagia. It is probably superior to endoscopy as a method for the identification of upper esophageal webs and Schatzki's rings and it is a safer way to identify pharyngoesophageal diverticula. Barium studies are superior to endoscopy for the identification of intramural lesions that do not involve the esophageal mucosa and esophageal compression by extraesophageal lesions like mediastinal tumors or a bone spur on a cervical vertebra.

The cine esophagram may also provide valuable clues to potential motor abnormalities underlying the symptom of dysphagia. It does so by providing a clear picture of bolus transport in the esophagus. The aperistalsis and failure of lower esophageal sphincter relaxation that are the hallmarks of achalasia can be identified by a cine esophagram. So can the spontaneous, repetitive and uncoordinated esophageal contractions that define esophageal spasm and presbyesophagus. The upper GI X-ray may also provide evidence for the presence of gastroesophageal reflux.

Endoscopic evaluation of the patient with dysphagia

While the utility of upper GI endoscopy as the first test in the evaluation of dysphagia is debated, there is little question that it is the best test for determining the nature of lesions obstructing the lumen of the esophagus. Endoscopy is particularly useful in the patient with dysphagia and heartburn. Endoscopy should be considered before barium studies for two reasons. First, endoscopy with biopsy is the most sensitive way to identify esophagitis since biopsies of the esophageal mucosa may demonstrate inflammation that is not apparent on endoscopic or radiographic examination of the mucosa. Second, complications of gastroesophageal reflux disease that cause dysphagia (peptic strictures or Schatzki's rings) can be treated with endoscopic techniques. Biopsies and cytological brushings should always be obtained as part of the endoscopic evaluation of intraluminal esophageal lesions obstructing the lumen of the esophagus. Endoscopy should always be performed on patients suspected of having achalasia to rule out a tumor of the cardia that mimics achalasia. Immunosuppressed patients who are suspected of an esophageal infection as the cause of dysphagia warrant an endoscopy for several reasons. First, radiographic studies may not identify the subtle mucosal changes induced by infectious agents. Second, biopsies and cultures are required to target therapies to treat specific infectious agents.

Manometry in the evaluation of the patient with dysphagia

Manometric techniques (Kahrilas et al 1994, Orlando 1993). Two manometric techniques are currently used in clinical practice: the perfused catheter and solid-state pressure sensors. The older and more widely used method is the perfused catheter which consists of a bundle of thin tubes. The tube is introduced into the pharynx or esophagus and placed at selected locations to measure the motor events induced by swallowing. When the flow of water through the lateral opening is occluded by contraction of the esophagus, the recorded pressure rises. The amplitude and timing of the pressure change reflect the force and timing of circular muscle contraction.

The other manometric method in common use employs solid-state pressure sensors placed at varying lengths along a flexible tube. Both methods provide reliable information regarding the timing and force of circular muscle contraction.

Manometry in the evaluation of oropharyngeal dysphagia. Standard manometric techniques are not very useful in the evaluation of oropharyngeal dysphagia because they cannot reliably record motor events in the pharynx and upper esophageal sphincter. Since these structures are not radially symmetrical, the direction in which the sensor faces greatly influences the recorded pressure. Thus, a powerful contraction in one axis may be feeble in another. Also, the pharynx shortens during swallowing while the recording device stays at a fixed point. This is particularly troublesome when trying to evaluate the upper esophageal sphincter because the recording port may slip out of the sphincter as it moves upward. This results in an artefactual drop in the sphincter tone.

Manometry in the evaluation of esophageal dysphagia. If careful radiographic studies and/or endoscopy fail to identify esophagitis or a lesion obstructing the lumen, esophageal manometry should be considered. Since abnormalities of esophageal motor function can cause dysphagia, esophageal manometry is widely used in the hope of identifying any motor disturbance underlying swallowing difficulties. However, the clinician should understand the low probability of finding a motor abnormality that will clearly explain dysphagia. Of all patients complaining of dysphagia with no obstructing lesion, 1–20% will have achalasia identified on manometry and 2–10% will have diffuse esophageal spasm (Ferguson et al 1981, Katz et al 1987). Both these disorders cause abnormal esophageal transit of the swallowed bolus and dysphagia. Up to 50% of patients with dysphagia with no mechanical lesion have non-specific motor abnormalities on esophageal manometry. In most cases these abnormalities do not appear to affect bolus transit in the esophagus, making their relationship to the symptom of dysphagia unclear.

Esophageal scintigraphy in the evaluation of dysphagia. Attempts have been made to use scintigraphic techniques as a way to evaluate esophageal motor function. The technique provides two pieces of information: whether the patient has gastroesophageal reflux and how well the esophagus is able to clear its intraluminal contents. The clinical applications and clinical value of the technique remain to be determined.

HEARTBURN – REFLUX ESOPHAGITIS

Heartburn is a very common symptom in the general population: 20–40% of the general population have heartburn once a month, 10–14% have heartburn once a week and 4–7% have daily heartburn.

Heartburn as a symptom most often indicates the presence of chronic mucosal inflammation in the distal esophagus. The inflammatory process is usually initiated and maintained by the reflux of gastric contents into the esophagus. Gastroesophageal reflux occurs either because the lower esophageal sphincter does not maintain adequate tone at rest or because it relaxes inappropriately, not only during swallowing. This allows the retrograde movement of gastric contents into the esophagus. This situation is exacerbated if esophageal peristalsis is disordered so that gastric contents are not cleared from the esophagus or if the motor function of the stomach is impaired so that it does not empty properly. Delayed gastric emptying increases the amount of time that noxious gastric contents may reflux into the esophagus. Heartburn is less frequently caused by infectious agents like *Candida albicans*, CMV or *Herpes* virus. In patients who do not take tablets with adequate amounts of fluids, the tablets can lodge in the distal esophagus to cause inflammation and heartburn.

Evaluation of the patient with heartburn

Historical features

The most important information to be obtained in the evaluation of the patient with heartburn comes from a careful history. Heartburn is most frequently described as a *burning* or *hot* sensation that is located in the midepigastrium near the xiphoid process or over the lower half of the sternum. Some patients describe heartburn as a 'sour stomach' or 'indigestion'. The symptom is almost never described as a sharp, crampy or squeezing pain. The severity of the heartburn does not predict the severity of the underlying pathological process.

The typical patient with heartburn has the symptom intermittently. Most exacerbations are related to practices by the patient that intensify the esophageal inflammation or promote gastroesophageal reflux. Smoking cigarettes or drinking alcohol promote reflux by decreasing the force of closure of the lower esophageal sphincter. Eating large, fatty meals increases reflux by several mechanisms. First, overeating increases the pressure gradient from the stomach to the esophagus. The result is increased reflux across the lower esophageal sphincter. Second, fats entering the duodenum decrease the force of closure of the lower esophageal sphincter and decrease the rate of gastric emptying. Coffee and other irritants like spicy foods and citrus juices also increase heartburn. When the patient is recumbent reflux episodes increase because gravity no longer counters the retrograde flow of intragastric contents across the lower esophageal sphincter. Finally, vomiting often aggravates heartburn.

Heartburn is often relieved by avoiding those aggravating factors described above. The avoidance of exacerbating factors is one arm of the treatment of heartburn. Most patients find that buffering agents like milk or antacids improve heartburn. Some even get relief by drinking water which presumably works by clearing acid from the distal esophagus.

Associated symptoms and illnesses

Dysphagia associated with heartburn indicates a complication arising from gastroesophageal reflux. These patients may also have mechanical lesions of the esophagus like esophageal cancer, peptic stricture or Schatzki's ring. Chronic gastroesophageal reflux may also give rise to esophageal motor abnormalities, like diffuse esophageal spasm, that are known to produce dysphagia. The presence of odynophagia most often indicates severe focal inflammation in the form of erosions or ulcers.

The coexistence of heartburn and respiratory symptoms, like chronic cough, hoarseness, laryngitis, asthma or recurrent pneumonias, should alert the clinician to the possibility that these symptoms are caused by gastroesophageal reflux. A number of historical clues may point to gastro-esophageal reflux as an etiologic factor in asthma. Reflux-related asthma usually starts in adulthood, is not associated with atopy, typically worsens at night and resists the usual therapies. If allowed to progress unchecked, chronic pulmonary injury from gastroesophageal reflux disease may lead to pulmonary fibrosis.

Patients may describe angina pectoris as heartburn. It is essential to take a careful history to distinguish the discomfort of esophageal inflammation from that of myocardial ischemia.

The therapeutic trial as a diagnostic test

Perhaps the simplest, safest and most cost-effective way to determine if heartburn is caused by gastroesophageal reflux is to perform a therapeutic trial with a proton pump inhibitor (Klauser et al 1993). These agents can nearly completely inhibit acid production by the stomach. Resolution of heartburn after 3–4 weeks of therapy with omeprazole at a dose of 40 mg per day is a good indicator that the heartburn comes from acid reflux. Failure of the therapeutic trial suggests that the symptom does not arise from acid reflux and should lead the clinician into a more extensive evaluation. This approach, while useful, should only be employed when the patient presents only with simple heartburn. Concurrent symptoms like dysphagia, odynophagia or chest pain are indicative of more serious problems that should be carefully evaluated.

Endoscopy in the evaluation of the patient with heartburn

Using endoscopy, the clinician is able to identify both obvious signs of esophageal inflammation, like esophageal ulcers or erosions, and subtle inflammatory changes of the esophageal mucosa that are not seen with other methods like the barium swallow. In addition, a visually normal esophageal mucosa does not rule out gastroesophageal reflux and esophagitis as the etiology for heartburn. Biopsies of apparently normal mucosa may demonstrate histologic changes, such as infiltration of the epithelium by eosinophils. Biopsies of erosions or ulcerations of the esophageal mucosa may give clues to the etiology of the inflammation. The identification of viral inclusion bodies or *Candida albicans* makes a diagnosis of a specific infectious esophagitis. For these reasons, all patients with heartburn who undergo endoscopy should have an esophageal biopsy.

Ambulatory intraesophageal pH monitoring in the evaluation of heartburn (Bozymski & Orlando 1993)

Ambulatory esophageal pH monitoring is a simple and widely used method that quantifies esophageal acid exposure (Chapter 6).

While there is little doubt that ambulatory pH monitoring identifies patients with abnormal gastroesophageal reflux (Mattox & Richter 1990), it does not prove that these patients have esophagitis. The diagnosis of esophagitis is made on the basis of symptoms and/or the presence of inflammation of the esophageal mucosa. In addition, the severity of heartburn depends upon the resistance of the esophageal mucosa to acid injury and the sensitivity of the sensory innervation of the esophagus as well as the intensity of esophageal acid exposure. This means that the severity of the symptom of heartburn does not necessarily correlate with the amount of esophageal acid exposure. For these reasons ambulatory pH monitoring should not be considered a first-line test for the evaluation of heartburn.

The main indication for ambulatory pH monitoring is the evaluation of patients with heartburn who have failed antireflux therapy. It can document the presence of excess esophageal acid exposure in patients after treatment with antisecretory drugs or after surgical antireflux procedures (Johnson & DeMeester 1974, Lieberman 1988). Failure to identify excessive esophageal acid exposure suggests that the heartburn does not arise from acid reflux. A small number of patients who do not respond to standard antireflux therapy may suffer from bile reflux esophagitis. Ambulatory pH monitoring is useful in identifying this subgroup. There are also a few patients with heartburn who have no endoscopic or histopathologic evidence of esophagitis, but who have an exquisite sensitivity to acid refluxed into the esophagus. Ambulatory pH monitoring can be useful in documenting the presence of excessive gastroesophageal reflux in these patients.

Esophageal manometry and the barium swallow in the evaluation of heartburn

Esophageal manometry and the barium swallow provide little information that helps in the evaluation or treatment of patients with simple heartburn. They may be useful in the evaluation of patients with heartburn before they undergo an antireflux procedure. The barium swallow documents the presence and extent of a hiatal hernia. Esophageal manometry identifies patients with esophageal motor abnormalities that interfere with the transit of the bolus from the esophagus to the stomach. The presence of a hiatal hernia or motor abnormality alters the surgical approach.

CHEST PAIN OF ESOPHAGEAL ORIGIN

Chest pain is a very disconcerting and anxiety-producing symptom because patients know it to be the primary symptom of a heart attack. Yet, some 10–30% of patients with suspected angina do not have demonstrable ischemic heart disease and 18–58% of this group are estimated to have pain of esophageal origin (Blackwell & Castell 1984, Kemp et al 1973). In practice this translates into the cardiologist ruling out coronary artery disease as the source of pain and referring the patient with 'non-cardiac chest pain' to a gastroenterologist.

Evaluation of the patient with chest pain

Historical features

As with other GI complaints, the most important information to be obtained in the evaluation of the patient with chest pain comes from a careful history and physical examination. The physician must remember that chest pain can arise from any of the organs within the chest or the chest wall. What is typically thought of as non-cardiac chest pain may be indistinguishable from angina pectoris. The pain is usually substernal in location and may be described as squeezing, a dull ache or heaviness. It may radiate into the neck, jaw or arm and may occasionally be brought on by exertion. If the chest pain has these characteristics or is associated with such symptoms as diaphoresis, shortness of breath or light-headedness, ischemic heart disease must be considered before any other diagnosis.

Chest pain arising from the musculoskeletal constituents of the chest wall is probably the most commonly misdiagnosed type of chest pain. This is a chronic pain that is often constant and dull in nature. It is usually least troublesome upon arising in the morning and worsens throughout the day. It is made worse by activity, particularly the use of the upper extremities. It is common for patients to complain of worsening pain after lifting or doing housework. When the pain becomes worse, it often does so precipitously, 'like someone throwing a switch or thrusting a knife into the chest'. Musculoskeletal chest pain is made better by rest, heat applied to the area and non-steroidal antiinflammatory medications. When this type of history is elicited it is important to do a careful musculoskeletal exam. The examiner should pay particular attention to palpation over the costochondral joints, the xiphoid and along the inferior margins of the lower ribs anteriorly. This often reproduces the pain of musculoskeletal origin. If the chest pain is musculoskeletal in origin, further GI evaluation should be abandoned and the pain should be treated appropriately. Examination of the chest wall may on occasion reveal the typical lesions of *Herpes zoster*.

Chest pain may also be either a functional symptom or related to other psychosocial pathology. Patients with panic disorder or anxiety disorders often complain of chest pain. A careful history demonstrates that episodes of chest pain occur most often when the patient is stressed. Associated symptoms may include shortness of breath, lightheadedness, numbness in the fingers and around the mouth and occasionally loss of consciousness. This set of symptoms should alert the clinician to the possibility that the patient has chest pain as part of a hyperventilation syndrome. It is often useful to ask the patient to hyperventilate when hyperventilation syndrome is suspected. The reversal of symptoms by rebreathing from a paper bag is an inexpensive and useful diagnostic test that is often enlightening to the patient. An inquiry into the social history, particularly regarding domestic violence or sexual abuse, may provide clues as to the functional nature of chest pain. Patients with psychosocial pathology as the source of their chest pain should not be subjected to an extensive esophageal work-up as that may only exacerbate their psychological problems. Instead, they should be reassured and referred for a psychological opinion.

The best discriminators of esophageal pain from other types of chest pain are the symptoms associated with the pain. Chest pain that occurs simultaneously with dysphagia, odynophagia, heartburn, nausea, vomiting, water brash or regurgitation is likely to be esophageal in origin. If it is brought on or worsened by drinking very cold liquids or eating ice cream, disorders of esophageal motor function like esophageal spasm may be the source of the pain. Overeating or the ingestion of acid foods like orange juice may produce chest pain in the patient with reflux esophagitis. It is in this group, patients with chest pain and symptoms of esophageal disease, that the clinician is most likely to identify a specific esophageal disorder as the source of chest pain. The work-up should focus on identifying the cause of those symptoms associated with chest pain for their discovery will almost always explain the chest pain.

Endoscopy in the evaluation of the patient with chest pain

Endoscopy is particularly useful in evaluating chest pain because it is the most sensitive way to identify esophagitis and diagnose other intraluminal lesions. While the endoscope does not identify specific esophageal motor abnormalities, an important factor in many motor disturbances is gastroesophageal reflux. Thus, the discovery of mucosal lesions, including esophagitis, should be considered an adequate explanation for non-cardiac chest pain and appropriate treatment should be instituted without further evaluation.

Esophageal manometry in the evaluation of chest pain

If endoscopy fails to identify a mucosal abnormality that might explain chest pain, esophageal manometry should be considered. Since abnormalities of esophageal motor function can cause pain, esophageal manometry is widely used in the hope of identifying a motor disturbance. While manometric abnormalities are prevalent in patients with chest pain, only a small percentage of these patients will have well-defined motor abnormalities like achalasia or diffuse esophageal spasm (Benjamin et al 1983, Ferguson et al 1981, Katz et al 1987, Traube et al 1983). Up to 50% of patients with non-cardiac chest pain have non-specific motor abnormalities of the esophagus that do not conform to the diagnostic criteria for achalasia or diffuse esophageal spasm. The most common of these abnormalities are the *nutcracker esophagus* (peristaltic contractions of very high amplitude) and the *hypertensive lower esophageal sphincter* (a lower esophageal sphincter with an abnormally high resting pressure that relaxes completely with swallowing). The high prevalence of these non-specific abnormalities in patients with chest pain as compared to normal healthy volunteers argues that the esophagus is the source of the pain. However, they are often recorded when the patient does not have pain, making a direct correlation between motor dysfunction and chest pain difficult. Thus, esophageal manometry is likely to diagnose a well-defined and specifically treatable disorder (achalasia or diffuse esophageal spasm) in a small minority of patients with non-cardiac chest pain.

Provocative testing with esophageal manometry. The poor correlation between manometrically proven abnormalities of esophageal motor function and chest pain prompts the use of provocative agents to provoke chest pains and motor abnormalities in patients with non-cardiac chest pain. Provocative testing is done either by the IV infusion of agents like edrophonium and cholinergic agonists or by the infusion of acid into the distal esophagus during manometry. Studies of this type have proven to be poor predictors of motor abnormalities that produce chest pain. They induce motor abnormalities that are temporally associated with pain in less than half of the patients studied and are known to produce non-specific motor abnormalities in normal individuals without chest pain (Benjamin et al 1983). The acid infusion test, also called the Bernstein test, may be the most useful of the provocative tests because it mimics a pathophysiologic state, the gastroesophageal reflux of acid. A positive Bernstein test, that is reproduction of typical chest pain by the infusion of 0.1 N HCl into the esophagus, is good evidence that the symptom of chest pain is caused by exposure of the esophageal mucosa to acid.

There is growing evidence that some patients with non-cardiac chest pain may have an abnormality of the afferent innervation to the esophagus. This abnormal innervation manifests as a decreased threshold for esophageal pain. To test this hypothesis, some investigators have dilated the esophagus with an intraluminal balloon as a stimulus. Up to

50% of patients with non-cardiac chest pain are reported to have typical chest pain reproduced by this method (Richter et al 1986).

Combined 24-hour ambulatory esophageal manometry and pH monitoring was developed several years ago in the hope that it would identify abnormal patterns of esophageal motility or gastroesophageal reflux in patients with non-cardiac chest pain. This did not prove to be the case. In a carefully constructed and thoughtfully analyzed study of patients with non-cardiac chest pain, Breumelhoff et al (1990) were able to

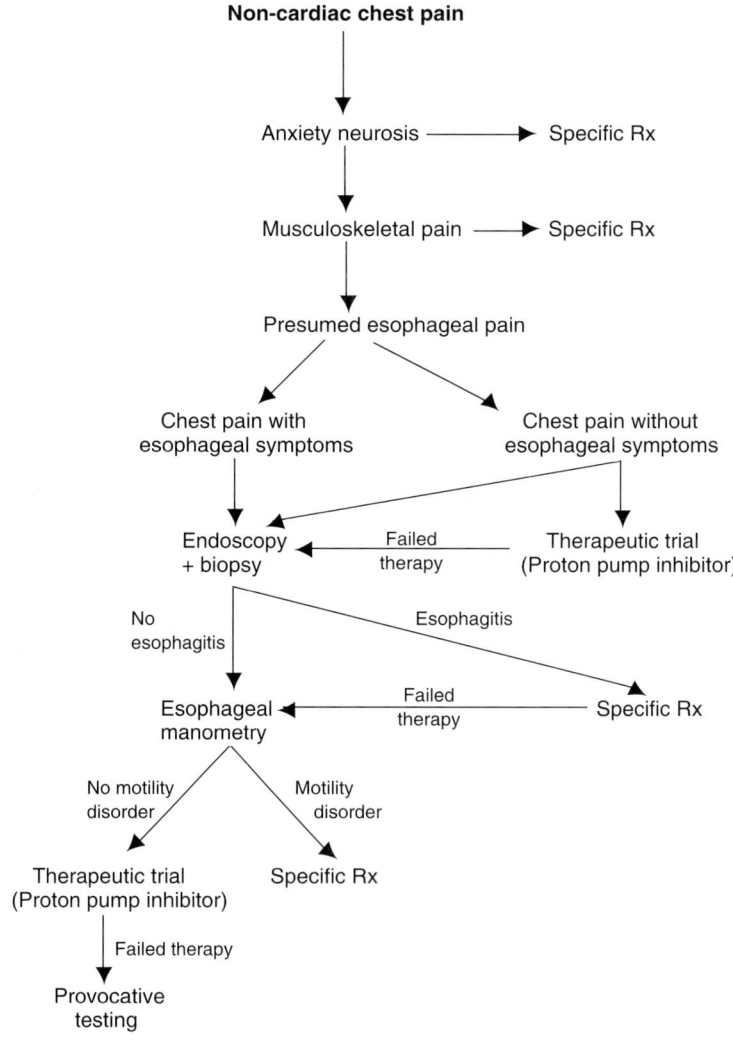

Figure 10.1 One approach to non-cardiac chest pain

correlate less than 20% of episodes of chest pain with gastroesophageal reflux and/or esophageal motor abnormalities. Soffer et al (1989) reported similar results and also found that very few reflux episodes (<5% of total reflux events) are associated with chest pain.

The therapeutic trial as a diagnostic test

As is the case with uncomplicated heartburn, it is reasonable to attempt a therapeutic trial using a proton pump inhibitor in patients with non-cardiac chest pain that is not associated with other symptoms. Resolution of chest pain after 3–4 weeks of therapy with omeprazole at a dose of 40 mg per day is a good indicator that the chest pain comes from acid reflux. Failure of the therapeutic trial suggests that the symptom does not arise from acid reflux and should lead the clinician into a more extensive evaluation. It is also reasonable to attempt a therapeutic trial in any patient with chest pain who has no endoscopic evidence of esophagitis or other esophageal lesions. Patients with chest pain and concurrent symptoms like dysphagia, odynophagia, nausea or vomiting need further evaluation.

Because the pathophysiologic mechanisms of non-cardiac chest pain remain unclear and are probably multifactorial, an unambiguous approach to its evaluation is not possible. In addition, algorithms meant to guide the clinician are likely to change as we learn more about these disorders.

REFERENCES

Benjamin S B, Richter J E, Cordova C M, Knuff T E, Castell D O 1983 Prospective manometric evaluation with pharmacologic provocation of patients with esophageal motility dysfunction. Gastroenterology 84: 893–901
Bieger D, Hopkins D A 1987 Viscerotopic representation of the upper alimentary tract in the medulla oblongata in the rat: the nucleus ambiguous. Journal of Comparative Neurology 262: 546–562
Blackwell J N, Castell D O 1984 Oesophageal chest pain: a point of view. Gut 25: 1–6
Bozymski E M, Orlando R C 1993 Ambulatory intraesophageal pH monitoring. In: Drossman D A (ed) Manual of gastroenterological procedures. Raven Press, New York, pp 50–55
Breumelhof R, Nadorp J H S M, Akkerman L M A, Smout A J P M 1990 Analysis of 24-hour esophageal pressure and pH data in unselected patients with noncardiac chest pain. Gastroenterology 99: 1257–1264
Christensen J, Conklin J L, Freeman B W 1973 Physiologic specialization at the esophagogastric junction in three species. American Journal of Physiology 225: 1265–1270
Code C F, Schlegel J F 1968 Motor action of the esophagus and its sphincters. In: Code C F (ed) Handbook of physiology, section 6: alimentary canal. Vol. IV: Motility. American Physiological Society, Washington DC, pp 1821–1839
Conklin J L, Christensen J 1994 Motor functions of the pharynx and esophagus. In: Johnson R L (ed) Physiology of the gastrointestinal tract. Raven Press, New York
Donner M W, Bosma J F, Robertson D L 1985 Anatomy and physiology of the pharynx. Gastrointestinal Radiology 10: 196–212

Doty R W 1968 Neural organization of deglutition. In: Code C F (ed) Handbook of Physiology, section 6: alimentary canal. Vol. IV: motility. American Physiological Society, Washington DC, pp 1861–1902

Du C, Murray J, Bates J, Conklin J L 1991 Nitric oxide: mediator of nonadrenergic noncholinergic hyperpolarization of opossum esophageal muscle. American Journal of Physiology 261: G1012–1016

Ferguson S C, Hodges K, Hersh T, Jinich H 1981 Esophageal manometry in patients with chest pain and normal coronary arteriogram. American Journal of Gastroenterology 75: 124–127

Goyal R K, Rattan S 1976 Genesis of basal sphincter pressure: effect of tetrodotoxin on lower esophageal sphincter pressure in opossum in vivo. Gastroenterology 71: 62–67

Holstege G, Graveland G, Bijker-Biemond C, Schudeboom I 1983 Location of motoneurons innervating soft palate, pharynx and upper esophagus. Anatomical evidence for a possible swallowing center in the pontine reticular formation. Brain Behavior and Evolution 23: 47–62

Johnson L F, DeMeester T R 1974 Twenty-four hour pH monitoring of the distal esophagus. A quantitative measure of gastroesophageal reflux. American Journal of Gastroenterology 62: 325

Kahrilas P J, Clouse R E, Hogan W J 1994 American Gastroenterological Association technical review on the clinical use of esophageal manometry. Gastroenterology 107: 1865–1884

Katz P O, Dalton C B, Richter J E, Wu W C, Castell D O 1987 Esophageal testing in patients with noncardiac chest pain or dysphagia. Annals of Internal Medicine 593–597

Kemp H G, Vokonas P S, Cohn P F, Gorlin R 1973 The anginal syndrome associated with normal coronary angiograms: report of a six year experience. American Journal of Medicine 54: 735–742

Klauser A G, Voderholzer W A, Muller-Lissner S A 1993 Is empiric acid suppression of diagnostic value in gastroesophageal reflux disease? Gastroenterology 104: A22

Lieberman D 1988 24-hour esophageal pH monitoring before and after medical therapy for reflux esophagitis. Digestive Diseases and Sciences 33: 166–171

Mattox H E, Richter J-E 1990 Prolonged ambulatory esophageal pH monitoring in the evaluation of gastroesophageal reflux disease. American Journal of Medicine 89: 345–356

Murray J, Du C, Ledlow A, Bates J N, Conklin J L 1991 Nitric oxide: mediator of nonadrenergic noncholinergic responses of opossum esophageal muscle. American Journal of Physiology 261: G401–406

Orlando R 1993 Esophageal manometry. In: Drossman D A (ed) Manual of gastroenterological procedures. Raven Press, New York, pp 36–49

Rattan S, Gidda J S, Goyal R K 1983 Membrane potential and mechanical responses to vagal stimulation and swallowing. Gastroenterology 85: 922–928

Richter J E, Barish C F, Castell D O 1986 Abnormal sensory perception in patients with esophageal chest pain. Gastroenterology 91: 845–852

Serio R, Daniel E E 1988 Electrophysiological analysis of responses to intrinsic nerves in circular opossum esophageal muscle. American Journal of Physiology 254: G107–116

Soffer E E, Scalabrini P, Wingate D L 1989 Spontaneous noncardiac chest pain: value of ambulatory pH and motility monitoring. Digestive Diseases and Sciences 34: 1651–1655

Sugarbaker D J, Rattan S, Goyal R K 1984 Mechanical and electrical activity of esophageal smooth muscle during peristalsis. American Journal of Physiology 248: G145–150

Traube M, Albibi R, McCallum R W 1983 High amplitude peristaltic esophageal contractions associated with chest pain. Journal of the American Medical Association 250: 2655–2659

11

Dyspepsia, nausea and vomiting

M. J. Benson

DYSPEPSIA

Definition

Although the term dyspepsia is widely used in clinical practice, it remains ill-defined. In recent years several working party reports have attempted to revise the definition (Barbara et al 1989, Drossman et al 1990, Talley et al 1991, Tytgat et al 1991). Based on their recommendations, dyspepsia may be defined as episodic or persistent upper abdominal pain or discomfort, localized to the epigastrium or upper abdomen and thought by the clinician to arise from the proximal gastrointestinal tract. In addition to this principal or dominant symptom, others may be present, including abdominal bloating and fullness, early satiety, anorexia, nausea, vomiting and heartburn. The symptoms may or may not be related to meals or exercise. It has also been suggested that symptoms should be present for several weeks or months before the term dyspepsia is applied (Talley & Phillips 1988).

Based on the outcome of clinical investigation, patients with dyspepsia can be divided into two groups. Approximately 50% of patients (Thompson 1984) have a clearly identifiable cause for their symptoms (organic dyspepsia) while the remainder do not (functional dyspepsia).

Prevalence

However defined, dyspepsia is one of the most common gastrointestinal complaints. The reported prevalence in the community in Northern European countries is between 19% and 41% (Knill-Jones 1991) and is 25% in the USA (Talley et al 1992).

Classification

Organic dyspepsia

The recognized causes of organic dyspepsia are shown in Box 11.1. Peptic ulcer disease, gastroesophageal reflux, biliary disease and drug-induced dyspepsia – in particular secondary to NSAIDs and alcohol – are the commonest causes.

Box 11.1 Organic causes of dyspepsia

Gastric and duodenal ulcer
Gastroesophageal reflux disease
Gastritis
• Granulomatous (idiopathic, Crohn's, sarcoidosis, TB, syphilis, fungal infection)
• Eosinophilic
• Hypertrophic (Ménétier's disease)
• Diffuse varioliform gastritis
Gastric neoplasm (carcinoma, lymphoma)
Biliary tract disease
• Cholelithiasis/choledocholithiasis
• Biliary dyskinesia/sphincter of Oddi dysfunction
Chronic pancreatitis
Pancreatic carcinoma
Malabsorption syndromes
Drugs (NSAIDs, aspirin, theophylline, potassium/iron supplements, alcohol)
Metabolic disorders
• Hyperthyroidism
• Hyperparathyroidism
• Addison's disease
Miscellaneous
• Ischemic heart disease
• Acute intermittent porphyria

Although some forms of gastritis are undoubtedly associated with dyspeptic symptoms, many patients with the most commonly occurring form, chronic non-erosive antral (type B) gastritis, may be asymptomatic. The prevalence of this type of gastritis increases with age, being present in the majority of the population by the sixth decade (Pettross et al 1988, Rauws et al 1988). It seems unlikely that this type of gastritis is a cause of dyspepsia (Dooley et al 1989, Bernersen et al 1992).

Sphincter of Oddi dysfunction is a rare cause of dyspepsia. It is due either to a primary motor abnormality of the sphincter of Oddi (sphincter of Oddi dyskinesia) or to papillary stenosis. It is usually encountered several years following cholecystectomy, particularly in middle-aged females, and presents with episodic biliary-type pain and is often accompanied by transiently elevated liver function tests.

Functional dyspepsia

Functional dyspepsia probably characterizes a heterogeneous group of patients with more than one underlying pathophysiological mechanism. It is possible to subdivide patients according to different symptom clusters that may reflect different underlying etiologies. Four main subgroups have been proposed (Drossman et al 1990, Talley et al 1991, Tytgat et al 1991): 'ulcer-like' dyspepsia, 'reflux-like' dyspepsia, 'dysmotility-like' dyspepsia and unspecified dyspepsia (Box 11.2).

Box 11.2 Symptom subgroups of functional dyspepsia (Talley 1991a)

'Ulcer-like' dyspepsia
Upper abdominal pain or discomfort and ≥2 of the following symptoms: pain relieved by food or antacids, periodic pain, postprandial pain, nocturnal pain waking patient from sleep.

'Reflux-like' dyspepsia
Upper abdominal pain or discomfort accompanied by heartburn or acid regurgitation.

'Dysmotility-like' dyspepsia
Upper abdominal pain or discomfort and ≥2 of the following symptoms: nausea or vomiting, early satiety or anorexia, postprandial abdominal bloating or distension, excessive bloating.

Unspecified dyspepsia
Upper abdominal pain or discomfort that does not fulfill the criteria for above subgroups.

The etiology of functional dyspepsia remains unknown. No clear association has been demonstrated with dietary, environmental or psychosocial factors or with acid hypersecretion (Talley 1991a). Recent studies have failed to demonstrate any significant increase in the prevalence of either chronic gastritis or *H. pylori* infection in functional dyspepsia when compared to an asymptomatic control population (Holtmann et al 1994). *H. pylori* infection is not associated with any specific symptom cluster (Goh et al 1991, Strauss et al 1990) and eradication does not necessarily correlate with improvement in symptoms (Patchet et al 1991). Based on available data, neither chronic gastritis nor *H. pylori* infection appear to be important etiological factors. Impaired gastric emptying, antral hypo-contractility and decreased visceral sensation have been reported, but whether a gastric motor and/or sensory abnormality is responsible for symptoms, even in a small subgroup, remains to be established (Malagelada 1991, Talley 1991a).

Discriminatory value of dyspeptic symptoms

Given the high prevalence of functional dyspepsia, the problem facing the clinician is differentiating patients with organic dyspepsia who require investigation from those with functional dyspepsia who do not. An organic cause may be suggested by the presence of certain clinical features (Richter 1991).

Peptic ulcer disease

The presence of vomiting and severe pain, relieved by food, is more common in peptic ulcer disease than in functional dyspepsia (Horrocks &

deDombal 1978, Talley & Piper 1986). The best discriminator, especially for duodenal ulcer disease, is the presence of nocturnal pain that awakens the patient from sleep, but while this is present in up to 70% of patients with duodenal ulceration and 33% of patients with gastric ulcer, it is also present in about 33% of patients with functional dyspepsia (Horrocks & deDombal 1978). Evidence of blood loss, particularly in older patients, suggests peptic ulcer disease.

Gastric carcinoma

A short history of unremitting pain, particularly in an elderly patient, is characteristic of gastric carcinoma. Anorexia and weight loss may also be present (Horrocks & deDombal 1978).

Biliary tract disease

Cholelithiasis is characterized by episodes of severe postprandial pain of constant intensity lasting several hours. Radiation to the back, an infrequent symptom in functional dyspepsia, may be a feature (Horrocks & deDombal 1978, Talley & Piper 1986). There may also be a history suggesting intermittent obstructive jaundice and/or abnormal liver biochemistry.

Pancreatic disease

Pain associated with chronic pancreatitis and pancreatic carcinoma is often non-specific but there may be several characteristic features including radiation to the back and an almost instantaneous aggravation by food. In addition, the pain may be eased by sitting forward or lying down and there may be associated steatorrhea or diabetes.

Despite these 'characteristic' features, accurate clinical diagnosis based on symptomatic assessment is often difficult (Healey & Rathbone 1987, Horrocks & deDombal 1978) and may be as low as 50% (Horrocks & deDombal 1975a). While the diagnostic accuracy may be increased by a structured questionnaire (Davenport et al 1985, Horrocks & deDombal 1975b), this approach has not been generally employed as it is too time consuming for routine clinical use. It was hoped that the subdivision of functional dyspepsia into symptom categories may improve diagnostic accuracy (Drossman et al 1990). Recent questionnaire-based studies have demonstrated considerable overlap between these various symptom subgroups and as a result this approach offers little or no diagnostic benefit (Talley et al 1992, 1993).

History and examination

Although it may be difficult to make a firm diagnosis based on symptoms, this does not imply that the history is of no importance. The clinician should ascertain the character, duration and periodicity of the symptoms together with the presence of any precipitating or relieving factors. The site of abdominal discomfort and any radiation should also be established. Other enquiries should be made about the known etiological factors in the organic causes of dyspepsia, for example smoking and consumption of alcohol and medications, with particular attention to self-medication with aspirin and non-steroidal antiinflammatory drugs.

Although physical examination may be normal, it is important to identify abnormalities suggesting an organic cause, including the presence of an abdominal mass, organomegaly, ascites, cachexia or peripheral lymphadenopathy.

Investigation strategy

The initial investigation should include routine hematological (full blood count, ESR) and biochemical (urea and electrolytes, liver function tests, serum calcium and phosphate and C-reactive protein) tests and in addition, thyroid function should be measured if clinically indicated. Any metabolic abnormality should be treated appropriately before proceeding with further investigation. The presence of a low hemoglobin or raised inflammatory indices should alert the clinician to a possible organic cause.

The choice of the initial diagnostic investigation should be dictated by a clinical impression as to the most likely cause of the symptoms based on the history and examination and results of screening investigations. A diagnostic algorithm is shown in Figure 11.1.

Investigation of the esophagus, stomach and proximal duodenum is usually the first to be performed. This can be achieved using either double contrast barium meal or endoscopy. While the accuracy of both methods is comparable (Brown et al 1978), endoscopy permits simultaneous biopsy to be performed and has become the investigation of choice. Endoscopy can be expected to demonstrate an identifiable lesion in over 50% of patients with dyspeptic symptoms deemed to be of sufficient severity to warrant investigation (Davenport et al 1985, Forbat et al 1987, Hallissey et al 1990). The diagnostic yield is age-dependent, being lower in younger patients (Forbat et al 1987) than in the elderly in whom the occurrence of major pathology, namely peptic ulceration and gastric carcinoma, is more common (Lockhart et al 1985).

Overall, the commonest endoscopic finding is esophagitis secondary to gastroesophageal reflux disease. Nevertheless, it is important to remember that up to 50% of patients, in whom reflux is the cause of symptoms, have

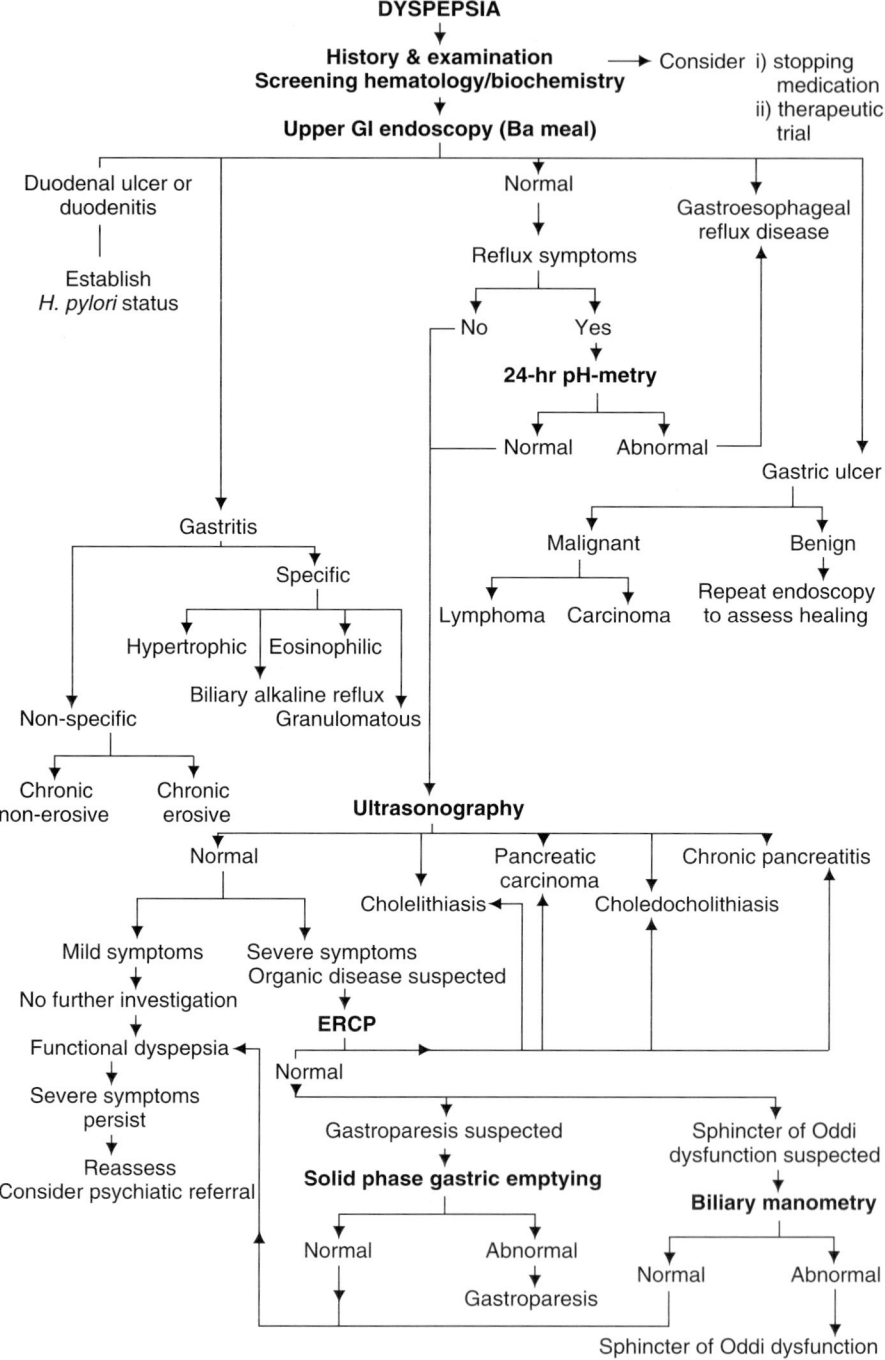

Figure 11.1 Diagnostic algorithm for dyspepsia

no detectable endoscopic abnormality of the esophageal mucosa (Joelsson & Johnsson 1989). However, clinical suspicion that reflux may be the cause of the symptoms is heightened if endoscopy demonstrates the presence of a hiatus hernia. Objective evidence of the presence of gastro-esophageal reflux causing symptoms can only be obtained by prolonged 24-hour pH-metry (see Chapters 1 and 6). Many physicians would employ a therapeutic trial with a proton pump inhibitor or H_2 blocker and only proceed to 24-hour pH-metry in those patients in whom the therapeutic trial afforded little or no symptomatic improvement.

Gastric ulcers should always be biopsied because of their malignant potential. With the strong association between *H. pylori* antral gastritis and duodenal ulcer disease (Dooley & Cohen 1988, Warren & Marshall 1983), an antral biopsy should be performed to look for the presence of the organism, either histologically or using the CLO urease test, in all patients with either erosive duodenitis or duodenal ulceration. In patients who also have diarrhea, distal duodenal biopsies should be taken to exclude a malabsorptive state. Areas of gastritis should also be biopsied to enable histological diagnosis.

Extraluminal organs, including the liver and pancreas, may be investigated either using ultrasonography or CT scan, both of which have a high sensitivity and specificity for detecting gallstones and pancreatic disease. Although the accuracy of a CT scan is slightly higher, it is usual to perform ultrasonography in the first instance as patient exposure to ionizing radiation is not involved and the technique is widely available and cheaper. CT scanning should be reserved for those instances when either ultrasound investigation was incomplete for technical reasons or was negative but underlying pancreatic or biliary disease is suspected. ERCP is the most sensitive and specific test for structural abnormalities of the pancreas and biliary tree but is invasive, expensive and involves ionizing radiation. As a diagnostic test, it should be reserved for the small number of cases where the index of clinical suspicion of pancreatobiliary disease is high, based on the history and/or serum biochemistry but where ultrasound and CT scan have revealed no abnormality. The role of endoscopic ultrasound (DiMagno et al 1982) and MRI scanning in the diagnosis of pancreatobiliary disease have yet to be established.

Cholelithiasis is a common finding and often asymptomatic and there-fore in the absence of other characteristic features, dyspepsia should not necessarily be attributed to gallstones. Chronic pancreatitis and pancreatic carcinoma can be diagnosed with a high degree of certainty with pan-creatic function testing (DiMagno et al 1977), but the usefulness of such testing has declined with the improved accuracy of radiological imaging. None of the available serological markers for pancreatic carcinoma are sensitive or specific enough to be used as a diagnostic test.

The above imaging techniques of the biliary tree lead to a definitive diagnosis in the majority of patients with biliary type pain, but cannot establish a firm diagnosis in cases of suspected sphincter of Oddi dysfunction. The cholangiogram obtained at ERCP may have provided some indirect evidence by demonstrating a dilated common bile duct ($\geq$12 mm), in the absence of a ductal stricture or calculi and/or delayed emptying of contrast medium into the duodenum. A non-invasive functional assessment of sphincter of Oddi activity can be obtained by real-time ultrasonography following a fatty meal (Daraweesh et al 1988), a bolus of secretin (Bolondi et al 1984) or by radioisotopic cholescintigraphy (Roberts-Thompson et al 1986). However, the sensitivity and specificity of these tests remain to be determined and their clinical role is currently ill defined. Endoscopic biliary manometry is the most objective test available for assessing sphincter of Oddi motor activity. There are four pathophysiological patterns:

1. elevated basal pressure ($\geq$40 mmHg);
2. rapid phasic activity;
3. excessive retrograde propagation ($\geq$50% of contractions);
4. paradoxical response to CCK-octapeptide with stimulation of activity rather than inhibition.

Gastroparesis typically presents with postprandial nausea and vomiting. In milder forms of the condition, the main symptom may be dyspepsia. With mild non-incapacitating symptoms, it is probably not worth undertaking quantitative assessment of gastric motor function unless there is nutritional compromise or the patient is known to have a systemic disease that may be complicated by gastroparesis (e.g. diabetes mellitus). This hypothesis is supported by the observation that some patients with functional dyspepsia have delayed gastric emptying, but improvement of gastric emptying with treatment with a prokinetic agent was not correlated to any symptom improvement (Corinaldesi et al 1987, Davis et al 1988, Jain et al 1989). Thus, mild abnormalities of gastric motor function may be unrelated to the symptoms.

Some patients with predominantly upper abdominal pain also have symptoms which suggest colonic dysfunction. In young patients, these symptoms are usually due to the irritable bowel syndrome. In older patients and in those where screening investigations reveal an anemia with normal upper gastrointestinal investigations, a double contrast barium enema examination is essential to exclude organic disease of the colon.

Deciding when not to investigate a patient with dyspepsia may present difficulties. The major source of unease is missing an occult gastric neoplasm. Gastric carcinoma in young patients under 45 years of age is rare (Forbat et al 1987). It seems reasonable, in young patients with dyspepsia with no signs or symptoms of organic disease, to postpone initial investigation until after a 4–6 week therapeutic trial of antacid or H_2 blocker together with relevant advice about smoking, alcohol consumption and drugs (Health and Public Policy Committee, American College of Physicians 1985). An alternative approach is to screen young patients for *H. pylori* using serology and then to offer empirical H_2 antagonists to those who are negative and to gastroscope those who are positive. Whether *H. pylori* eradication is indicated for dyspepsia with no detectable mucosal lesion apart from non-erosive gastritis remains controversial.

Management

Patients with peptic ulcer disease should be treated with a course of antiulcer therapy (either H_2 blocker or proton pump inhibitor). For *H. pylori*-positive patients with erosive duodenitis or duodenal ulceration, treatment should also include eradication therapy. A repeat endoscopy should be performed following treatment when a gastric ulcer has been diagnosed because of the potential for occult malignancy. Gastritis, with the possible exception of chronic non-erosive gastritis, should be treated as indicated by histology. Lymphoma and carcinoma should be further assessed using CT scanning prior to a decision on subsequent management, i.e. surgery ± chemotherapy ± radiotherapy or surgery ± chemotherapy respectively.

In patients with chronic pancreatitis, management is directed at pain relief and treatment of any pancreatic insufficiency with enzymatic supplementation. A similar approach applies where pancreatic carcinoma has been diagnosed in addition to further assessment for either surgery and/or chemotherapy. Patients with choledocholithiasis should undergo therapeutic ERCP to remove the ductal calculi.

Medical treatment for sphincter of Oddi dysfunction has proved disappointing but an endoscopic sphincterotomy may produce prolonged symptomatic improvement (Geenen et al 1989). The therapeutic role of the endoscopic papillary balloon dilatation has yet to be established.

Patients with functional dyspepsia may or may not require any specific therapy. Their major concern is an underlying organic cause for symptoms. Once reassured that no serious pathology is present and advised regarding the avoidance of possible precipitating factors, many patients accept their symptoms, which are usually mild, and do not need or want further medication (Talley & Phillips 1988).

For patients with intractable symptoms, various therapeutic agents including antacids, H_2 blockers and prokinetic agents have been employed; 30–60% of patients show a placebo response to prescribed therapies (Talley & Phillips 1988). The development of 'targeted' therapeutic strategies is further compounded by the fact that functional dyspepsia represents a heterogeneous group whose etiopathogenesis is poorly understood. The symptom subgroups of 'ulcer-like', 'reflux-like' and 'dysmotility-type' dyspepsia have been used as a basis for different treatment regimes. However, the usefulness of this approach to determine management is questionable due to the large overlap of symptoms between the various subgroups (Talley et al 1992, 1993). The use of antacids is not indicated as they offer no symptomatic benefit other than a placebo effect (Gotthard et al 1988, Nyrén et al 1986). Data on the effectiveness of H$_2$ blockers are contradictory, but there is evidence to suggest that patients with 'reflux-like' and to a lesser extent 'ulcer-like' dyspepsia are most likely to be afforded symptomatic improvement (Gotthard et al 1988, Talley et al 1986). Based on these data, it would seem reasonable to use H$_2$ blockers only in patients in these subgroups.

The role of prokinetic agents has not been fully established but available data suggest that both domperidone and cisapride improve symptoms (Talley 1991b). Symptomatic improvement is not necessarily correlated to improvement of gastroduodenal motor activity (Corinaldesi et al 1987, Davis et al 1988, Jain et al 1989). Although long-term studies are still required, prokinetic agents should be considered for patients with 'dysmotility-like' and perhaps 'reflux-like' dyspepsia. Due to the overlap between the symptom subgroups, if treatment with an H$_2$ blocker is ineffective, a prokinetic agent should be tried and vice versa. The data on the use of sucralfate and bismuth in functional dyspepsia are inconclusive. *H. pylori* eradication has not been shown to result in any convincing symptomatic improvement (Talley 1991a) and cannot be recommended as a useful therapeutic maneuver in the management of functional dyspepsia.

NAUSEA AND VOMITING

Definition

Nausea describes the sensation that precedes vomiting, although vomiting may not necessarily occur. Nausea is often associated with hyper-salivation. The term may also be used to describe a variety of other sensations including early satiety, abdominal fullness, anorexia and a dislike of food.

Vomiting is defined as the forceful expulsion of gastric or intestinal contents through the mouth. This is effected by a coordinated reflex motor response involving both somatic and visceral musculature and is often preceded by retching in which a similar motor response occurs without the expulsion of upper gastrointestinal contents.

Regurgitation and rumination may be confused with vomiting. Two features allow regurgitation of stomach contents into the mouth to be distinguished from vomiting: the absence of accompanying nausea and lack of somatic motor response. The causes for this symptom include mechanical or functional obstruction of the esophagus and free gastro-esophageal reflux. Rumination is the repetitive regurgitation of small amounts of food into the mouth soon after a meal. The regurgitated food bolus is usually reswallowed. This is a common self-limiting condition in young children but may also occur in adults. No mechanical or physio-logical abnormality of the esophagus has been identified and it is thought to represent an acquired behavioral response. Rumination may become more prominent during periods of stress, while in others it represents a voluntary and often pleasurable act.

Pathophysiology

Current understanding of the pathophysiology of nausea and vomiting is based on data obtained primarily from the cat (Borison & Wang 1953). A schematic representation of the mechanisms involved is shown in Figure 11.2. While not specifically tested, similar mechanisms are believed to apply in man.

Two anatomically and functionally distinct areas within the medulla are involved in the vomiting response, the vomiting center and the chemotrigger zone. The former is located within the reticular formation and receives excitatory afferent activity, primarily via the vagus nerve, from visceral nociceptors located in the gastrointestinal tract, peritoneum, mesenteric vasculature, biliary ducts, pharynx and heart. The vomiting center also receives other excitatory afferent inputs from higher centers within the central nervous system. These pathways may be involved in

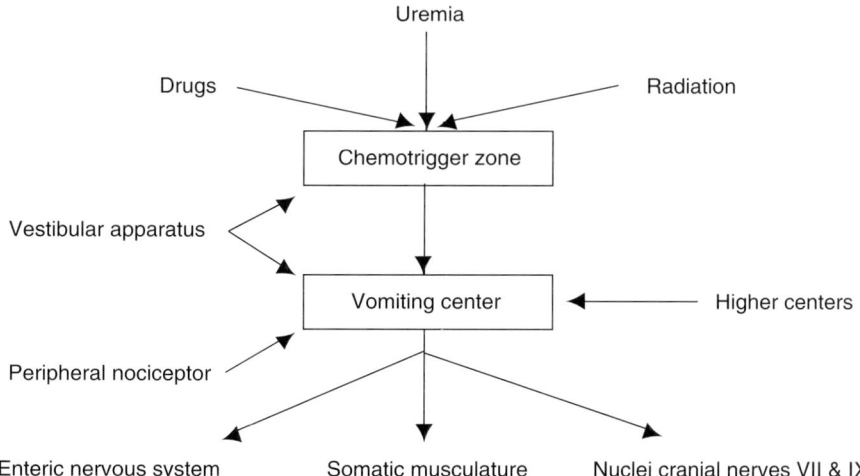

Figure 11.2   Schematic representation of the pathophysiology of nausea and vomiting

nausea and vomiting thought to be functional (e.g. psychogenic) in origin or precipitated by 'noxious' olfactory, gustatory and visual stimuli. The chemotrigger zone is situated in the area postrema in the floor of the fourth ventricle and is activated by direct chemical stimulation. Once activated, the chemotrigger zone produces a neurally mediated excitation of the vomiting center. The chemotrigger zone is involved in nausea and vomiting associated with drugs (e.g. opiates, digoxin) and uremia (Borison et al 1984), radiation sickness (Alexander et al 1989) and possibly motion sickness (Borison et al 1984).

The major efferent pathway from the vomiting center goes to the somatic musculature involved in vomiting, the diaphragm, abdominal wall and intercostal muscles. In addition, there are visceral vagal efferent pathways responsible for the characteristic gastroduodenal motor response observed during nausea and vomiting, namely a reduction in antral phasic and tonic activity and orad propagated proximal small bowel phasic activity that is responsible for the reflux of intestinal contents into the stomach immediately prior to emesis. The motor nuclei of both VII and XI cranial nerves are activated, explaining the increase in salivation observed during nausea and vomiting.

History and examination

While the duration of symptoms is readily established from the history, the patient's description of severity is often exaggerated in terms of both frequency and volume of vomitus. When evaluating cases of acute nausea and vomiting, the presence or absence of coexistent abdominal pain may help in formulating a differential diagnosis. In the absence of pain, the underlying etiology may be infectious (e.g. viral gastro-enteritis), neurological (e.g. labyrinthitis, headache) or drug related. The presence of abdominal pain as a predominant symptom suggests an acute surgical cause for the symptoms (e.g. small bowel obstruction, acute cholecystitis).

It is not uncommon for patients to complain of chronic vomiting when in fact they are experiencing either regurgitation or rumination. These symptoms have a different differential diagnosis, investigation and sub-sequent management and it is therefore important to ascertain the exact nature of the symptom by careful questioning.

In patients with chronic vomiting, the temporal relationship between emesis and the ingestion of food can provide helpful clues in establishing the underlying cause. Vomiting that occurs during or early in the post-prandial period, i.e. within 1 hour of the meal, is characteristic of a functional underlying cause, in particular psychogenic vomiting and eating disorders. However, this association is not diagnostic as a similar pattern of emesis is often observed in patients with a peripyloric peptic ulcer. When vomiting occurs up to several hours after eating meals, it is likely that the underlying cause is impaired gastric emptying due to either gastric outflow obstruction or gastroparesis. In such circumstances, it is essential to inquire about a previous history of peptic ulcer disease as this is the most likely cause of impaired emptying (Kozoll & Meyer 1964). Vomiting occurring soon after waking is commonly observed in pregnancy but may also be a feature of uremia, alcohol abuse or raised intracranial pressure. Vomiting without associated nausea may suggest raised intracranial pressure and has been described as 'projectile'; however, this term is difficult to define accurately, lacks both sensitivity and specificity and is best avoided.

Information about the possible underlying cause may also be obtained from the content and odour of the vomitus. The clinician should inspect the vomitus, if possible, rather than rely upon the patient's description. The presence of undigested food is suggestive of regurgitation. Consistently large volumes of vomitus together with the presence of partly digested food imply impaired gastric emptying, especially if the last meal was several hours prior to emesis. Where gastric stasis is due to mechanical obstruction at or proximal to the pylorus, the vomitus may not contain bile. However, the presence of bile in the vomitus is not a specific feature because bile may be regurgitated from the duodenum into the stomach in sufficient quantities to stain the vomitus, irrespective of the cause. An unusually heavy load of bile may occur in patients who have had previous gastric surgery. Vomitus with a feculent odor suggests either chronic small bowel obstruction with secondary bacterial overgrowth or a gastrocolic fistula.

Other important considerations are the drug history, including alcohol consumption, and the presence of coexistent disease known to be complicated by nausea and vomiting (e.g. diabetes mellitus). Neurological symptoms of recent onset may suggest a lesion within the central nervous system as a cause for the symptoms.

Although the clinical examination is often normal, important physical signs should be sought. The presence of abdominal tenderness or succussion splash may be valuable in differential diagnosis. Neurological examination including fundoscopy should be performed and lying and standing blood pressure should be measured to look for postural hypotension. The latter may provide some indication of the severity of the vomiting and may also alert the clinician to the presence of an autonomic neuropathy.

Differential diagnosis

Acute nausea and vomiting

The major causes of acute nausea and vomiting are shown in Box 11.3. Intraabdominal causes are usually associated with severe pain and

---

Box 11.3 Causes of acute nausea and vomiting

Infection
- Gastroenteritis
- Hepatitis
- Herpes virus (CMV, HSV, VZV) in immunocompromised patients

Small bowel obstruction
- Mechanical
  — Adhesions
  — Volvulus
  — Obstructed hernia
  — Tumor
- Functional
  — Postoperative ileus
  — Paralytic ileus

Acute pancreatitis/acute cholecystitis

Drugs
- Antibiotics
- Opiates
- Chemotherapeutic agents

CNS origins
- Labyrinthitis
- Headache
- Head injury

---

present as acute 'surgical' emergencies. The investigation and subsequent surgical management of these conditions are beyond the scope of this chapter. Infectious causes are usually clinically apparent as symptoms settle either spontaneously or following treatment. In general, such cases require no further investigation. Similarly, drug-induced nausea and vomiting is usually obvious from the history and resolves on withdrawal of the offending drug.

Chronic nausea and vomiting

There are many causes of chronic nausea and vomiting. The following discussion is limited to those conditions in which nausea and/or vomiting usually represent a prominent feature of the presenting 'symptom complex'. It is worth noting that conditions which characteristically present with dyspepsia may on occasion present with nausea and vomiting and vice versa.

The major causes of chronic nausea and vomiting are shown in Box 11.4.

Pregnancy. Nausea and vomiting are common in pregnancy. Nausea occurs in approximately 90% of all pregnancies while vomiting occurs in

---

Box 11.4 Causes of chronic nausea and vomiting

Gastric outflow obstruction
- Mechanical
  - — Gastric malignancy
  - — Chronic peptic ulcer disease
  - — Duodenal carcinoma
  - — Crohn's disease
  - — Pancreatic disease
- Functional
  - — Gastroparesis
  - — Diabetes mellitus
  - — Scleroderma
  - — Anorexia nervosa
  - — Idiopathic
  - — Postgastric surgery

Intestinal pseudoobstruction
- Amyloidosis
- Diabetes mellitus
- Familial visceral neuropathy/myopathy
- Hypothyroidism
- Scleroderma

Raised intracranial pressure

Drugs

Psychogenic causes
- Anorexia nervosa
- Bulimia

Metabolic/endocrine causes
- Hypothyroidism
- Addison's disease
- Hyper/hypocalcemia
- Uremia

Pregnancy
- Nausea and vomiting of pregnancy
- Hyperemesis gravidarum

---

approximately 50%. Symptoms may begin soon after the missed period, before the pregnancy is diagnosed.

Approximately three per 1000 pregnancies are complicated by severe vomiting (hyperemesis gravidarum), with the mother developing both fluid and electrolyte disturbances and nutritional deficiencies. Symptoms start early in the pregnancy and usually resolve spontaneously by the end of the third trimester. The cause of this condition is not clear, but it may be part of an underlying psychosomatic disorder.

Mechanical obstruction.

Gastric outflow obstruction. Gastric emptying may be impaired by any mechanical lesion compromising the patency of the lumen of the distal stomach or proximal small bowel. The commonest cause for outlet obstruction, accounting for approximately 80% of cases, is scarring from chronic pyloric channel or duodenal ulcer disease (Kozoll & Meyer 1964). Obstruction may also occur as the result of inflammatory edema from an acute ulcer with underlying scarring causing subcritical impairment of gastric outflow. Other causes of outflow obstruction include eosinophilic and granulomatous gastritis, gastric antral neoplasm (e.g. carcinoma or lymphoma), adult hypertrophic pyloric stenosis, gastric bezoars, superior mesenteric artery syndrome, duodenal neoplasms and inflammatory strictures. Patients may present with upper abdominal fullness and a characteristic pattern of vomiting. The stomach may become atonic and grossly distended, causing left-sided abdominal pain.

Small bowel obstruction. Partial small bowel obstruction due to either a tumor or an inflammatory stricture may cause chronic nausea and vomiting. Vomiting occurs after a meal and is even more delayed than vomiting due to gastric outlet/high duodenal obstruction. Patients often present with accompanying abdominal pain and bloating that is characteristically relieved by vomiting.

Functional obstruction – gastroparesis. Gastroparesis describes the condition in which gastric motor activity is impaired with consequent delayed gastric emptying. Gastroparesis has become increasingly recognized as a cause of hitherto unexplained nausea and vomiting.

Gastroparesis may be classified as being primary (idiopathic) or secondary to gastric surgery or systemic disease (Box 11.5). Irrespective of the underlying cause, gastroparesis gives rise to variable symptoms; while some patients may experience only mild chronic dyspeptic symptoms (bloating, early satiety, nausea), others have symptoms indistinguishable from those of mechanical outflow obstruction.

Idiopathic. This represents the largest group. The onset of symptoms is usually insidious although in a small proportion of patients, the appearance of symptoms is preceded by a 'flu-like' illness, suggesting a possible viral etiology. The clinical course is equally variable, symptoms spontaneously remitting after several months in some patients while continuing or worsening in others.

Secondary. Symptomatic gastric stasis is a well-recognized if uncommon complication of gastric surgery. It occurs after subtotal gastrectomy or operations which have included a truncal or selective vagotomy. The pathogenesis of this problem is poorly understood. Following vagotomy, antral contractile activity is reduced (Malagelada et al 1980), and while this may contribute to delayed emptying of solids, it cannot explain delayed emptying after antrectomy and vagotomy or subtotal gastrectomy, where the antrum has been surgically removed.

The Roux-en-Y procedure may also be complicated by gastric stasis.

Box 11.5   Classification of gastroparesis

1 Idiopathic

2 Secondary
   - Postsurgical
     Distal gastric resection and vagotomy
   - Visceral myopathy
     Primary visceral myopathy (familial, non-familial)
     Connective tissue disease (scleroderma, dermatomyositis, systemic lupus erythematosus)
     Muscular dystrophies (myotonia dystrophica, progressive muscular dystrophy)
     Infiltrative diseases (amyloidosis)
   - Visceral neuropathy
     Primary neuropathy (familial, non-familial)
     Primary autonomic dysfunction (Shy–Drager syndrome, idiopathic hypotension)
     Diabetes mellitus
     Postviral
   - Drugs
     Adrenergic agonists
     Dopaminergic D_2 agonists
     Cholinergic antagonists
     Opioids
     Cytotoxic agents
   - Metabolic/endocrine
     Hypoparathyroidism
     Hypothyroidism
     Pheochromocytoma
     Uremia
   - Miscellaneous
     Paraneoplastic
     Small-cell carcinoma of lung
     Radiation injury

This is thought to be due to retrograde peristalsis developing in the jejunal arm causing a functional impairment to gastric emptying through the gastrojejunostomy (Miedema & Kelly 1991). Symptoms are difficult to treat and often surgical reversal of the Roux-en-Y is required.

Diabetic gastroparesis usually occurs in patients with long-standing poorly controlled insulin-dependent diabetes, particularly where other complications of the disease are present (e.g. autonomic neuropathy, retinopathy, nephropathy). Delayed gastric emptying occurs in approximately 20% of insulin-dependent diabetics. Most are asymptomatic and the prevalence of symptomatic gastroparesis has been estimated as less than 1% (De Ponti et al 1987). Although some patients experience persistent nausea and vomiting, the more usual clinical picture is that of episodes of nausea and vomiting lasting for several days or weeks before gradually resolving. In the intervening periods, patients may be relatively symptom free.

Motility studies have demonstrated postprandial antral hypomotility (Abell et al 1988) and increased pyloric tonic and phasic activity and proximal small bowel dysmotility (Mearin et al 1986). The functional consequence of the former observation is a reduction of the grinding effect of the antrum on solid food particles, while the latter increases resistance to flow of the gastric contents into the duodenum. Both these effects act to delay gastric emptying. The precise pathogenesis of these findings is not fully understood. Diabetic gastroparesis is generally believed to be the result of an autonomic neuropathy although not all patients have clinical evidence of this (Keshavarzian et al 1987).

Connective tissue disorders may be complicated by gastroparesis, which most commonly occurs in progressive systemic sclerosis. Gastroparesis is a relatively late complication and nausea and vomiting may be overshadowed by those symptoms resulting from impaired motility in other regions of the gastrointestinal tract, namely gastroesophageal reflux, bacterial overgrowth secondary to small bowel dysmotility and constipation. Early in the disease process, gastrointestinal symptoms are thought to arise from a neuropathy while later in the disease the smooth muscle can be involved, giving rise to a myopathy.

Other causes are listed in Box 11.5 and represent well-recognized but rare causes of gastroparesis.

Central nervous system disorders. Raised intracranial pressure may present with nausea and vomiting. There is usually accompanying headache and alteration of conscious state. Peripheral neurological signs and papilledema may also be present.

Functional disorders

Eating disorders. Anorexia nervosa and bulimia are relatively common neuropsychiatric disorders affecting 5–10% of the young female population (Kurtzman et al 1989). Patients suffering from anorexia present with weight loss but may also complain of a variety of gastrointestinal symptoms including nausea and vomiting, together with early satiety, bloating and constipation. In anorexia, delayed solid-phase gastric emptying has been demonstrated (McCallum et al 1985) but this is likely to be secondary to central nervous system stress effects or to be a direct consequence of malnutrition rather than a primary abnormality (Rigaud et al 1988). In bulimia, vomiting is one of the major symptoms and up to 50% of patients have electrolyte disturbances, usually hypokalemic hypochloremic alkalosis, as a consequence of vomiting (Halmi 1987). No characteristic pathological or physiological findings are associated and diagnosis is based on identifying characteristic behavioral patterns.

Psychogenic vomiting. Psychogenic vomiting typically occurs in young women. Patients give a history of chronic vomiting which may be accompanied by severe abdominal pain. Vomiting tends to be associated with meals, occurring during or shortly after the meal and is rarely preceded by nausea. There is often an underlying emotional disturbance (Wruble et al 1982) but rarely is there an underlying psychiatric disturbance (Muraska et al 1990).

Cyclic vomiting. This condition is characterized by paroxysmal attacks of nausea and vomiting lasting up to several days and may be associated with fever, headache or abdominal pain. Recovery tends to be spontaneous and patients are completely well between episodes. The condition usually resolves around the time of puberty, but it may persist into early adulthood. The pathogenesis of the condition is unclear. Evidence for an underlying psychological abnormality is contradictory (Abell et al 1988, Reinhart et al 1977).

Investigation strategy

As with the investigation of dyspepsia, the first investigation should include a routine hematological (full blood count, ESR) and biochemical profile (urea and electrolytes, liver function tests, serum calcium and phosphate, C-reactive protein) together with thyroid function tests. In all female patients of childbearing age, a serum or urinary β-HCG estimation should be requested to exclude pregnancy. Several biochemical abnormalities, including hypercalcemia, hypokalemia, hyperglycemia, ketoacidosis and hypothyroidism, can either cause or contribute to chronic nausea and vomiting. These should be corrected and the symptomatic response monitored before any further investigation is undertaken. Likewise, any possible role of any medication should be evaluated by discontinuing the drug, if possible, before further investigation is arranged.

Selecting further diagnostic tests depends on the clinical impression formulated from the history and examination. A diagnostic algorithm is shown in Figure 11.3.

In circumstances where clinical signs are few, the next investigation should be aimed at excluding a pathological lesion, e.g. peptic ulcer or gastritis in the upper GI tract. This can be achieved by either a double contrast barium meal or upper GI endoscopy. The relative merits of these two investigations have already been considered.

If endoscopy is negative and especially if the history is suggestive of a psychogenic cause, a CT scan should be done to exclude intracranial pathology. If normal, no further investigation is warranted. For patients with recent onset of neurological signs and symptoms, a CT brain scan is mandatory.

The clinical investigation of symptoms secondary to mechanical or non-mechanical obstruction is complex. Tests to detect anatomical abnormalities and physiological dysfunction are required.

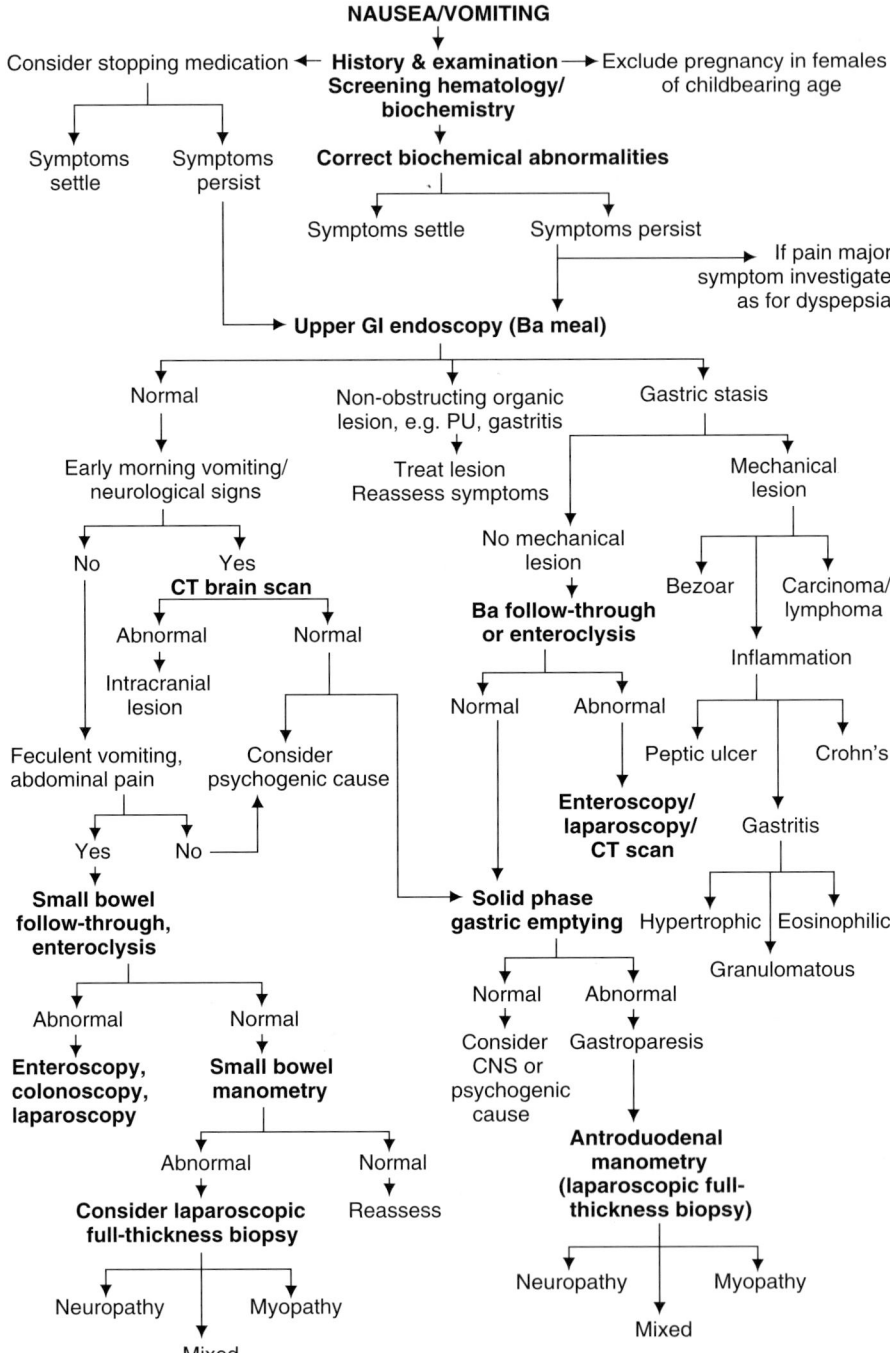

Figure 11.3 Diagnostic algorithm for chronic nausea and vomiting

Gastric stasis

If gastric stasis is suspected, indirect evidence for the diagnosis can be obtained from a plain abdominal X-ray which may demonstrate massive gastric enlargement with the stomach occupying the entire left side of the abdomen. An upper GI barium study will identify the site of any obstruction, may suggest the nature of the underlying cause and, unlike routine upper GI endoscopy, also permits visualization of the distal duodenum. If a lesion is identified, subsequent upper GI endoscopy with biopsy should be performed. Due to the risk of pulmonary aspiration, endoscopy is best performed following a 24–48 hour period of gastric aspiration and/or gastric lavage. Neither ultrasonography nor CT scan are first-line investigations in patients with gastric outflow obstruction. However, both can be useful in obtaining further information in patients with an extrinsic obstructive cause.

Symptoms of gastric stasis in the absence of a demonstrable mechanical lesion suggest gastroparesis. Gastric emptying of both solids and liquids is controlled by integration of fundal tone, antral phasic activity, pyloric phasic and tonic activity and phasic activity of the proximal duodenum (Meyer 1991) and physiological dysfunction of one or more of these may cause symptomatic delayed gastric emptying. For a clinical diagnosis of gastroparesis to be made, the impairment of gastric motor activity must be demonstrated. This may be investigated either by measuring gastric emptying to assess overall function or by measuring phasic and contractile activity to identify the underlying pathophysiological abnormality.

Radioisotopic scintigraphy has become the 'gold standard' for studying gastric emptying (see Chapter 2). It has superseded conventional radiological methods (e.g. barium meal or 'barium burger' meal) since, in addition to involving exposure to lower doses of ionizing radiation, it permits quantitative evaluation of gastric emptying. Measurement of solid emptying is more sensitive than that of liquid emptying in detection of underlying pathophysiology (Lin & Meyer 1991). A possible explanation for this is that solid emptying requires vigorous antral phasic activity to both grind food particles and propel them through the pylorus. In contrast, liquid emptying may be virtually independent of phasic motor activity, with liquids passing into the duodenum along a pressure gradient created by tonic contractile activity in the fundus or by gravity.

Several other techniques permit quantitative assessment of gastric emptying, namely applied potential tomography (Avill et al 1987), gastric impedance (Sutton et al 1985), real-time ultrasonography (Holt et al 1986) and magnetic resonance imaging (Schwizer et al 1992). Both applied potential tomography and gastric impedance are based on the principle that passage of an electrical current through the trunk is related to the electrical resistance of the intervening tissues. Intragastric contents with a different resistance to that of the surrounding tissues will modify the overall resistance to the flow of electric current. Therefore changes in electrical impedance, measured over the upper abdomen, provide an indirect measure of the change in volume of the stomach (Spyrou & Castillo 1993). The major limitations of these two methods are that only liquid emptying can be measured and reproducibility is poor. Similarly, real-time ultrasonography and MRI are restricted to liquid meals. Although of potential clinical interest because they do not require ionizing radiation, further development of these methods is required before they can be employed as a clinical diagnostic test.

Gastric emptying studies identify patients with gastric stasis, but provide little information about the underlying cause. Further data may be obtained by direct measurement of gastric and proximal small bowel motor activity. Although several non-invasive techniques are currently being developed, the method of choice remains intraluminal manometry. Short duration stationary manometry allows study of antral, pyloric and duodenal responses to eating, but prolonged ambulant manometry is required to characterize small bowel motility. Manometry enables the magnitude and temporospatial relationships of individual contractions to be quantified and provides objective data on the site and type of physiological disturbance. Abnormalities may be classified as myopathic, neuropathic or mixed. In the myopathic group, the contractile amplitude is reduced while the pattern of contractile activity is normal. In the neuropathic group the contractile amplitude is normal but the phasic activity is abnormally propagated (Camilleri 1993).

Patients found to have a myopathic process should be screened for a connective tissue disorder. If a chronic inflammatory condition is present, rectal biopsy should be performed to exclude amyloid. If neuropathic changes are present, autonomic function tests should be performed. If no clinical evidence for this can be found, it can be assumed that the neuropathy is confined to the enteric nervous system. The pathophysiologic classification on the basis of intraluminal studies is indirect and definitive confirmation of an enteric myopathy or neuropathy can only be obtained by histological examination of full-thickness biopsies of the gut wall. Such biopsies can now be obtained laparoscopically but should be limited to those patients with severe refractory symptoms in whom it is considered that a more definite diagnosis will be helpful to the overall management.

Small intestinal obstruction

Barium contrast radiology is the investigation of choice. Small bowel enema (or enteroclysis) is more sensitive than barium meal follow-through (Gurian et al 1982) but is less well tolerated by patients and is more time consuming. A reasonable approach would be to perform a barium meal follow-through and proceed to enteroclysis if results are negative or inconclusive. Obstructing lesions within the terminal ileum can usually be reached by colonoscope and biopsied. The recent development of push-enteroscopy enables biopsies to be obtained from lesions in the proximal jejunum (Davies et al 1995), but a large proportion of the small bowel remains inaccessible endoscopically. Even without histological diagnosis, the management of symptomatic small bowel tumors is surgical excision. In the case of a presumed inflammatory lesion a more conservative approach is desirable. The major differential diagnosis is between Crohn's disease, tuberculosis and lymphoma. Radiological appearances may favor one of these (e.g. short multiple strictures in tuberculosis), but if diagnostic uncertainty persists, then laparoscopy and peritoneal biopsy may prove helpful. If any doubt remains, a tissue diagnosis should be obtained at laparotomy.

In the absence of mechanical obstruction of the small bowel, intestinal pseudoobstruction should be excluded. Functional assessment can be made of small bowel motor activity by measuring small bowel transit rates using radioscintigraphy. The diagnostic value is poor because of marked intrinsic variability. Manometric abnormalities of the small bowel have been described in chronic idiopathic pseudoobstruction (Camilleri 1993) and myopathic and neuropathic causes may be distinguished. When the manometric data are inconclusive but the diagnosis is strongly suspected, particularly in the presence of an associated systemic disease, a definitive diagnosis may be obtained by histological examination of a full-thickness biopsy.

Management

The management of peptic ulceration and gastritis has already been considered. Where active peptic ulcer disease is complicated by gastric outflow obstruction, initial management should be medical with either H_2 blockers or proton pump inhibitors. Although the acute ulcer may heal, symptomatic stasis persists as a consequence of severe scarring of the gastric outflow tract due to chronic peptic ulceration and operative intervention is often required. Gastric outflow obstruction caused by other inflammatory lesions (e.g. granulomatous gastritis, Crohn's disease) should be treated medically in the first instance, in the expectation that the inflammation will settle and the patient's symptoms resolve. If significant symptoms persist, surgery should be considered. The management of obstruction due to malignancy or extramural lesions is surgical. Symptomatic gastric bezoars may be removed endoscopically in a piecemeal fashion (Rider et al 1984) or surgically if this fails. A similar approach may be adopted for partial obstruction of the small bowel.

Gastroparesis should initially be managed by treating any underlying cause and by dietary manipulation. Patients should be advised to consume frequent small meals. Solid foodstuffs with a high content of indigestible material are best avoided because of the risk of bezoar formation. Liquid nutrient meals may be required in patients with severe gastroparesis because of an inability to empty solids from the stomach. If these conservative measures fail, treatment with prokinetics should be considered. Prokinetic agents (e.g. domperidone, cisapride and erythromycin) can increase gastric emptying in gastroparetic patients, although their long-term therapeutic effectiveness has yet to be fully established. These drugs act by increasing the release of neurotransmitters within the enteric nervous system and, perhaps not surprisingly, are most effective in circumstances where there is an underlying neuropathy, while patients with a myopathy are unlikely to respond to this treatment. Prokinetics also improve symptoms in postoperative gastroparesis, except in the 'Roux stasis syndrome', while the outcome of further surgical management is unpredictable and generally disappointing. The 'Roux stasis syndrome' is difficult to manage and often the only treatment is surgical reversal of the Roux-en-Y anastomosis.

In circumstances where symptoms are severe and intractable, nutritional support may be necessary. If the motor abnormality is restricted to the stomach, enteral jejunal feeding via either a nasojejunal tube or a feeding jejunostomy is possible. If both small bowel and gastric motor activity are abnormal, as is often the case in a myopathic process, this treatment often fails and home parenteral nutrition may be required. The outcome after surgical drainage procedures is usually disappointing and they are best avoided.

The management of intestinal pseudoobstruction is similar to that outlined for gastroparesis. It is possible to manage milder forms with dietary manipulation, advising the patient to take small, frequent, low-residue meals. Prokinetics may be of some benefit when a neuropathy is suspected. Symptoms may be exacerbated by secondary bacterial overgrowth. This may respond to cyclical broad-spectrum antibiotics. Patients with severe symptoms who do not respond to these measures usually require home parenteral nutrition. Occasionally, surgical resection or bypass is indicated when the disease process appears localized (e.g. megaduodenum).

Early morning sickness associated with pregnancy does not usually require any specific therapy. Patients with hyperemesis gravidarum require fluid and electrolyte replacement together with supportive psychotherapy. Psychotherapy may also be of benefit in patients with psychogenic vomiting. Cyclical vomiting and vomiting secondary to eating disorders are usually refractory to any specific treatment and are best managed by simple supportive means.

REFERENCES

Abell T L, Kim C H, Malagelada J-R 1988 Idiopathic cyclic nausea and vomiting – a disorder of gastrointestinal motility. Mayo Clinic Proceedings 63: 1169–1175

Alexander E, Siddon R L, Loeffler J S 1989 The acute onset of nausea and vomiting following stereotactic radiosurgery: correlation with total dose to area postrema. Surgical Neurology 32: 40–44

Avill R, Mangnal Y F, Bird N C et al 1987 Applied potential tomography. A new, noninvasive technique for measuring gastric emptying. Gastroenterology 92: 1019–1026

Barbara L, Camilleri M, Corinaldesi R et al 1989 Definition and investigation of dyspepsia. Consensus of an international ad hoc working party. Digestive Diseases and Sciences 34: 1272–1276

Bernersen B, Johnsen R, Bostad L, Straume B, Sommer A-I, Burhol P G 1992 Is *Helicobacter pylori* the cause of dyspepsia? British Medical Journal 34: 1276–1278

Bolondi L, Gaiani S, Gullo L, Labo G 1984 Secretin administration in duct dilatation of the main pancreatic duct. Digestive Diseases and Sciences 19: 802–808

Borison H L, Wang S C 1953 Physiology and pharmacology of vomiting. Pharmacological Review 5: 193–207

Borison H L, Borison R, McCarthy L E 1984 Role of the area postrema in vomiting and related functions. Federal Proceedings 43: 2955–2958

Brown P, Salmon P R, Burwood R J, Knox A J, Clendinnen B G, Read A E 1978 The endoscopic, radiological and surgical findings in chronic duodenal ulceration. Scandinavian Journal of Gastroenterology 13: 557–560

Camilleri M 1993 Study of human gastroduodenojejunal motility: applied physiology in clinical practice. Digestive Diseases and Sciences 38: 785–794

Corinaldesi R, Stanghellini V, Raiti C, Rea E, Salgemini R, Barbara L 1987 Effect of chronic administration of cisapride on gastric emptying of a solid meal and on dyspeptic symptoms in patients with idiopathic gastroparesis. Gut 28: 300–305

Daraweesh R M A, Dodds W J, Hogan W J et al 1988 Efficacy of quantitative hepatobiliary scintigraphy and fatty meal sonography for evaluating patients with suspected partial common bile duct obstruction. Gastroenterology 94: 779–786

Davenport P M, Morgan A G, Darborough A, deDombal F T 1985 Can preliminary screening of dyspeptic patients allow more effective use of investigational techniques? British Medical Journal 290: 217–220

Davies G R, Benson M J, Gertner D G, van Someren R N M, Rampton D S, Swain C P 1995 The clinical role of 'push-type' enteroscopy. Gut 37: 346–352

Davis R H, Clench M H, Mathias J R 1988 Effects of domperidone in patients with chronic unexplained upper gastrointestinal symptoms: a double blind, placebo-controlled study. Digestive Diseases and Sciences 33: 1505–1511

De Ponti F, Fealy R D, Malagelada J-R 1987 Gastrointestinal syndromes due to diabetes mellitus. In: Dyck P J, Thomas P K, Ashury A K, Winegrad A I, Porte D Jr (eds) Diabetic neuropathy. W B Saunders, Philadelphia, p 155

DiMagno E P, Malagelada J-R, Taylor W F, Go V L W 1977 A prospective comparison of current diagnostic tests in pancreatic carcinoma. New England Journal of Medicine 297: 737–742

DiMagno E P, Regan P T, Clain J E 1982 Human endoscopic ultrasonography. Gastroenterology 83: 824–829

Dooley C P, Cohen H 1988 The clinical significance of *Campylobacter pylori*. Annals of Internal Medicine 108: 70–79

Dooley C P, Cohen H, Fitzgibbons P L, Bauer M, Appleman M D, Perez-Perez G I, Blaser M J 1989 Prevalence of *Helicobacter pylori* infection and histologic gastritis in asymptomatic persons. New England Journal of Medicine 321: 1562–1566

Drossman D A, Thompson G W, Talley N J et al 1990 Identification of subgroups of functional bowel disease disorders. Gastroenterology International 3: 159–172

Forbat L N, Gribble R J, Baron J H 1987 Gastrointestinal endoscopy in the young. British Medical Journal 295: 365

Geenen J E, Hogan W J, Dodds W J, Toouli J, Venu R P 1989 The efficacy of endoscopic sphincterotomy in postcholecystectomy patients with sphincter of Oddi dysfunction. New England Journal of Medicine 320: 82–87

Goh K L, Parasakthi N, Peh S C, Wong N W, Lo Y L, Puthucheary S D 1991 *Helicobacter pylori* infection and non-ulcer dyspepsia: the effect of treatment with colloidal bismuth subcitrate. Scandinavian Journal of Gastroenterology 26: 1123–1131

Gotthard R, Bodemar G, Brodin U, Jönsson K-A 1988 Treatment with cimetidine, antacid or placebo in patients with dyspepsia of unknown origin. Scandinavian Journal of Gastroenterology 23: 7–18

Gurian L, Jendrzejewski J, Katon R, Bilbao M, Cope R, Melnyk C 1982 Small bowel enema – an underutilised method of small bowel examination. Digestive Diseases and Sciences 27: 1101–1108

Hallissey M T, Allum W H, Jewkes A J, Ellis D J, Fielding J W L 1990 Early detection of gastric cancer. British Medical Journal 301: 513–515

Halmi K A 1987 Anorexia and bulimia. Annual Review of Medicine 38: 373–780

Health and Public Policy Committee, American College of Physicians 1985 Endoscopy in the evaluation of dyspepsia. Annals of Internal Medicine 102: 266–269

Healey R V, Rathbone B J 1987 Dyspepsia: a dilemma for doctors? Lancet ii: 779–782

Holt S, Cervantes J, Wilkinson A, Kirk Wallace J H 1986 Measurement of gastric emptying rate in humans by real time ultrasonography. Gastroenterology 90: 918–923

Holtmann G, Goebell H, Holtmann M, Talley N J 1994 Dyspepsia in healthy blood donors. Pattern of symptoms and association with *Helicobacter pylori*. Digestive Diseases and Sciences 39: 1090–1098

Horrocks J C, deDombal F T 1975a Computer aided diagnosis of 'dyspepsia'. American Journal of Digestive Diseases 20: 397–406

Horrocks J C, deDombal F T 1975b Diagnosis of dyspepsia using data collected by a 'physician's assistant'. British Medical Journal 2: 421–423

Horrocks J C, deDombal F T 1978 Clinical presentation of patients with 'dyspepsia'. Gut 19: 19–26

Jain R, Ducrot F, Ruskone A et al 1989 Symptomatic, radionuclide and therapeutic assessment of chronic idiopathic dyspepsia. A double-blind placebo controlled evaluation of cisapride. Digestive Diseases and Sciences 34: 657–664

Joelsson B, Johnsson F 1989 Heartburn – the acid test. Gut 30: 1523–1528

Keshavarzian A, Iber F L, Vaeth J 1987 Gastric emptying in patients with insulin-requiring diabetes mellitus. American Journal of Gastroenterology 82: 29–35

Knill-Jones R P 1991 Geographical differences in the prevalence of dyspepsia. Scandinavian Journal of Gastroenterology 26 (Suppl 182): 17–24

Kozoll D D, Meyer K A 1964 Obstructing gastroduodenal ulcers: general factors influencing incidence and mortality. Archives of Surgery 88: 793

Kurtzman F D, Yager J, Landsver J, Wiesmeier E, Bodurka D C 1989 Eating disorders among selected female student populations at UCLA. Journal of the American Dietetic Association 89: 45–53

Lin H C, Meyer J H 1991 Disorders of gastric emptying. The physiology of gastric motility and gastric emptying. In: Yamada T (ed) Textbook of gastroenterology Vol I. J B Lippincott, Philadelphia, pp 1213–1234

Lockhart S P, Schofield P M, Gibble R J, Baron J H 1985 Upper gastrointestinal endoscopy in the elderly. British Medical Journal 290: 283

Malagelada J-R, Rees W D W, Mazzolta L J, Go V L W 1980 Gastric motor abnormalities in diabetic and postvagotomy gastroparesis: effect of metoclopramide and bethanecol. Gastroenterology 78: 286–293

Malagelada J-R 1991 Gastrointestinal motor disturbances in functional dyspepsia. Scandinavian Journal of Gastroenterology 26 (Suppl 182): 29–32

McCallum R W, Grill B B, Lange R, Planky M, Glass E E, Greenfeld D G 1985 Definition of gastric emptying abnormality in patients with anorexia nervosa. Digestive Diseases and Sciences 30: 713–722

Mearin F, Camilleri M, Malagelada J-R 1986 Pyloric dysfunction in diabetics with recurrent nausea and vomiting. Gastroenterology 90: 1919–1925

Meyer J H 1991 The physiology of gastric motility and gastric emptying. In: Yamada T (ed) Textbook of gastroenterology, Vol I. J B Lippincott, Philadelphia, pp 137–157

Miedema B W, Kelly K A 1991 The Roux operation for postgastrectomy syndromes. American Journal of Surgery 161: 256–261

Muraska M, Mine K, Matsumoto K, Nakai Y, Nakagawa T 1990 Psychogenic vomiting: the relation between patterns of vomiting and psychiatric diagnosis. Gut 31: 526–528

Nyrén O, Adami H-O, Bates S, Bergström R, Gustavsson S, Loof L, Nyberg A 1986 Absence of therapeutic benefit from antacids or cimetidine in non-ulcer dyspepsia. New England Journal of Medicine 314: 339–343

Patchett S, Beattie S, Leen E, Keane C, O'Moraine C 1991 Eradicating *Helicobacter pylori* and symptoms of non-ulcer dyspepsia. British Medical Journal 303: 1238–1240

Pettross C W, Appleman M D, Cohen H, Valenzuela J E, Chandrasoma P, Laine L A 1988 Prevalence of *Campylobacter pylori* and association with antral mucosal histology in subjects with and without upper gastrointestinal symptoms. Digestive Diseases and Sciences 33: 649–653

Rauws E A J, Langenberg W, Houthoff H J, Zanen H C, Tytgat G N J 1988 *Campylobacter pylori*-disassociated chronic active antral gastritis. Gastroenterology 33: 649–653

Reinhart J B, Evans L, McFadden D L 1977 Cyclic vomiting in children: seen through the psychiatrist's eyes. Pediatrics 59: 371

Richter J E 1991 Stress and psychologic and environmental factors in functional dyspepsia. Scandinavian Journal of Gastroenterology 26 (Suppl 182): 40–46

Rider J A, Foresti-Lorenti R F, Garrido J, Puletti E J, Rider D L, King A H, Bradley S P 1984 Gastric bezoars: treatment and prevention. American Journal of Gastroenterology 79: 357–359

Rigaud D, Bedig G, Merrouche M, Vulpillat M, Bonfils S, Apfelbaum M 1988 Delayed gastric emptying in anorexia nervosa is improved by completion of a re-nutrition program. Digestive Diseases and Sciences 8: 919–925

Roberts-Thomson I C, Toouli J, Blanchett W, Lichtenstein M, Andrews J T 1986 Assessment of bile flow by radioscintigraphy in patients with biliary type pain after cholecystectomy. Australia and New Zealand Journal of Medicine 16: 788–793

Schwizer W, Maeke H, Fried M 1992 Measurement of gastric emptying by magnetic resonance imaging. Gastroenterology 103: 369–376

Spyrou N M, Castillo F D 1993 Electrical impedance measurements. In: Kumar D, Wingate D (eds) An illustrated guide to gastrointestinal motility, 2nd edn. Churchill Livingstone, London, pp 276–289

Strauss R M, Wang T C, Kelsey P B et al 1990 Association of *Helicobacter pylori* infection with dyspeptic symptoms in patients undergoing gastroduodenoscopy. American Medical Journal 89: 464–469

Sutton J A, Thompson S, Sobnack R 1985 Measurement of gastric emptying rates by radioactive isotope scanning and gastric impedance. Lancet i: 898–900

Talley N J 1991a Non-ulcer dyspepsia: myths and realities. Alimentary and Pharmacological Therapeutics 5 (Suppl 1): 145–162

Talley N J 1991b Drug treatment in functional dyspepsia. Scandinavian Journal of Gastroenterology 26 (Suppl 182): 47–56

Talley N J, Phillips S F 1988 Non-ulcer dyspepsia: potential causes and pathophysiology. Annals of Internal Medicine 108: 865–879

Talley N J, Piper D W 1986 Comparison of the clinical features and illness behaviour of patients presenting with dyspepsia of unknown cause (essential dyspepsia) and organic disease. Australia and New Zealand Journal of Medicine 16: 352–359

Talley N J, McNeil D, Hayden A, Piper D W 1986 Randomised, double-blind, placebo-controlled crossover trial of cimetidine and pirenzepine in non-ulcer dyspepsia. Gastroenterology 91: 149–156

Talley N J, Colin-Jones D, Koch K L, Koch M, Nyrén O, Stanghellini V 1991 Functional dyspepsia: a classification with guidelines for diagnosis and management. Gastroenterology International 4: 145–160

Talley N J, Zinsmeister A R, Schleck C D, Melton L J 1992 Dyspepsia and dyspepsia subgroups: a population-based study. Gastroenterology 102: 1259–1268

Talley N J, Weaver A L, Tesmer D L, Zinsmeister A R, 1993 Lack of discriminant value of dyspepsia subgroups in patients referred for upper endoscopy. Gastroenterology 105: 1378–1386

Thompson W G 1984 Non-ulcer dyspepsia. Canadian Medical Association Journal 130: 565–569

Tytgat G N J, Heading R C, Knill-Jones R P, Richter J E, Malagelada J-R, Nyrén O, Talley N J 1991 Towards an understanding of dyspepsia. An update and consensus from an international working party. Scandinavian Journal of Gastroenterology 26 (Suppl 182): 1–74

Warren J R, Marshall B 1983 Unidentified curved bacilli on gastric epithelium in active chronic gastritis. Lancet i: 1273–1275

Wruble L D, Rosenthal R H, Webb W L Jr 1982 Psychogenic vomiting: a review. American Journal of Gastroenterology 77: 318–321

12

Abdominal pain

J. Christensen

SPECIFIC FEATURES OF ABDOMINAL PAIN

The character of abdominal pain

The quality or character of abdominal pain can strongly suggest the nature of the responsible pathological process. Pains are difficult to describe, however, and patients' vocabularies may not be adequate. If the patient does not volunteer a description the examiner can fruitfully press for a description by offering terms or phrases from which the patient can choose. Offered a wide selection, patients may choose terms which can then be pursued for further description, but some patients will refuse all descriptions. Abdominal pains thus can be classified in three categories which have different implications: *bright pains, dull pains and undifferentiated pains*.

Bright pains are those which patients describe with such terms as 'hot', 'burning', 'sharp', 'knifelike', 'stabbing' or 'sour'. Bright pains nearly always reflect a mucosal pathology.

Dull pains are those which patients may describe as 'dull', 'squeezing', 'cramping', 'like something too big' or 'like something moving around'. These pains seem more difficult for people to describe, but such descriptors usually indicate an origin either in a solid organ or in the muscular walls of the gastrointestinal tract.

Undifferentiated or indescribable pains are those which cannot be described by either bright or dull terms or cannot be described at all ('just a pain') or are described as an 'ache' or a 'soreness'. Such pains often arise in solid organs. Pancreatic pain, for example, is almost always indescribable and abdominal wall pain often is. Pain referred to the abdomen in myocardial ischemia and in pneumonia or pulmonary embolus is also usually indescribable.

The severity of pain can be judged by asking patients to rate it on a 1–10 scale, by asking them to compare it to a commonly experienced pain such as a labor pain or by asking how it limits activities. How does it affect work, play, sleep and rest? The latter, as a functional assessment of severity, may be the more nearly objective measure of severity.

The location of abdominal pain

The location of abdominal pain suggests the organ of origin. Some abdominal pains radiate so that they have both *primary* and *secondary sites* (Figs 12.1, 12.2). Usually, the pain appears first and is most severe at the primary site, but not always. The radiations or projections of abdominal

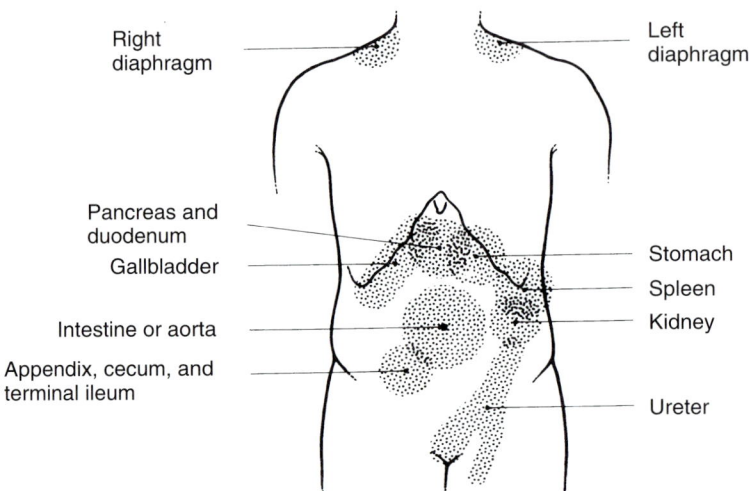

Figure 12.1 Anterior view showing primary and secondary sites of pain from various organs.

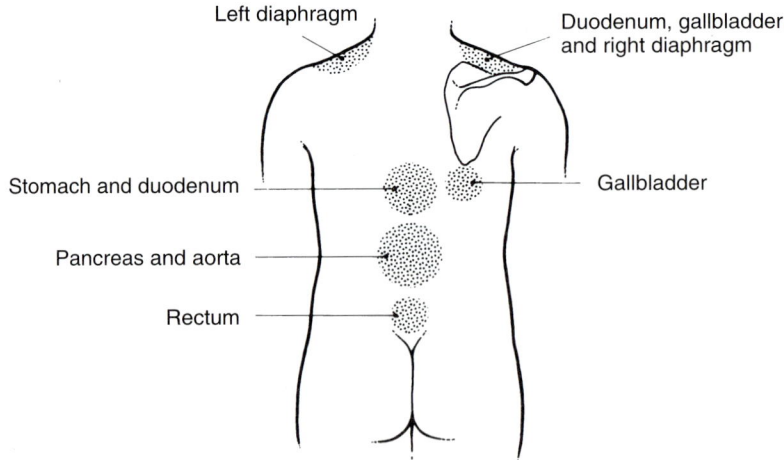

Figure 12.2 Posterior view showing sites of radiation or projection of pains of abdominal origin.

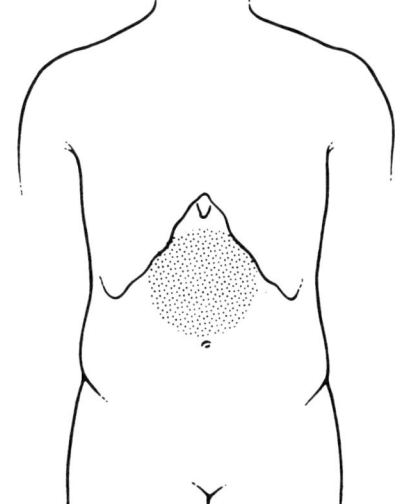

1. Pancreatitis
2. Duodenal ulcer
3. Gastric ulcer
4. Cholecystitis
5. Pancreatic carcinoma
6. Hepatitis
7. Intestinal obstruction
8. Appendicitis (early)
9. Subphrenic abscess
10. Pneumonia
11. Pulmonary embolus
12. Myocardial pain

Figure 12.3 The commonest causes of pain in the epigastrium.

pains mainly reflect the shared sensory innervations of various parts of the body but visceral pains can be poorly localized so location of pain is often quite misleading.

Primary epigastric pain usually arises from the organs located there, pancreas, stomach, duodenum or liver (Fig. 12.3). Pancreatic pain often projects straight through to the back, to the midline in the lumbar region (Fig. 12.4). Pain from the stomach and duodenum do so less often and seem to be a little higher in the back when they do so. Liver pain often projects into the chest, mainly on the right. Sometimes thoracic disease produces mainly epigastric pain. This can be true of myocardial ischemia, pulmonary inflammation and esophagitis.

Primary pain in the right hypochondrium usually arises from the gallbladder, duodenum, pancreas, liver or (rarely) colon (Fig. 12.5). Gallbladder pain often projects straight through to a point just below the tip of the right scapula. Much less often, it can project to the base of the neck on the right side. This is the location of pain referred from the right diaphragm. Pain from the liver commonly projects across the abdomen toward the left side and sometimes projects into the right flank.

Primary pain in the left hypochondrium usually signifies an origin in the spleen, less often in the stomach, rarely in the left hepatic lobe or colon (Fig. 12.6). Splenic pain sometimes radiates to the base of the neck on the left, the projection site for the left diaphragm, and it may radiate to the left flank.

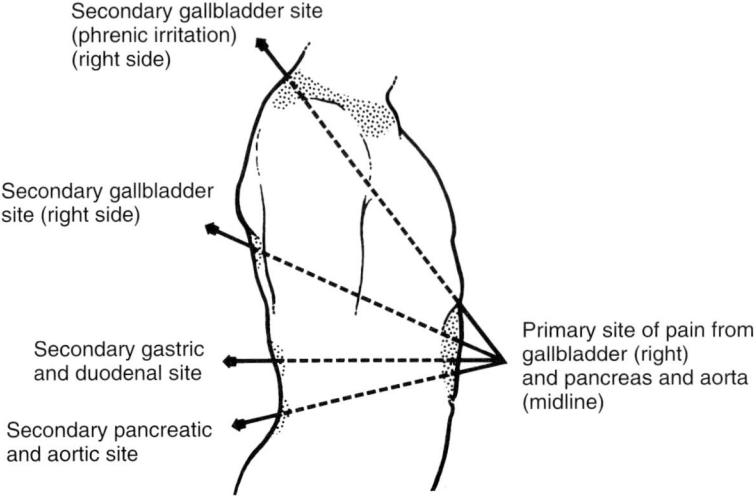

Figure 12.4 Epigastric pains radiating to the back often differ slightly in the level to which they seem to project.

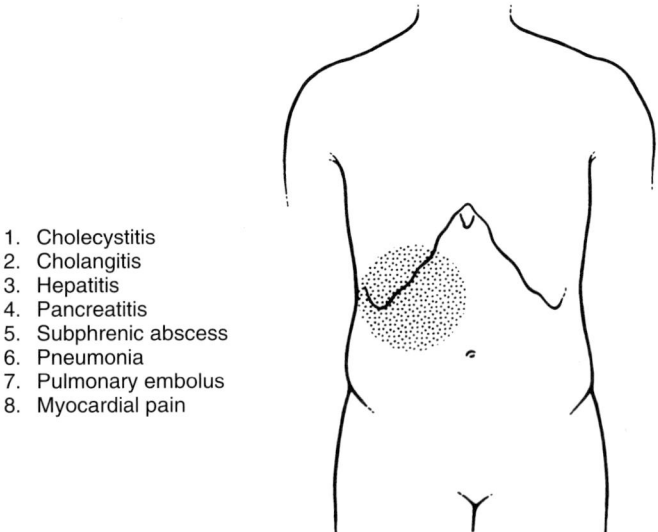

1. Cholecystitis
2. Cholangitis
3. Hepatitis
4. Pancreatitis
5. Subphrenic abscess
6. Pneumonia
7. Pulmonary embolus
8. Myocardial pain

Figure 12.5 The commonest causes of pain in the right hypochondrium.

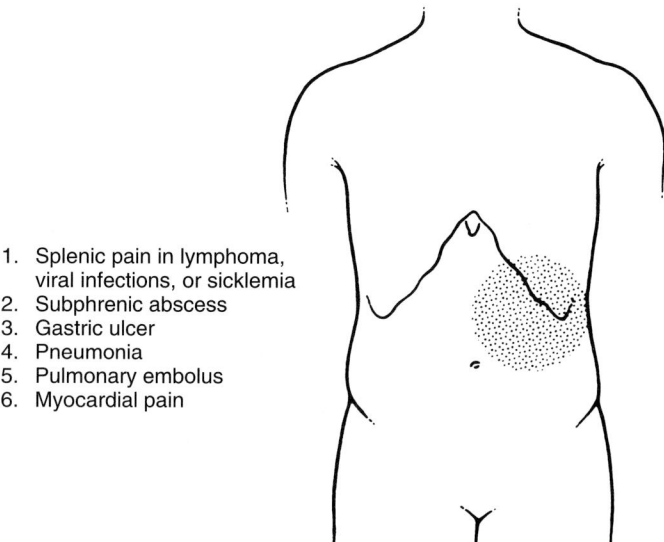

1. Splenic pain in lymphoma, viral infections, or sicklemia
2. Subphrenic abscess
3. Gastric ulcer
4. Pneumonia
5. Pulmonary embolus
6. Myocardial pain

Figure 12.6 The commonest causes of pain in the left hypochondrium.

Primary pain in the periumbilical region most commonly arises from the small intestine, the aorta or the pancreas (Fig. 12.7). Small intestinal pain seems almost never to project to the back whereas pain from the other organs often does. Projection of a periumbilical pain to the back usually signifies an origin in retroperitoneal structures.

Primary pain in the flanks usually arises from the kidneys, but it may arise from an abnormally placed gallbladder or the colon on the right or from the left colon on the left (Fig. 12.8). Renal pain often seems to project laterally around the flank to the back but colonic pain does not (Fig. 12.9). Ureteral pain projects down over the abdomen toward or into the genitalia (Fig. 12.1). Colonic pain usually spreads diffusely toward the midline anteriorly.

Primary pain in the inguinal areas and suprapubic region may be colonic in origin but more often signifies ureteral, renal or adnexal origins (Fig. 12.10). Rarely, gastric pain may be perceived in the lower abdomen.

The chronology of abdominal pain

The onset of the pain, its timing and its circumstances may provide major clues to the nature of the pathological process. If the character and location of the pain have not changed since the onset, the process itself probably has not changed.

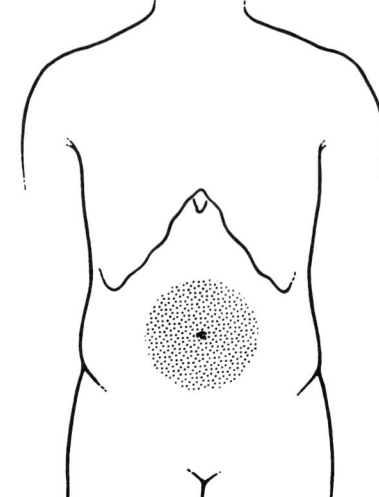

1. Pancreatitis
2. Pancreatic carcinoma
3. Intestinal obstruction
4. Aortic aneurysm
5. Appendicitis (early)

Figure 12.7 The commonest causes of pain in the periumbilical region.

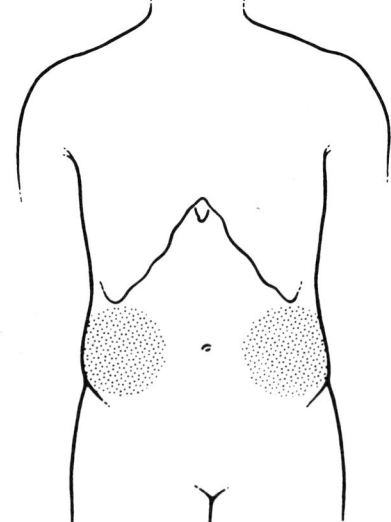

1. Kidney stone
2. Pyelonephritis
3. Perinephric abscess
4. Colonic cancer

Figure 12.8 The commonest causes of pain in the flanks.

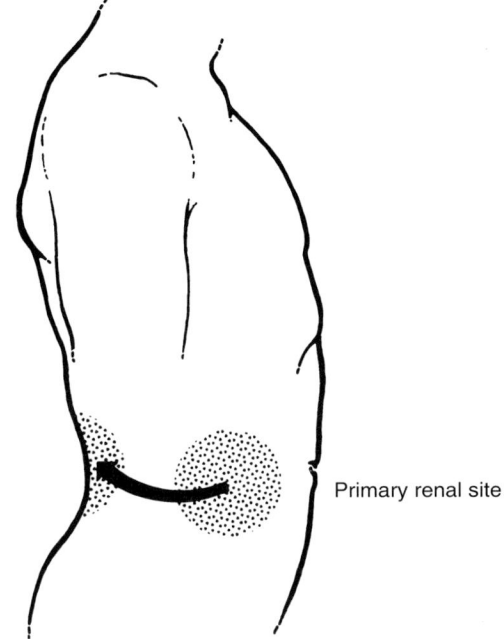

Figure 12.9 A frequent pattern of radiation of renal pain.

Primary renal site

1. Colonic diseases
2. Appendicitis (right side)
3. Diverticular disease (left side)
4. Salpingitis
5. Cystitis
6. Ovarian cyst
7. Ectopic pregnancy
8. Mittelschmerz

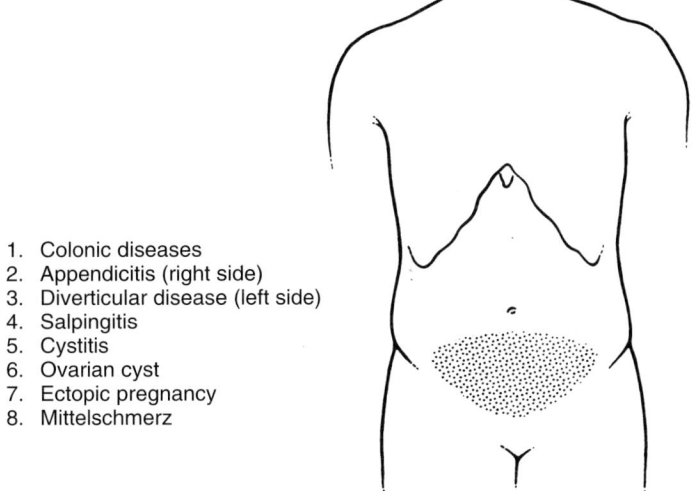

Figure 12.10 The commonest causes of pain in the suprapubic and inguinal areas.

The circumstances of the onset can be most helpful. If none are volunteered, the examiner can suggest some – an injury or accident, a period of emotional or physical stress, an operation, the use of an unusual drug or an unusually large drug dosage, a large meal or a period of fasting.

There are many reputed or real associations between diseases and the circumstances of onset of pain. Some common ones are the association of gastric and esophageal inflammation with the use of non-steroidal anti-inflammatory agents, the association of idiopathic inflammatory bowl disease with severe physical or emotional stress and the association of pancreatitis with abdominal trauma or refeeding after a prolonged fast. When the onset of a complaint is remote, patients may forget these circumstances so the matter must be specifically brought up by the examiner.

The progress of abdominal pain reflects the progress of the pathological process. Very few abdominal pains are truly constant; most exhibit changes in intensity which can be described as crescendo, decrescendo or waxing and waning. True constancy is approached by only a few conditions, pancreatic carcinoma, dissection of an abdominal aneurysm and referred pain of cardiac or pulmonary origin, for example.

Most gastrointestinal pains come and go, some with daily recurrences, others at longer intervals or episodes. One should ask the duration of episodes as well as frequency. *Daily pains* may reflect the exacerbation of some constant pathological process by a normal daily event, such as eating or defecation. *Episodic pains* suggest, instead, a pathological process that is itself episodic, such as the passage of a gallstone.

Aggravating factors in abdominal pain

The analysis of the factors that aggravate an abdominal pain can go far to confirm impressions both about the organ of origin and about the nature of the pathological process. The most important aggravating factors to explore are eating and drinking in general, the ingestion of specific foods or beverages, the taking of medicines, defecation, body position and physical activity.

When *eating and/or drinking* in general increase the pain, the pain is usually found to be arising from an organ prominently stimulated by eating – the esophagus, stomach, pancreas, biliary tract or intestine, but not the liver or colon. If the pain worsens within 20–30 minutes of the act, it is likely to be the proximal parts of the tubular gut that are responsible, rather than the distal regions or the accessory organs. The length of delay is suggestive: pain coming on without delay is likely to be esophageal while greater delays characterize pain of gastric and intestinal origin. Pancreatic and biliary pain may not come on for 45 minutes after eating because of the time required for the production of the hormones of intestinal origin that stimulate these organs.

Patients commonly notice *specific foods or beverages* that seem particularly to exacerbate abdominal pains. Such information can be most helpful in confirming the impression of upper gastrointestinal inflammation, where the commonest offenders are coffee, alcohol, spicy foods and fruit juices. One should ask specifically about them. Often, patients with incomplete distal intestinal obstruction (from adhesions or strictures) may notice exacerbation of the pain after the ingestion of large quantities of high-fiber foods. Some, like bran cereals and celery, are obvious but others, such as raw fruits, mushrooms, raw vegetables, peanuts and water chestnuts, are not.

Defecation can exacerbate pain of colonic origin. In asking about this, the questioner must not confuse pain from the movement of the fecal mass with pain from the contraction of the abdominal wall muscles. In patients with painful abdominal wall pathology, 'bearing down' or straining at stool can be very painful and so suggest visceral disease to those who do not think long about the meaning of the association.

Some *body positions* exacerbate abdominal pain. The pain in a patient with a partially obstructed viscus, for example, often seems to be worse with the torso fully extended or the abdomen compressed.

Similarly, *activity* makes certain pains worse. Pancreatic pain, for example, often worsens with walking, climbing stairs or riding in a car over bumpy road, all consistent with the mechanism explained in Chapter 1 for the jar test.

Relieving factors in abdominal pain

While patients commonly have much to say about aggravating factors in abdominal pain, they often neglect mentioning relieving factors. It is just as important to know what has worked as it is to know what has not worked. The questioner should remember specifically to cover four areas — eating, medicines, defecation and body position.

The relief of abdominal pain by *eating* or *drinking* strongly suggests upper gut pain, classically that of duodenal ulcer. The effectiveness of buffer antacids in relieving pain strongly correlates with upper gut inflammation. Relief of pain with defecation sometimes characterizes pain of colonic origin.

Relief by certain *activities* or *body positions* is sometimes striking. The avoidance of motion and the assumption of the fetal position are strongly associated with pain of retroperitoneal (mainly pancreatic) origin. Restlessness, the constant seeking of one position or another, frequently occurs in pains arising from the hollow viscera.

Some patients apply *heat* to the abdomen in the hope of finding relief. The benefit is most striking in pain arising in the abdominal wall.

Associated symptoms in abdominal pain

The interpretation of abdominal pain can be greatly facilitated by the associated gastrointestinal symptoms such as weight loss, nausea and vomiting, diarrhea, constipation, blood in the stools, jaundice, bloating and belching. Some patients fail to mention them so they must be specifically asked about.

Weight loss always signifies either a reduced caloric intake or an increased caloric loss. Increased loss can arise from fever or malignancy. Although pains made worse by eating should reduce caloric intake, patients may unconsciously circumvent this result by taking frequent small meals, by avoiding specific offending foods or by taking increased quantities of calorically dense foods. Such maneuvers do not work in caloric loss from fever or malignancy nor do they compensate in the weight loss of intestinal ischemia.

Nausea and vomiting accompany many causes of abdominal pain but not all. They are commoner in upper gut disease, except for esophageal disease, than in colonic disease. These symptoms seem especially to reflect the distension of a hollow organ, but they also often accompany rapid hepatic enlargement.

Diarrhea accompanying abdominal pain points especially to the pancreas, small intestine and colon as the sources of the pain. Patients who take large quantities of buffer antacids for inflammatory disease of the upper gut often fail to recognize that this practice can cause diarrhea.

Constipation with abdominal pain signifies an origin in colonic disease or in any condition producing ileus. The failure to pass gas is a major sign of both ileus and colonic obstruction.

Blood in the stools with abdominal pain only signifies that mucosal disruption characterizes the responsible pathological process. The absence of blood in the stool on testing does not speak strongly against occult bleeding unless the test is negative in at least three successive stools.

Jaundice accompanying abdominal pain usually means that the source lies in the pancreatobiliary system, but not always. Patients with Gilbert's syndrome can become jaundiced with fasting or fever associated with other kinds of abdominal pain. Hemolysis associated with various disorders, especially sickle cell disease, can also produce mild jaundice associated with abdominal pain.

Bloating is the sensation of abdominal distension. It usually signifies obstruction of the tubular gut, though it may also reflect an ileus of any cause.

Belching, with or without bloating, frequently accompanies the pain of esophagitis and it may be the major complaint rather than heartburn.

INVESTIGATION OF ABDOMINAL PAIN

With so many diagnostic modalities available, the choice of tests to investigate abdominal pain is not easy. Efficiency in diagnosis not only assures speed but also minimizes costs and patient discomfort. The choice of tests must be guided by the conclusions reached through the application of logic to the facts uncovered in the clinical interview and examination.

The three categories of abdominal pain

A simple classification should always occupy the mind of the physician examining a case of abdominal pain. He must think of three general categories of pain: *organic visceral pain, organic parietal pain (abdominal wall pain)* and *non-organic pain.*

Organic visceral pain (Fig. 12.11)

Organic visceral pain always comes to mind first and, for gastro-enterologists, should constitute the principal category of pain to investigate. The concept should be supported by historical or physical evidence to suggest an organ of origin. It is especially the *location* of pain that suggests the originating organ, but the other five features of the pain

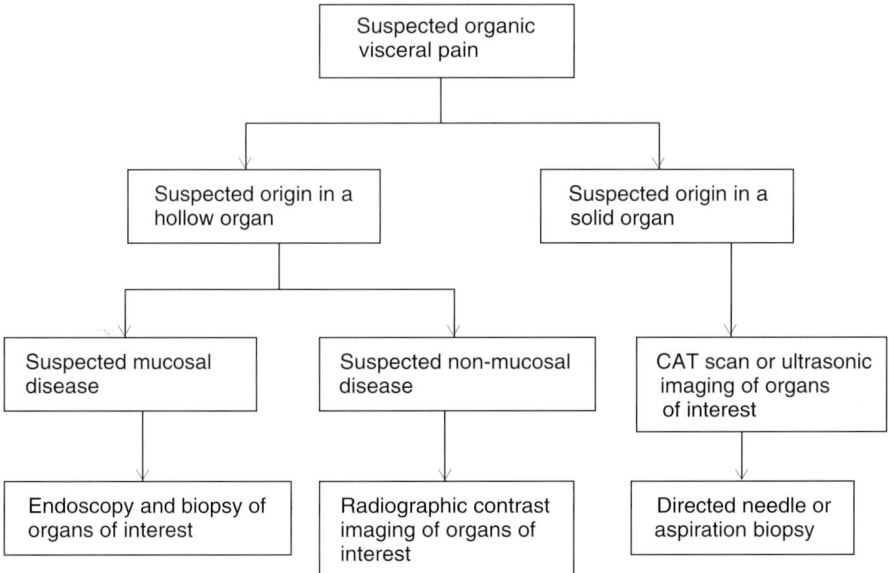

Figure 12.11 An algorithm for the use of objective diagnosis in cases of suspected organic visceral pain.

should support or, at least, not tend strongly to refute the initial impression of the organ of origin. The first tests should be directed to a specific and sensitive investigation of that organ.

The hollow viscera

When any of the hollow viscera are to be studied, the kind of test depends to some degree upon the nature of the pathological process suspected. Most cases of abdominal pain arise from mucosal disease, especially inflammation, and an impression of such a process can be supported by other features of the pain, especially its *character*, the *aggravating* and *relieving factors* and the *associated symptoms*.

When mucosal disease, tumor or inflammation is suspected, the most sensitive and specific assessment of the process comes from *endoscopic inspection* and *endoscopically-directed biopsy*. However, when the features of the pain suggest some other process, like obstruction or motor dysfunction, *radiographic imaging* of the organ is more likely to be fruitful as the first step, though endoscopic imaging and biopsy may be necessary as a second investigation. This distinction, it seems obvious, arises from the fact that the endoscope, while giving the clearest possible image of the mucosa, is not very sensitive to changes in the gross morphology of the organ, its size, its displacement, its deformities, thickenings in its walls or its movements. Radiographic imaging, in contrast, shows these latter features of an organ more clearly but reveals mucosal lesions comparatively poorly.

The solid viscera

Where the organ of origin is suspected to be a solid organ, the liver, spleen, pancreas or a retroperitoneal structure, the first test should constitute an attempt to image these abdominal structures as sensitively and specifically as possible. The modern techniques of *cross-sectional imaging* (computerized axial tomography, the CAT scan) and *ultrasound* meet such needs. Neither method provides very sensitive information about the hollow viscera mainly because these are mobile, but the relative immobility of the solid viscera makes them amenable to visualization by the CAT scan and the ultrasound probe.

Neither technique is flawless. Especially in regard to the identification of stones in the pancreatobiliary ducts or the morphology of these ducts, the ultrasound probe and the CAT scan can and do miss major disease. Thus, in this specific instance, *endoscopic retrograde connulation* of the pancreatobiliary system with the injection of radiographic contrast media is often the first choice in diagnostic evaluation, despite the greater cost, effort, skill and risks involved as compared to non-invasive imaging techniques.

When imaging has provided evidence for disease in a solid organ, biopsy, which is so easy at endoscopy, is usually required for specific diagnosis because specific therapy requires histologic evidence. This can be done by conventional needle biopsy from the liver in diffuse liver disease. When malignancy or another focal lesion is suspected, fine needle aspiration guided by computerized tomography can be used in any organ to obtain biopsy material.

Organic parietal pain (Fig. 12.12)

When features of the clinical history and physical examination suggest that the origin of abdominal pain lies in the abdominal wall, further investigations are rarely helpful. The presence of a convincingly positive

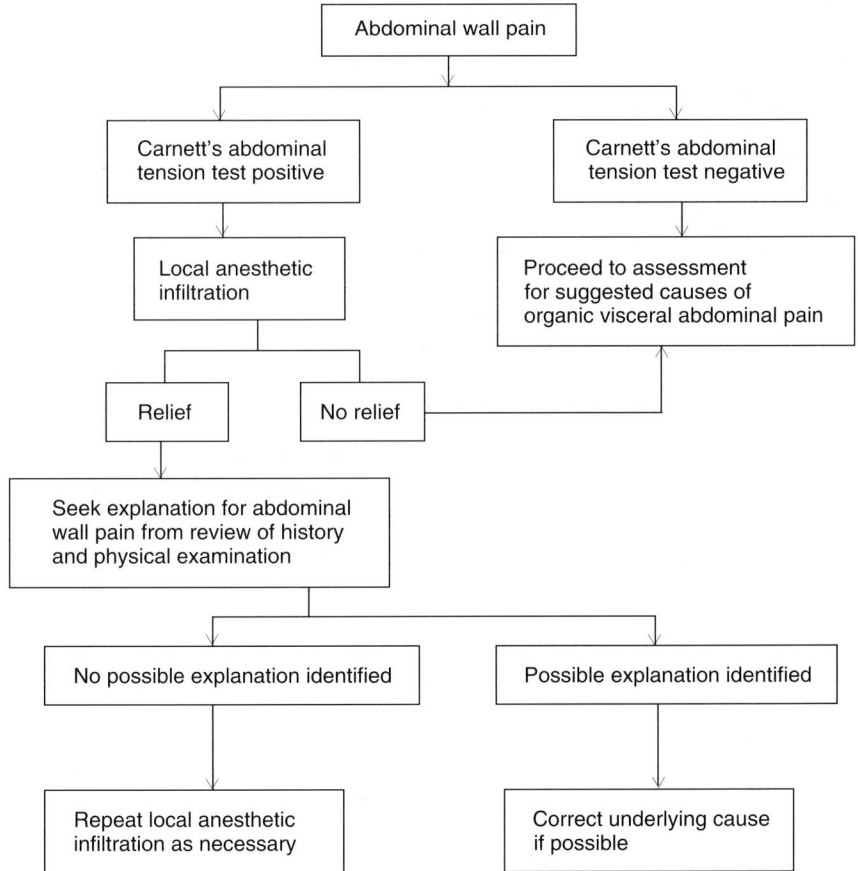

Figure 12.12 An algorithm for the investigation of suspected abdominal wall, or parietal, abdominal pain.

abdominal tension test (Carnett's test) as described in Chapter 1 can be all that is needed for diagnosis. When there is reason to suspect a concealed abdominal wall hernia or a mass lesion in the abdominal wall that needs biopsy, a CAT scan may show it. But most cases of abdominal wall pain represent a sensory neuropathy and proof of that lies in showing that local anesthesia abolishes the pain. Thus, in conventional practice, points of tenderness thought to represent 'trigger points' in the abdominal wall can be infiltrated with a local anesthetic or a mixture of a local anesthetic and corticosteroid. When the infiltration produces complete relief of pain and tenderness within seconds or minutes, that result confirms the parietal origin of the pain.

Non-organic pain

Abdominal pain is a not infrequent consequence or accompaniment of emotional illness. Indeed, the distinction of organic from non-organic abdominal pain is the most common problem in outpatient gastro-enterology. The 'functional' (meaning 'non-organic') syndromes, including pain syndromes, remain among the most common diagnoses made in the practice of medicine. Their diagnosis is one of exclusion; that is, the plausible organic causes of any particular pain syndrome must be ruled out to make such a diagnosis. Such diagnoses cannot be made strictly objectively since the decision as to what must be ruled out is not always strictly definable. The clinical problem facing the physician is the question of how far he must go in testing to conclude that organic explanations do not exist for an abdominal pain in any single case.

The more fruitful approach in such cases is for the physician to initiate a brief psychological assessment at the outset in every case where the findings on interview and examination do not strongly suggest an organic cause (either visceral or parietal). Evidence for emotional illness as a cause or factor in abdominal pain gathered at the outset might prevent the extensive 'testing' that is so commonly done to 'rule out' a long list of organic diseases in such cases. While some psychological assessment should occur in every case, of course, the possibility that an emotional illness contributes prominently to abdominal pain can profitably be developed early and pursued in situations where the routine work-up before testing has failed to raise much suspicion of organic illness.

Put more simply, an experienced gastroenterologist who strongly suspects a specific organic diagnosis at the end of the history and physical examination usually finds himself very close to the mark after the objective testing is done. When he does not strongly suspect a specific organic diagnosis at that point, the likelihood of non-organic abdominal pain is high and that possibility should be pursued from that moment. Obviously, accuracy in this decision process improves with experience.

FURTHER READING

Christensen J L 1987 Bedside logic in diagnostic gastroenterology, Churchill Livingstone, New York

Davenport H 1982 Physiology of the digestive tract, 5th edn. Year Book Medical Publishers, Chicago

DeGowin E L, DeGowin R L 1994 Bedside diagnostic examination, 6th edn. Macmillan, New York

Engle G L, Morgan W L (eds) 1973 Interviewing the patient. W B Saunders, Philadelphia

Gelin L-E, Nyhus L M, Condon R E (eds) 1969 Abdominal pain: a guide to rapid diagnosis. J B Lippincott, Philadelphia

Granger D N, Barrowman J A, Kvietys P R 1985 Clinical gastrointestinal physiology. W B Saunders, Philadelphia

Greenberger N J (ed) 1986 Gastrointestinal disorders: a pathophysiologic approach, 3rd edn. Year Book Medical Publishers, Chicago

Johnson L 1985 Gastrointestinal physiology, 3rd edn. C V Mosby, St Louis

Judge R D, Zuidema G D (eds) 1982 Clinical diagnosis: a physiological approach, 4th edn. Little, Brown, Boston

Silen W 1983 Cope's early diagnosis of the acute abdomen, 16th edn. Oxford University Press, New York

13

Bloating and wind

S. S. C. Rao

INTRODUCTION

'Doctor, I am full of gas' and 'I have terrible wind' are complaints that are frequently encountered in the gastrointestinal clinic. The actual prevalence of such problems has not been assessed because patients may use many terms to describe their symptoms such as 'belching', 'burping', 'eructation', 'bloating', 'sick to my stomach', 'nausea', 'cramps', 'loud bowel sounds', 'gas', 'wind' and 'flatus'. These symptoms can herald the onset of such organic syndromes as malabsorption, gastrointestinal obstruction, bacterial overgrowth and parasitic infestation and they can represent anxiety-related bowel dysfunction. The clinical challenge is to identify a cause so as to provide relief of symptoms. This section reviews the pathophysiology of gas production in the gut and discusses a diagnostic and therapeutic approach for this complex group of symptoms.

SOURCES AND COMPOSITION OF GASTROINTESTINAL GAS

There are four important sources of gas production within the gut (Strocchi & Levitt 1993, Tomlin et al 1991):

1. air that has been swallowed;
2. CO_2 produced by the interaction of gastric acid with food, bicarbonate or alkaline secretions;
3. gas produced by bacterial fermentation of food residues, particularly in the colon;
4. diffusion of gas between the gastrointestinal lumen and the blood.

It is not clear how much air reaches the stomach from swallowing (Strocchi & Levitt 1993). In two studies, the composition of gases found in the stomach were fairly consistent; N_2 79%, O_2 17% and CO_2 14% (Kantor 1918, Levitt & Bond 1968). In contrast, the composition of flatus was extremely variable; N_2 23–80%, O_2 0.1–23%, H_2 0.06–47%, CH_4 0–26% and CO_2 5.1–29% (Kirk 1949, Levitt & Bond 1968, Tomlin et al 1991). There is general agreement, however, that the normal gastrointestinal tract contains approximately 200 mL of gas (Bedell et al 1956, Roth 1985, Tomlin et al 1991), although the volume released is influenced by the diet. A brief

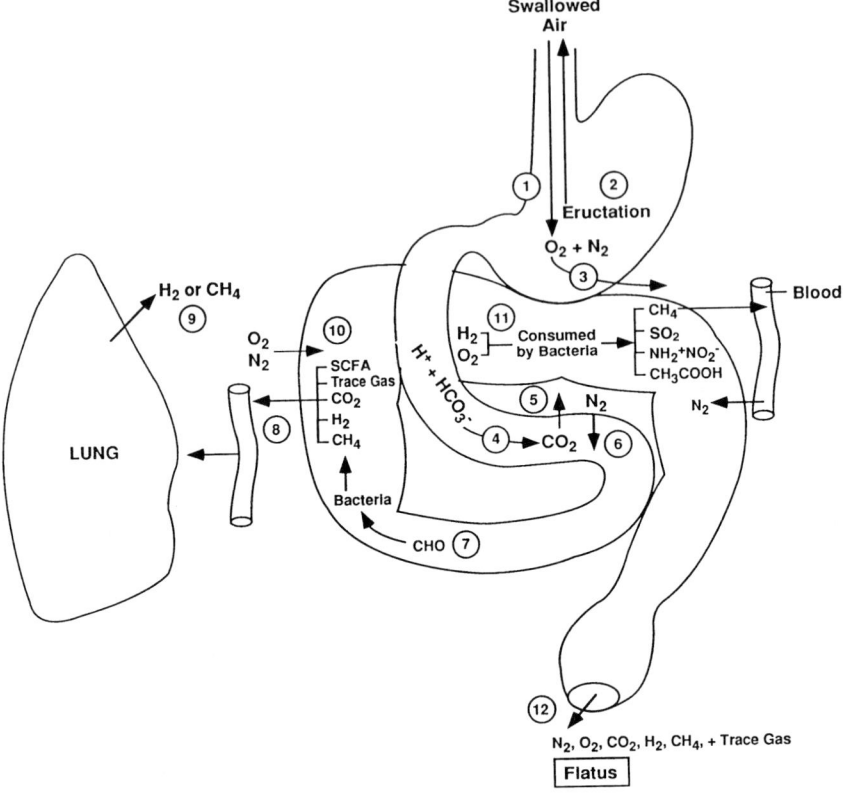

Figure 13.1   This shows the sources for gas production in man. 1) Air is swallowed. 2) A substantial portion is regurgitated (eructation). 3) O_2 and N_2 diffuse into the blood. 4) CO_2 is produced by the interaction of H^+ and HCO_3^-. 5) CO_2 diffuses into the blood. 6) N_2 diffuses into the lumen. 7) Unabsorbed carbohydrate (CHO) residues arrive in the colon and are fermented by anaerobic bacteria to produce SCFA and $H_2 + CO_2 + CH_4$ + trace gases. 8) A proportion of these gases diffuse into the blood. 9) H_2 and CH_4 are excreted through the lungs. 10) $O_2 + N_2$ are consumed by colonic bacteria. 11) H_2 and O_2 are also consumed by colonic bacteria to produce CH_4, SO_2 and other gases, some of which are absorbed. 12) The remaining gases are expelled with stools or as flatus (Figure modified and adapted with permission from Strocchi & Levitt 1993).

description of the important gases found in the gut and their possible sources follows. (Fig. 13.1).

Nitrogen (N_2) and oxygen (O_2)

It is well known that these gases are present in high concentrations in atmospheric air. Analysis of the composition of gases from the stomach has revealed concentrations of N_2 similar to that found in the atmosphere, suggesting that the predominant source of this gas is swallowed air. It has been estimated that approximately 10–20 cc of air is swallowed with each bolus of food or drink (Kahrilas et al 1988). This air is normally present in the dead space of the pharyngeal cavity and becomes entrapped within the bolus during a voluntary swallow to be propelled into the stomach (Kahrilas et al 1988). Since, there is little or no diffusion of N_2 between the gastrointestinal lumen and the blood, the predominant source of N_2 found in the gut or in flatus is that which is swallowed with air. In contrast, oxygen diffuses freely between the blood and the gastrointestinal lumen and consequently its concentration may vary depending on the amount of air swallowed and the metabolic processes occurring within the gut.

Hydrogen (H_2)

Germ-free rats (Levitt et al 1968), newborn infants and mammalian cells (Engel & Levitt 1970) do not produce H_2. However, hydrogen is produced within hours after bacterial colonization of the human gut. In Man, the colon is the primary site for H_2 production. It has been estimated that between 30 and 150 g of carbohydrate normally escapes digestion in the small bowel and reaches the colon every day (Cummings 1984). This unabsorbed carbohydrate serves as substrate for fermentation by colonic anaerobic bacteria and H_2 is produced by this process. Dietary constituents such as fruits and vegetables (legumes) contain high concentrations of unabsorbable oligosaccharides. Similarly flours made from wheat, oats, potatoes and corn also contain significant amounts of unabsorbable polysaccharides that could serve as sources of H_2. Endogenous substances such as glycoproteins may also serve as substrates for H_2 production (Perman & Modler 1982). The net volume of H_2 excreted from the body (breath and flatus) depends on the amount of H_2 produced in the colon and the volume consumed by bacteria within the gut (Strocchi & Levitt 1993, Strocchi et al 1992). These two processes are further influenced by many other factors (Box 13.1). In addition, conditions that are associated with carbohydrate malabsorption, such as lactase deficiency, may also increase the volume and rate of H_2 production. Ordinarily, most of the H_2 produced in the colon is either consumed by

---

Box 13.1 Factors that influence hydrogen metabolism in the colon (modified with permission from Strocchi & Levitt 1993)

Absolute H_2 Production $\rightarrow$	H_2 Consumption $\rightarrow$	Net H_2 Excretion
• H_2-producing bacteria	• H_2-consuming bacteria	• H_2 excreted in flatus
• Fermentable substrates	• H_2 tension of colonic contents	• H_2 excreted in breath
	• Location of H_2-consuming bacteria	
	• Substrate fermentability	
	• Colonic pH	

colonic metabolic processes or eliminated as flatus. Only 14–21% is absorbed into the bloodstream and eliminated through the lungs (Levitt 1969) (see Fig. 13.1).

Methane (CH$_4$)

Methane is also a product of the intracolonic metabolism of unabsorbed carbohydrate residues. The following reaction summarizes methano-genesis and also explains how H$_2$ is consumed during this process: $4\,H_2 + CO_2 \rightarrow CH_4 + 2\,H_2O$ (Miller & Wolin 1982). As can be seen, 5 moles of gas are used in order to produce 1 mole of CH$_4$. Thus, methanogenesis serves as a mechanism for reducing the volume of gas produced in the colon. Approximately one-third of the world's population has high concentrations of methanogenic flora in the colon (Bond et al 1971). This appears to be a familial trait influenced by environmental rather than by genetic factors (Patel et al 1986). The prevalence of methanogenic flora is higher among Mexicans than among Caucasians living in the USA. The latter have a higher prevalence than Asians from India (Patel et al 1986). The precise reason for such geographical variations is not known. Similarly, it is unclear why children under the age of 3 years do not have detectable levels of methane in alveolar air (Peled et al 1985). While hydrogen-generating anaerobes are located throughout the colon, the methanogens are found predominantly in the left colon (Strocchi et al 1992).

Subjects who produce large amounts of methane may have stools that consistently float in water. This occurs because some of the methane produced in the colon becomes entrapped within stool and this process reduces the density of stool below that of water (Levitt 1972). The buoyancy of stool is largely determined by its gas content rather than by its fat content (Levitt & Duane 1972).

Carbon dioxide (CO$_2$)

Most of the carbon dioxide produced within the gut is found in the upper intestine. The gas is formed during neutralization of acid by bicarbonate and by other alkaline secretions in the gut (Levitt 1972, Perman & Salzburg 1992). Up to 2 litres of carbon dioxide may be produced within 24 hours (Levitt 1972). Other sources for carbon dioxide production include intestinal digestion of fat and protein. Hence, a large meal that is rich in fat and protein can produce significant amounts of carbon dioxide but most of this is absorbed from the small bowel. Thus, although large amounts are produced in the upper gut very little is excreted in flatus. Like other gases, the bulk of carbon dioxide that is present in flatus is derived from bacterial fermentation of dietary substrates in the colon (Strocchi & Levitt 1993).

Gas and odor

Those gases which are the major components of flatus do not have an odor. The unpleasant odor is believed to be related to sulfur-containing compounds such as methanethiol and dimethyl sulfide which are present only in trace quantities in feces (Moore et al 1987).

CLINICAL CONDITIONS ASSOCIATED WITH BLOATING AND WIND

Although patients use diverse terms to describe their problem, for clinical purposes it is useful to consider the various conditions associated with bloating and wind under the following three categories:

1. Belching/eructation;
2. Bloating/distension;
3. Flatulence.

Belching/eructation

This symptom may be defined as the involuntary and sometimes noisy regurgitation of air from the stomach and through the mouth.

Pathophysiology

This physiological event appears to be initiated by an abrupt increase in intraabdominal pressure followed by relaxation of the lower esophageal sphincter and retrograde passage of gas into the esophagus. This leads to the formation of an isobaric gastroesophageal cavity. The abrupt increase in esophageal pressure causes relaxation of the upper esophageal sphincter and the passive escape of gas into the mouth (Kahrilas et al 1986). This sequence is followed by a primary peristaltic contraction in the esophagus which restores esophageal pressures to basal levels (Kahrilas et al 1986).

The occasional belch that occurs during or following a meal expels gas from the stomach and is a normal physiological event. In some patients, excessive belching may result from one of the medical problems listed in Box 13.2. In others, the symptom may represent habit. Many patients who complain of chronic excessive belching appear to have an emotional disorder and can be shown to aspirate air into the esophagus before each belch. Most of the aspirated air may never reach the stomach and in fact is regurgitated immediately, leading to the development of a cycle of belching–aspiration–belching. Nonetheless, it is always important to exclude organic dysfunction before attributing the symptom to anxiety-related aerophagia.

Box 13.2 Common causes of excessive belching

1. Aerophagia
2. Gastroesophageal reflux disease or peptic ulcer disease
3. Hiatal hernia
4. Hypersalivation from chewing gum
5. Smoking
6. Drinking carbonated fluids
7. Anxiety with hyperventilation
8. Gastroparesis
9. Gastric outlet obstruction
10. Poorly fitting dentures
11. Esophageal retention secondary to stricture or achalasia
12. Pregnancy
13. Asthma and chronic obstructive pulmonary disease
14. Postnasal drip and related rhinolaryngeal problems

Management

The first step is to identify an underlying organic disorder. A detailed history, physical examination and relevant investigations should normally help to establish or exclude a pathophysiological basis for the symptoms. Patients with medical conditions such as gastroesophageal reflux disease or gastritis may respond to antacids or antisecretory drugs. Patients who smoke, chew gum constantly or drink carbonated beverages in excess may benefit from breaking these habits. Patients with anxiety and hyperventilation may benefit from treatment with anxiolytics or psychotherapy.

If common medical problems can be excluded, measures to counter aerophagia should be pursued. The approach to aerophagia should include a detailed evaluation of swallowing patterns and may require video fluoroscopy. Postnasal drip and rhinolaryngeal problems may predispose to excessive belching.

In patients with chronic belching counseling regarding the aerophagia–belching cycle, reassurance regarding the benign nature of the problem and encouragement to impose self-restraint and develop control of the habit by overcoming their urge to belch can all prove effective. Although belching may not cease, an understanding of the benign nature of the problem may reduce distress.

Symptomatic relief may be obtained from the use of preparations containing simethicone, although their effectiveness has never been established objectively. In patients with an inability to belch, preparations containing peppermint oil or agents that reduce lower esophageal sphincter tone such as nitrates or calcium channel blockers may be helpful. A single case of a patient with an inability to belch secondary to a failure of the upper esophageal sphincter to relax and associated with severe postprandial chest pain has been reported (Kahrilas et al 1987).

Since the upper esophageal sphincter relaxes in response to a voluntary swallow, efforts to relieve this problem could include postural and biofeedback swallowing techniques (Kahrilas et al 1988a).

Bloating/distension

Many patients complain that garments do not fit and that friends and relatives have noticed a distended abdomen. Although 40–50% of patients presenting with this symptom may not have demonstrable dysfunction, the rest may have a recognizable cause for complaint. Box 13.3 provides a list of common conditions that can cause bloating or distension.

Pathophysiology

In one study of bloating in irritable bowel syndrome, 74% of patients and none of the controls reported abdominal pain and distension coinciding with the arrival of meal residues in the colon (Cann et al 1983). This temporal relationship has led to the widely held notion that bloating may arise from excessive production of intestinal gas during fermentation of meal residues in the gut. However, in such cases, radiographic examinations have often failed to document more gas than normal and a recent study using CAT scanning also failed to demonstrate excess gas (Maxton et al 1991).

A systematic analysis of the intestinal gas contents using the argon gas washout technique showed that the mean volume of gas in 18 patients with bloating and in ten normal subjects was 176 mL vs 199 mL and the mean composition of gases was similar (Lasser et al 1975). However, the patients differed from normals in that more of the infused gas refluxed back into the stomach and they complained of abdominal pain more frequently than normals (Lasser et al 1975). This suggests that many of these patients may have either disturbed motility of the gut or visceral hyperalgesia with increased sensitivity of the viscera to luminal distension. The observation that the bowel does not contain more gas does not rule out the possibility that these patients produce excess gas. Some patients may expel gas as soon as it is generated and thereby evade clinical detection (Read 1987). This hypothesis is supported by the observation that gas can pass rapidly through the gut with a mouth to anus transit time of 15–20 minutes (Levitt 1971).

Syndromes associated with bloating/distension

A number of syndromes have been described in association with bloating.

Gas-bloat syndrome may occur in 25–50% of patients following gastric fundoplication for a hiatal hernia (Hocking et al 1982, Walls & Gonzales

---

Box 13.3 Common causes of bloating/distension

1. Idiopathic
2. Gastric disorders
   - Peptic ulcer disease
   - *Helicobacter pylori* gastritis
   - Gastroparesis
   - Gastric bezoar
   - Gastric outlet obstruction/gastric cancer
3. Small bowel disorders
   - Lactose malabsorption
     — Primary
     — Secondary: bacterial overgrowth, celiac disease, giardiasis, tropical sprue, Whipple's disease, *Taenia* and other parasitic infestation
   - Sucrose/fructose malabsorption
   - Bacterial overgrowth
   - Parasites: giardiasis, hookworm, tapeworm
   - Fat malabsorption
   - Pneumatosis cystoides intestinalis
   - Crohn's disease
   - Chronic intestinal pseudoobstruction
   - Visceral neuropathy/myopathy
   - Systemic sclerosis/muscular dystrophy
   - Small intestinal obstruction/stricture/lymphoma/carcinoma
4. Colonic disorders
   - Constipation: slow transit constipation, obstructive defecation
   - Inflammatory bowel disease
   - Amebiasis and other parasitic infestations
   - Hirschsprung's disease
   - Chronic intestinal pseudoobstruction
   - Bacterial/viral and parasitic infections
   - Diverticular disease
   - Colon cancer
5. Miscellaneous
   - Cholelithiasis
   - Drugs: narcotics, anticholinergics, antidiarrheals, kaolin compounds, lomotil, loperamide, calcium channel blockers, psyllium supplements (Metamucil, etc.)
   - Hypothyroidism
   - Diabetes mellitus
   - Ingestion of carbonated beverages
   - Chewing gum, particularly those containing sorbitol
   - Food intolerance
   - Acute or chronic liver disease
   - Aerophagia

1977). It stems from the inability to belch and so expel gas from the stomach following a meal. Usually, the problem resolves with time and only rarely requires surgical revision (Rossetti & Hell 1977). Patients with a total laryngectomy may also develop this problem, which usually occurs when they are learning esophageal speech. In this form of verbalization, patients are taught to swallow air by relaxing the upper esophageal sphincter and then to expel this through the mouth to form speech (Maddock et al 1949).

Hepatic/splenic flexure syndrome may arise from the entrapment of gas at the hepatic and splenic flexures (Macella et al 1952) and sometimes the descending/sigmoid colon junction. The pain induced by overstretching the viscera may be referred to the shoulder, chest, back, neck, thigh or legs. Many patients with this problem are constipated and have anxiety or emotional distress. The patient's symptoms may be reproduced during double contrast radiography or flexible colonoscopy. Symptomatic relief may be obtained from treating constipation and providing emotional support.

Magenblase syndrome arises from the progressive and excessive accumulation of air swallowed during the course of a day, resulting in marked postprandial epigastric fullness and bloating, particularly after the evening meal. Symptoms are often relieved by belching (Roth 1985).

History and physical examination in patients with bloating/distension

The most important step in the evaluation of a patient with bloating is to obtain a detailed history. In particular, the inquiry should focus on the time and duration of symptoms and the presence of other associated gastrointestinal disturbances. The history should include a detailed dietary assessment with particular attention to recent changes in dietary habits and to the association of symptoms with the ingestion of dairy products, fructose, sucrose or sorbitol, beans or fatty foods. The relationship of symptoms to meals and defecation is also important. The history of smoking, alcohol consumption, the ingestion of carbonated drinks and the use of chewing gum should be obtained.

A history of psychiatric disturbances such as anxiety or depression and the presence of metabolic disorders such as diabetes and hypothyroidism is important. A history of weight loss, nocturnal gastrointestinal symptoms, vomiting or diarrhea suggest an organic cause. The drug history may point to agents which delay gastrointestinal transit or alter motility. A family history of celiac disease, inflammatory bowel disease, lactose intolerance or other food allergies and intolerances can provide important clues regarding the nature of the underlying problem.

The patient must be examined carefully for evidence of weight loss, anxiety, hyperventilation and aerophagia. A cursory abdominal examination may suggest a distended abdomen, but a more careful appraisal may reveal an exaggerated lumbar lordosis with consequent protuberance of the belly. Such non-gaseous distension of the abdomen due to exaggerated lumbar lordosis is the mechanism for abdominal distension in pseudocyesis. Flexion of the hips of the supine patient abolishes both the lordosis and the distension, quickly confirming the diagnosis.

The abdomen must be carefully examined to exclude organomegaly, signs of intestinal obstruction and ascites. Patients who appear anxious, have cold skin and who avoid eye contact and wince easily to gentle palpation, may have an anxiety-related bowel disorder.

Standard investigations in patients with bloating/distension

Many medical problems can cause bloating or distention. The primary goal in investigating a patient should be to either confirm or refute specific problems suggested by the history and the physical examination, not to embark on a crusade to exclude every possible gastrointestinal ailment.

Conventional blood tests such as CBC, ESR, urea and electrolytes, liver function tests, thyroid function, calcium and glucose measurements are useful to investigate underlying metabolic dysfunctions or serious organic diseases. Fresh stool samples (at least three) must be examined for ova/parasites, stool culture and presence of *Giardia* antigen. A serology for *E. histolytica* may also be useful. Tests for *Helicobacter pylori* may help to identify this as a cause of bloating and dyspepsia. The IgA endomysial antibody test is useful in patients with suspected celiac disease.

An ultrasound examination of liver, gallbladder and pancreas and/or pelvic structures may prove useful. Plain X-rays of the abdomen may show excessive fecal loading. Upper endoscopy with biopsy and an aspirate from the small bowel for bacterial culture may be useful. Similarly, an upper GI series with a small bowel follow-through, a barium enema or colonoscopy with biopsy may help.

Special investigations (breath tests) in patients with bloating/distension

During the last two decades, breath analysis for hydrogen and for methane have become important tools to investigate carbohydrate malabsorption, bacterial overgrowth and mouth-to-cecum transit time (King & Toskes 1983, Read et al 1980, Solomons 1984). This simple test consists of administering an oral dose of a carbohydrate that is suspected of causing the patient's symptom, for example lactose, and measuring the breath H_2 responses.

In healthy subjects, most of the ingested carbohydrate is digested and absorbed in the small bowel. However, between 30–150 g may not be salvaged and it reaches the colon (Cummings 1984). This unabsorbed carbohydrate is fermented by colonic anaerobic bacteria to short chain fatty acids, hydrogen and other gases which are then absorbed rapidly together with salt and water (Ruppin et al 1983). The following equation (Cummings 1984, Miller & Wolin 1982) summarizes the anaerobic breakdown of carbohydrate:

$$34.5\ C_6H_{12}O_6 \Rightarrow 64\ SCFA + 23.75\ CH_4 + 34.23\ CO_2 + 10.5\ H_2O.$$

As little as 2 g of carbohydrate reaching the colon may produce an appreciable increase in breath hydrogen values (Levitt 1969). In addition to the amount of carbohydrate residue reaching the colon, a number of other factors may also influence H_2 production (see Box 13.1). Most of the hydrogen produced in the colon is either utilized by the colonic mucosa or expelled as flatus. Only 14–21% is absorbed into the blood perfusing the colon and expired through the lung during a single pass (Levitt 1969) (see Fig. 13.1). Thus, an assessment of the concentration of H_2 in alveolar air provides a simple and non-invasive method of detecting carbohydrate malabsorption.

The H_2 breath test has been widely used for the detection of lactose malabsorption, and has superseded other methods such as the serial measurement of blood glucose levels (Newcomer et al 1975) or the serial measurement of serum galactose and urinary galactose levels (Lerch & Riebrand 1991). The H_2 breath test may be more reliable than the glucose blood test for lactose malabsorption (DiPalma & Narvaez 1988, Newcomer et al 1975). A typical H_2 breath profile in a patient with lactose malabsorption is shown in Figure 13.2. The lactose-H_2 breath test is positive in about 90% of patients with lactose malabsorption. However, between 5 and 15% of patients with lactose malabsorption may have a false negative H_2 breath test and many of these may have an acidic pH in the colon, methanogenic flora or a deficiency of H_2-producing bacteria in the colon (Strocchi & Levitt 1992). Other causes are listed in Box 13.3. A recent study compared the sensitivity and specificity of H_2 breath analysis with $^{13}CO_2$ lactose breath test (Hiele et al 1988). The H_2 breath test had a sensitivity,

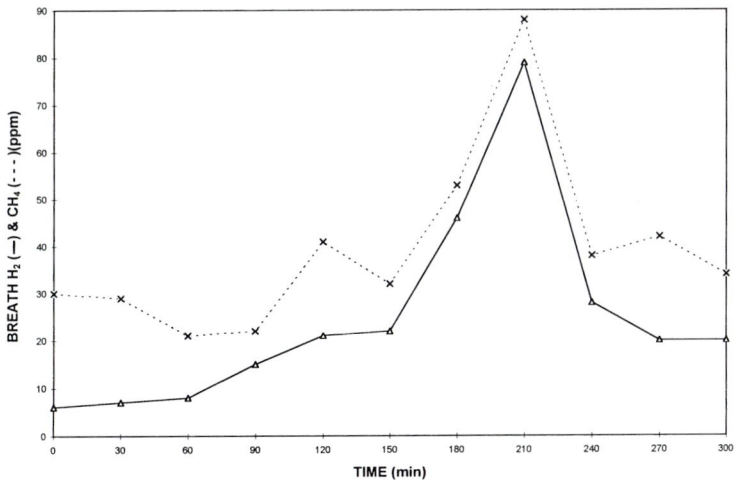

LACTOSE BREATH TEST

Figure 13.2   A typical breath H_2 and CH_4 profile in a patient with lactose malabsorption, after ingestion of 25 g of lactose. A significant rise in breath H_2 and CH_4 values can be seen after 2.5 hours.

LACTOSE BREATH TEST

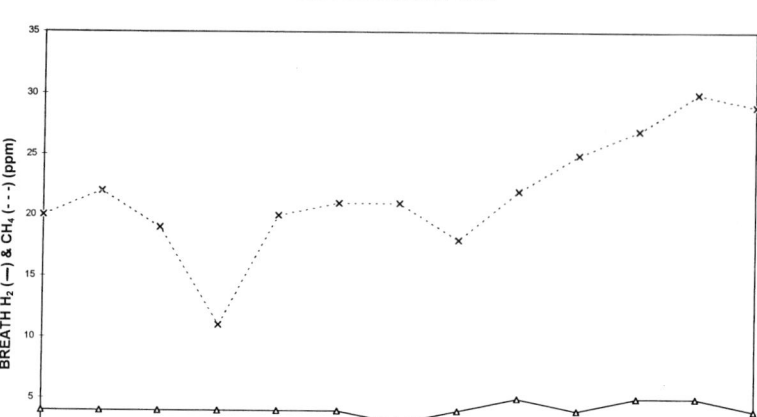

Figure 13.3 A typical breath H_2 and CH_4 profile in a patient with lactose malabsorption, illustrating the usefulness of measuring CH_4 in breath samples. This patient, a methane producer, had high basal levels of CH_4 that rose significantly after 4 hours of lactose ingestion.

specificity and accuracy of 73%, 89% and 83% as compared to 84%, 96% and 91% for the $^{13}CO_2$ lactose.

Approximately 15–30% of people have methanogenic flora. Following the ingestion of unabsorbable carbohydrate, the breath H_2 values may not rise in these subjects and instead the CH_4 values may increase. In one study of 166 subjects with a negative lactose-H_2 breath test, 57/166 (34%) were found to be methane excretors and 25/166(15%) showed a significant rise in CH_4 levels after lactose ingestion (Corazza et al 1991). Because colonic metabolism of disaccharide may produce H_2 alone, CH_4 alone or both gases, simultaneous measurements of H_2 and CH_4 should improve the sensitivity and specificity of the breath analysis tests for carbohydrate malabsorption. An example of a patient in whom breath H_2 values did not change but where CH_4 analysis was useful to establish lactose intolerance is shown in Figure 13.3.

Treatment

The management of a patient with bloating/distension depends on the underlying cause. Patients with lactose malabsorption benefit from the complete elimination or the restriction of lactose. Educating the patient with the help of a dietitian is most useful since lactose is present in many popular foods and is often not recognized by the patient. Patients with a mild deficiency may benefit from lactase supplements (Lactaid®, McNeil

Pharmaceuticals; Dairy-ease®, Sterling Health). The incubation of milk with lactase may also be helpful. However, it is important to warn the patients that they may not obtain complete relief of symptoms, since either the digestion of lactose is incomplete or it is difficult to estimate the dose of enzyme that is required to digest the lactose in a given quantity of milk. Similarly, lactase enzyme tablets may improve tolerance of a lactose-containing meal but is not a panacea for all patients with lactose intolerance. Hence, enzyme supplementation serves as an adjunct to dietary discretion, not as a substitute for it. Non-dairy synthetic drinks such as Coffee-mate® (Carnation, Nestle) may be recommended as a useful substitute for milk.

Patients with secondary lactose intolerance require treatment of the underlying condition. A gluten-free diet for celiac disease, metronidazole or tinidazole for giardiasis or oxytetracycline for tropical sprue may improve tolerance to lactose. Patients with intolerance to other carbohydrates such as fructose, sucrose and sorbitol must be advised to avoid foods containing these carbohydrates. Patients with bacterial overgrowth may benefit from antibiotics. In those patients who require prolonged courses of treatment with antibiotics, it is advisable to rotate these drugs at monthly intervals to reduce antibiotic resistance.

Patients with constipation and bloating may benefit from fiber supplementation, increased oral fluids, exercise, bowel retraining, stool softeners and laxatives. Prokinetic drugs may be useful in patients with a motor disorder (Johnson 1971, Van Outryve et al 1991). Patients who suffer from bloating with beans may obtain relief from α-galactosidase (Beano®, A.K. Pharma) (Solomons et al 1991). The benefit from activated charcoal tablets remains controversial (Hall et al 1981, Jain et al 1986, Potter et al 1985, White et al 1991).

The avoidance of offending foods such as beans, cabbage, lentils, Brussels sprouts, nuts and legumes may reduce bloating and gas production. High fiber diets, particularly those containing bran and fiber supplements such as psyllium products (Metamucil, Citrucel, Fibercon), may cause bloating which abates with time. Patients with refractory symptoms may benefit from elimination diets (Jones et al 1982). Patients maintain a strict log of symptoms and foods consumed over a period of one month. This diary is then reviewed to identify food items that may have provoked symptoms. If food items are recognized as troublesome, they are eliminated.

Patients in whom an underlying cause is not identified may respond to reassurance together with drugs that bring about symptomatic relief. Some patients may benefit from antispasmodics such as mebeverine HCL, dicyclomine, hyoscine or peppermint oil (Weber & McCallum 1992). Despite the widespread usage of such agents, controlled trials are lacking and the evidence for benefit is unclear. It has been claimed that exercise helps bloating, but apart from a single report which showed that rocking in a rocking chair relieved gaseous discomfort following cesarean section (Thomas et al 1990), there has been little evidence to support this form of therapy (Strocchi & Levitt 1993). Hypnotherapy with self-hypnosis may benefit some patients (Whorwell et al 1987).

In refractory patients, balloon distension of the small bowel may reveal visceral hyperalgesia suggesting that these patients are hypersensitive to normal amounts of gas within the gut.

Flatulence

The passage of excessive gas from the anus, particularly gas with an unpleasant odor, is a frequent source of embarrassment to many patients.

Pathophysiology

Flatus usually comprises nitrogen (N_2), oxygen (O_2), carbon dioxide (CO_2), hydrogen (H_2), methane (CH_4) and trace amounts of a few other gases. However, the concentration of each gas within a single emission or during the course of a day or between individuals is extremely variable (Tomlin et al 1991). The daily volume of flatus production may range from 475 to 1500 cc (median 600–700 cc) (Kirk 1949, Tomlin et al 1991) (Fig. 13.4). Unlike previous studies of flatus collection (Beazell & Ivy 1941, Calloway & Burroughs 1969), a more physiological 24-hour collection revealed that flatus is produced during both day and night and during sleep, but the mean volume at night is 16 mL/h, about half that produced during the day, 34 mL/h (Tomlin et al 1991). A greater amount of flatus is produced after meals than at other times and the flatus that is produced more rapidly contains a larger proportion of gases produced by fermentation (Tomlin et al 1991).

A major diagnostic problem in a patient with flatulence is to determine if the patient is producing excessive amounts of gas or is unusually sensitive to normal amounts of flatus. The average number of flatus emissions in a normal subject is variable. In one study the median value was eight episodes/day (Tomlin et al 1991), while in another a mean of 13.6 ± 6 (1 SD) episodes per day were observed (Strocchi & Levitt 1993). It is generally believed that <25 episodes/day is normal (Perman & Salzburg 1992). A more frequent passage of flatus may suggest excess gas production, although frequency is only a rough guide to the volume generated.

The causes of excess flatus are similar to those that induce excess bloating (see Box 13.3). In addition, patients with incontinence of feces or flatus may also complain of flatulence. A fiber-rich diet significantly increases flatus production, whereas a fiber-free diet virtually eliminates it

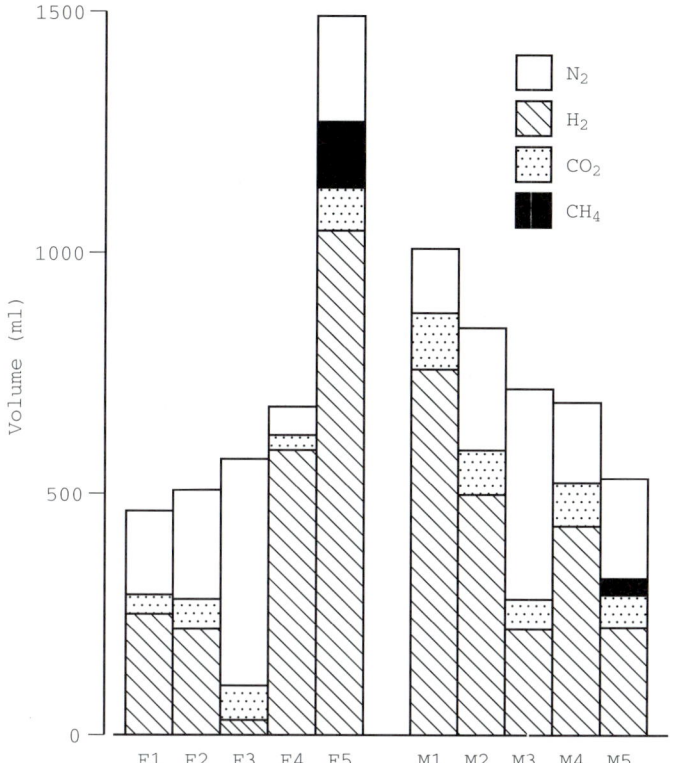

Figure 13.4   The individual values for the total volume of flatus collected from 10 normal subjects over a period of 24 hours (modified with permission from Tomlin et all 1991)

(Tomlin et al 1991). This suggests that, at least in most normal subjects, the major source of flatus is bacterial fermentation in the colon. The presence of excess amounts of flatus may suggest either malabsorption of carbohydrate (lactase deficiency) or an imbalance between gas-producing and gas-consuming bacteria in the colon (Strocchi et al 1992). In addition to methanogenic bacteria, the colon has sulfate-reducing bacteria which also consume H_2:

$$SO_4^{2-} + 4 H_2 \longrightarrow S^{2-} + 4 H_2O \text{ (Gibson 1990).}$$

It is believed that most individuals only harbor one of the two types of bacteria, that is, methanogenic or sulfate-reducing, in the colon (Strocchi et al 1992). The finding that breath H_2 levels are lower in patients who excrete CH_4 (Bjorneklett & Jenssen 1982) and that methanogenic bacteria (Strocchi et al 1992) consume H_2 more efficiently than sulfate-reducing bacteria suggests that methanogenesis may be a more efficient way to handle gas production in the colon.

Management

There has been no systematic assessment of drugs that might reduce flatus production or alter the odor of flatus, although several compounds have been suggested. Activated charcoal, administered prior to a meal, has been advocated (Hall et al 1981, Jain et al 1986), although its mechanism of action is not known. Simethicone may act by altering the surface tension and the elasticity of mucus-coated gas bubbles. This causes the smaller bubbles to break down and coalesce (Bernstein & Kasich 1974, Bernstein & Schwartz 1974). Its usefulness and efficacy remain to be established (Perman & Salzburg 1991). More recently a chlorophyllin copper complex (DERIFIL®, Rystan Co Inc, Little Falls, New Jersey), an agent which reduces fecal odor in patients with ileostomy, has been suggested as a useful adjunct to antiflatus therapy, particularly in patients with incontinence to flatus (Young & Beregi 1980, O'Connell 1968). Controlled trials are, however, lacking. Patients with incontinence to flatus may benefit from bowel retraining using biofeedback techniques to improve rectal sensation, anal tone and rectoanal coordination (Rao et al 1994). This may allow them to regain better control of flatus expulsion. A diet low in lactose, starch and legumes and a fiber-free diet reduce flatus production (Tomlin et al 1991). However, compliance with such a diet is poor.

REFERENCES

Beazell J M, Ivy A C 1941 The quantity of colonic flatus excreted by the normal individual. American Journal of Digestive Diseases 8: 128–129
Bedell G N, Marshall R, Dubois A B, Harris J H 1956 Measurement of the volume of gas in the gastrointestinal tract. Journal of Clinical Investigation 35: 336–345
Bernstein J E, Kasich A M 1974 A double-blind trial of simethicone in functional disease of the upper gastrointestinal tract. Journal of Clinical Pharmacology 14: 617–623
Bernstein J E, Schwartz S R 1974 An evaluation of the effectiveness of simethicone in acute upper gastrointestinal distress. Current Therapeutic Research 16: 617–620
Bjorneklett A, Jenssen E 1982 Relationship between hydrogen (H_2) and methane (CH_4) production in man. Scandinavian Journal of Gastroenterology 17: 985–992
Bond J H, Engel R R, Levitt M D 1971 Factors influencing pulmonary methane excretion in man. Journal of Experimental Medicine 133: 572–588
Bond J H, Levitt M D 1977 Use of breath hydrogen (H_2) in the study of carbohydrate absorption. Digestive Diseases 22: 379–382
Calloway D H, Burroughs S E 1969 Effect of dried beans and silicone on intestinal hydrogen and methane production in man. Gut 10: 180–184

Calloway D H, Murphy E L, Bauer D 1969 Determination of lactose intolerance by breath analysis. American Journal of Digestive Diseases 14: 811–815

Cann P A, Read N W, Brown C, Hobson N, Holdsworth C D 1983 The irritable bowel syndrome (IBS). Relationship of disorders in the transit of a single solid meal to symptom patterns. Gut 24: 405–411

Corazza G R, Strocchi A, Sorge M, Benati G, Barahona M T, Gasbarrini G 1991 The measurement of breath methane (CH_4) must be combined with hydrogen (H_2) measurement in the diagnosis of carbohydrate malabsorption (abstract). Italian Journal of Gastroenterology 23: A516

Cummings J H 1981 Short chain fatty acids in the human colon. Gut 22: 763–779

Cummings J H 1984 Colonic absorption: the importance of short chain fatty acids in man. Scandinavian Journal of Gastroenterology 19: 89–99

DiPalma J A, Narvaez R M 1988 Prediction of lactose malabsorption in referral patients. Digestive Diseases and Sciences 33: 303–307

Engel R R, Levitt M D 1970 Intestinal tract gas formation in newborns (abstract). In: Program for Meeting of American Pediatric Society and Society for Pediatric Research, 266

Gibson G R 1990 Physiology and ecology of sulfate-reducing bacteria (review). Journal of Applied Bacteriology 69: 769–797

Hall R G Jr, Thompson H, Strother A 1981 Effects of orally administered activated charcoal on intestinal gas. American Journal of Gastroenterology 75: 192–196

Hickey C A, Calloway D H, Murphy E L 1972 Intestinal gas production following ingestion of fruits and fruit juices. American Journal of Digestive Diseases 17: 383–389

Hiele M, Ghoos Y, Rutgeerts P, Vantrappen G, Carchon H, Eggermont E 1988 $^{13}CO_2$ breath test using naturally ^{13}C-enriched lactose for detection of lactose deficiency in patients with gastrointestinal symptoms. Journal of Laboratory and Clinical Medicine 112: 193–200

Hocking M P, Maher J W, Woodward E R 1982 Definitive surgical therapy for incapacitating 'gas-bloat' syndrome. American Surgeon 48: 131–133

Hyams J S 1983 Sorbitol intolerance: an unappreciated cause of functional gastrointestinal complaints. Gastroenterology 84: 30–33

Jain N K, Patel V P, Pitchumoni C S 1986 Activated charcoal. l Gas: a double-blind study. Annals of Internal Medicine 105: 61–62

Johnson A G 1971 Controlled trial of metoclopramide in the treatment of flatulent dyspepsia. British Medical Journal 2: 25–26

Jones A V, McLaughlin P, Shorthouse M, Workman E, Hunker J O 1982 Food intolerance, a major factor in the pathogenesis of irritable bowel syndrome. Lancet ii: 1115–1117

Kahrilas P J, Dodds W J, Denk D 1986 Upper esophageal sphincter function during belching. Gastroenterology 91: 133–140

Kahrilas P J, Dodds W J, Hogan W J 1987 Dysfunction of the belch reflex - a cause of incapacitating chest pain. Gastroenterology 93: 818–822

Kahrilas P J, Logemann J A, Shoh V, Ha T 1988 Upper esophageal sphincter opening and modulation during swallowing. Gastroenterology 97: 1467–1478

Kantor J L 1918 A study of atmospheric air in the upper digestive tract. American Journal of Medical Science 155: 829–856

King C E, Toskes P P 1983 The uses of breath tests in the study of malabsorption. Clinics in Gastroenterology 12: 591–610

Kirk E 1949 The quantity and composition of human colonic flatus. Gastroenterology 12: 782–794

Lasser R B, Bond J H, Levitt M D 1975 The role of intestinal gas in functional abdominal pain. New England Journal of Medicine 293: 524–526

Lerch M, Riebrand H C 1991 Concordance of indirect methods for the detection of lactose malabsorption in diabetic and nondiabetic subjects. Digestion 48: 81-88

Levitt M D 1969 Production and excretion of hydrogen gas in man. New England Journal of Medicine 281: 122–127

Levitt M D 1971 Volume and composition of human intestinal gas. New England Journal of Medicine 284: 1394–1398

Levitt M D 1972 Intestinal gas production. Journal of the American Dietary Association 60: 487–496

Levitt M D, Bond J H 1968 Volume, composition and source of intestinal gas. Gastroenterology 59: 921–929

Levitt M D, Duane W C 1972 Floating stools – flatus versus fat. New England Journal of Medicine 286: 973-975

Levitt M D, French P, Donaldson R M 1968 Use of hydrogen and methane excretion in the study of the intestinal flora (abstract). Journal of Laboratory and Clinical Medicine 72: 988–989

Levitt M D, Lasser R B, Schwartz J S, Bond J H 1976 Studies of a flatulent patient. New England Journal of Medicine 295: 260–262

Macella T E, Dworken H J, Biel F J 1952 Observations on the splenic flexure syndrome. Annals of Internal Medicine 37: 543–552

Maddock W G, Bell J L, Tremaine M J 1949 Gastrointestinal gas. Annals of Surgery 130: 512–537

Maxton D G, Martin D F, Whorwell P J, Godfrey M 1991 Abdominal distension in female patients with irritable bowel syndrome: exploration of possible mechanisms. Gut 32: 662–664

Miller T L, Wolin M J 1982 Enumeration of *Methanobrevibacter smithii* in human species. Archives of Microbiology 131: 14–18

Moore J G, Jessop L D, Osborne D N 1987 A gas chromatographic and mass spectrometric analysis of the odor of human feces. Gastroenterology 93: 1321–1329

Newcomer A D, McGill D B, Thomas P J, Hofmann A F 1975 Prospective comparison of indirect methods for detecting lactose deficiency. New England Journal of Medicine 293: 1232–1236

O'Connell I 1968 A useful adjunct for odor control in malodorous surface lesions and incontinence. Journal of the Central Islip State Hospital 2: 23–26

Patel V P, Jain N K, Pitchumoni C S 1986 Factors affecting fasting breath hydrogen levels in healthy adults. A study in two continents. American Journal Gastroenterology 81: 771–773

Peled Y, Gilant, Liberman E, Bujanover Y 1985 The development of methane production in childhood and adolescence. Journal of Pediatric Gastroenterology and Nutrition 4: 575–579

Perman J A, Modler S 1982 Glycoproteins as substrates for production of hydrogen and methane by colonic bacterial flora. Gastroenterology 82: 911–917

Perman J A, Salzburg D M 1992 Approach to the patient with gas and bloating. In: Yamada T (ed) Textbook of gastroenterology, J B Lippincott, Philadelphia, pp 681–691

Potter T, Ellis C, Levitt M D 1985 Activated charcoal: in vivo and in vitro studies of effect on gas formation. Gastroenterology 88: 620–624

Rao S S C, Welcher K, Happel J 1994 Can biofeedback therapy improve anorectal function in patients with fecal incontinence? Gastroenterology 107: A1245

Ravich W J, Bayless T M, Thomas M 1983 Fructose: incomplete intestinal absorption in humans. Gastroenterology 84: 26–39

Read N W 1987 Irritable bowel syndrome (IBS). Definition and pathophysiology. Scandinavian Journal of Gastroenterology 22: 7–13

Read N W, Miles C A, Fisher D et al 1980 Transit of a meal through the stomach, small intestine and colon in normal subjects and its role in the pathogenesis of diarrhea. Gastroenterology 79: 1276–1282

Read N W, Al-Janabi N M, Bates T E 1985 Interpretation of the breath hydrogen profile obtained after ingesting a solid meal containing unabsorbable carbohydrate. Gut 26: 834–842

Rossetti M, Hell K 1977 Fundoplication for the treatment of gastroesophageal reflux in hiatal hernia. World Journal of Surgery 1: 439–444

Roth J L A 1985 Gaseousness. In: Berk J E, (ed) Bockus gastroenterology. W B Saunders, Philadelphia, pp 142-166

Ruppin H, Bar-Meir S, Soergel K H, Wood C M, Schmitt M G Jr 1983 Absorption of short chain fatty acids by the colon. Gastroenterology 78: 1500–1507

Solomons N W 1984 Evaluation of carbohydrate absorption: the hydrogen breath test in clinical practice. Clinical Nutrition 3: 71–78

Solomons N, Vasquez A, Grazioso C 1991 Orally-ingested, microbial alpha-galactosidases produce effective in vivo, intraintestinal digestion of the bean oligosaccharide rattinose. Gastroenterology 100: A251

Strocchi A, Levitt M D 1992 Factors affecting hydrogen production and consumption by human fecal flora: the critical roles of hydrogen tension and methanogenesis. Journal of Clinical Investigation 89: 1304–1311

Strocchi A, Levitt M D 1993 Intestinal gas. In: Sleisenger, Fordtran, Scharschmidt, Feldman (eds) Gastrointestinal disease: pathophysiology, diagnosis and management. Vol. 1, 5th edn. W B Saunders, Philadelphia, pp. 1035–1042

Strocchi A, Corazza G R, Gasbarrini G 1992 Recent advances in hydrogen metabolism in man. Journal of Italian Gastroenterology 24: 207–211

Sutalf L O, Levitt M D 1979 Follow-up of a flatulent patient. Digestive Diseases and Sciences 24: 652–654

Thomas L, Ptak H, Giddings L S, Moore L, Oppermann C 1990 The effects of rocking, diet modifications and antiflatulent medication on postcesarean section gas pain. Journal of Perinatal and Neonatal Nursing 4: 12–24

Tomlin J, Lowis C, Read N W 1991 Investigation of normal flatus production in healthy volunteers. Gut 32: 665–669

Van Outryve M, Milo R, Toussaint J, Van Eeghem P 1991 'Prokinetic' treatment of constipation-predominant irritable bowel syndrome: a placebo controlled study of cisapride. Journal of Clinical Gastroenterology 13: 49–57

Walls A D F, Gonzales J G 1977 The incidence of gas-bloat syndrome and dysphagia following fundoplication for hiatus hernia. Journal of the Royal College of Surgeons of Edinburgh 22: 391–394

Weber F H, McCallum R W 1992 Clinical approaches to irritable bowel syndrome. Lancet ii: 1447–1452

White J G, Hightower N C, Riggs M, Dyck W P 1991 Does activated charcoal relieve gas symptoms – a placebo controlled study. Gastroenterology 100: A261

Whorwell P J, Prior A, Colgan S M 1987 Hypnotherapy in severe irritable bowel syndrome: further experience. Gut 28: 423–425

Young R W, Beregi J S 1980 Use of chlorophyllin in the care of geriatric patients. Journal of the American Geriatric Society 28: 46–47

14

Diarrhea

J. A. Murray

INTRODUCTION

Diarrhea is both a common medical problem and a universal experience. Despite the commonplace nature of diarrhea, there can be much disparity, not only between lay people but also among professionals, in what is meant by diarrhea. Those who complain of diarrhea may be referring to an increased frequency of stool, a liquid or unformed stool, a sense of urgency to defecate or mucus with and coating an otherwise normal stool. Some persons may refer to fecal incontinence as diarrhea. Of course, it is much more likely that one will be incontinent of liquid than of solid stool.

A significant diarrheal episode may be defined as more than two loose stools per day for more than 3 days. The weight of a normal stool ranges from 102–195 g/day for men and from 31–81 g/day for women. A widely accepted definition of diarrhea is a stool weight of greater than 250 g/day, at which point most patients will experience a change in stool habit and a noticeable increase in stool volume. Most patients are able to estimate the volume of the stool that they have passed. High volume diarrhea usually results in the passage of large quantities of liquid stool every hour or even more frequently.

Stool is the end product of digestion. It reflects not only the waste products of ingested material but the end result of complex processes involving the digestive tract, its accessory organs (liver, pancreas and salivary glands) and the colonic microflora. Normal stool is mainly water (60–80%) containing bacteria, non-digestible fiber, gas, sloughed mucosal cells, bile pigment (the main determinant of color) and various organic compounds resulting from bacterial fermentation (often responsible for odor).

The volume of oral intake is not simply concentrated but is first greatly expanded by the addition of large volumes of secretions. These secretions come from the salivary glands, gastric mucosa, pancreas, bile and intestinal mucosa itself. The daily oral intake, 2 L, is supplemented by 5 L from pancreatobiliary secretion and 2 L from gastrointestinal secretion. This volume is easily handled by the intestine and colon. Intestinal volume is a function of the osmotic properties of the chyme. Digestive enzymes break down complex carbohydrates, proteins and fats to smaller, more osmotically active substances. The sugars and amino acids are rapidly and actively absorbed. Water and sodium passively equilibrate across the intestinal epithelium balancing plasma and fecal osmolality. Motor activity of the intestine serves to mix and slow passage of chyme to allow time for this process to occur. If less of these osmotically active substances is absorbed, more water is retained in the lumen. The Na^+ moves out of the lumen down the osmotic gradient.

The colon has an absorptive capacity reserve of up to 5 liters per day. When the absorptive capacity is overwhelmed by a volume that either exceeds its reserve absorptive capacity or that arrives at a rate that exceeds its retentive capacity, the result is the passage of liquid stools. Defective absorption and rapid transit may also produce diarrhea. The combination of an increased input to the colon and a reduced absorptive capacity will result in severe diarrhea. The site as well as mechanisms involved in diarrhea both affect the volume of diarrhea.

The most severe diarrhea occurs in cholera where the small intestinal mucosa produces such large quantities of secretion, 10–20 liters per day, that the colon's maximum absorptive capacity of 5 liters is overcome, resulting in a tremendous loss of fluid and electrolytes. Proximal colonic disease results in diarrhea of up to 1–1.5 liters daily. Disease limited to the left side of the colon tends to produce soft small stools. Purely rectal disease may produce increased frequency of formed stools. There are, however, some exceptions to these generalizations. Villous adenomas of the colon may secret large volumes of potassium and water (Tjandra 1990).

HISTORY

A detailed history is the essential first step in a proper evaluation. A careful inquiry into the nature, frequency, timing and duration of diarrhea and the presence of urgency is essential. The patients should be asked to describe the characteristics of the stool. Most are able to provide at least a minimal description of the color, consistency and odor of the stool. The patient's description of the stool does not substitute for the physician's examination of the stool. The pale gray stools of steatorrhea are characterized by a pungent odor often commented on by family members. The presence of visible blood in the stools suggests an inflammatory, neoplastic or vascular process in the colon. The consistency of a diarrheal stool may vary from liquid to soft or unformed in nature. Buoyancy suggests either excessive fat due to malabsorption or gas due to fermentation in the stool. Some patients who complain of diarrhea do not have diarrhea but pass frequent well-formed stools. Sometimes these are pellety and hard or similar to toothpaste and occur as a result of an undefined motor or functional bowel disorder or a low-fiber diet.

Timing of diarrhea

The timing of stools may also be important. Nocturnal diarrhea that awakens the patient suggests an organic rather than a functional cause. Diarrhea that occurs solely at night in a diabetic patient suggests autonomic dysfunction. A diarrheal episode that occurs mainly following meals suggests malabsorption or maldigestion. However, due to the presence of the gastrocolic reflex, the ingestion of food may precipitate a diarrheal episode even in patients with colonic disease.

The nature of the onset of diarrhea may be revealing. An abrupt onset suggests an infective process or, in the elderly patient with bloody diarrhea, should raise the suspicion of an ischemic process affecting the colon. Other inflammatory illnesses may occasionally have an acute onset. Inflammatory conditions are also apt to present in the postnatal period, particularly inflammatory bowel disease and celiac disease. This likely coincides with the relatively abrupt reversal of the immune suppression related to pregnancy.

The diarrhea may usefully be categorized into acute (less than 3 weeks duration) or chronic (>3 weeks) diarrhea. This distinction is important because of the different etiologies. There are some exceptions to this. For example, ulcerative colitis can begin suddenly mimicking infectious diarrhea.

Associated symptoms

A careful inquiry into the presence of associated symptoms may help sharpen the diagnostic focus.

Weight loss

Appreciable weight loss is significant in either acute or chronic diarrhea. In acute diarrhea, weight loss usually reflects dehydration. The loss of more than 10% of body weight indicates severe dehydration. Weight loss in chronic diarrhea suggests chronic nutritional imbalance, due to increased metabolism from a chronic inflammatory or neoplastic state, diminished ingestion to avoid food-induced symptoms, loss of appetite or malabsorption. Nausea and vomiting are unhelpful in identifying a cause of diarrhea. The presence of significant vomiting can make dehydration more profound and rehydration more difficult.

Abdominal pain

Abdominal pain either before, during or after the diarrheal episode is common. The abrupt onset of severe abdominal pain with diarrhea in an elderly person with a history of vascular disease suggests acute ischemia. A history of chronic recurring abdominal pain suggests Crohn's disease. Chronic cramping abdominal pain and/or lower back pain may also be a feature of anxiety-induced bowel dysfunction. The pain related to diverticular disease and its complication, diverticulitis, is usually located in the left lower quadrant. Though the rare proximal colonic diverticulum may perforate, it usually is not associated with an alteration in bowel habit.

Tenesmus

Tenesmus is the intense and unproductive sensation of the urge to defecate which cannot be suppressed. This sensation almost always reflects rectal involvement in the underlying disease process.

Miscellaneous symptoms

Perianal itching suggests fecal leakage. Generalized malaise, fever and chronic fatigue suggest an inflammatory or neoplastic process. The occurrence of bone pain, arthritis or arthralgias suggest inflammatory bowel disease, celiac disease or Whipple's disease. Neurologic abnormalities might be caused by a malabsorptive disease.

Factors modifying diarrhea

Diet

Patients with chronic diarrhea often try extensive dietary manipulation or restriction in an attempt to control symptoms. Many patients with lactose intolerance successfully identify the offending agent. Other food-induced diarrheas such as seen in gluten-sensitive enteropathy, disaccharide intolerance or sorbitol ingestion may not be apparent. The patient should be questioned about the use of sugar-free chewing gum, diabetic or fruit sugar-sweetened foods as well as any perceived association between the ingestion of the food substance and the diarrhea. Fasting is not often tried voluntarily but one expects all but the severe toxic and hormonally-induced diarrheas to be diminished by fasting. The passage of >300 cc of stool in a fasting patient prompts the search for hormonal causes of secretory diarrhea (Afzalpurkar et al 1992). Complete cessation of diarrhea with fasting suggests a malabsorptive or maldigestive diarrhea.

Patients may become convinced that they are allergic to multiple foods. Food-related symptoms may be due to many mechanisms with classic IgE-mediated allergy being the least common as confirmed by objective measures. Diarrhea can also be due to a non-IgE-mediated allergic pheno-

---

Box 14.1   Mechanisms of food reactions

T-cell mediated	Celiac disease
Delayed hypersensitivity response	Milk protein allergy
Maldigestion	Lactose
	Fructose
	Sucrose
	Sorbitol
	Cellulose
	Raffinose
Pharmacological	Caffeine
	Tartrazine
IgE mediated	Shellfish
Mast cell mediated	Nuts
Anaphylaxis	Other proteins

---

menon, to pharmacologic effects or to maldigestive responses to a common ingredient in the offending foods (Box 14.1). However, urticarial or angioedematous responses to foods are more common. Typical offending agents include shellfish, nuts and other proteins (Crowe & Perdue 1992).

Anxiety

Diarrhea of all causes may be exacerbated by anxiety. Where anxiety is the only precipitant for diarrheal stools, one should be suspicious of a functional or anxiety-induced diarrhea.

Medication history

A careful medication history is essential as current or recent medications may result in diarrhea. The most common cause of acute diarrhea in the hospital setting is antibiotic-related. Many other drugs may cause iatrogenic diarrhea (Box 14.2). Drug-induced diarrhea (with the exceptions of pseudomembranous colitis and chemotherapy-associated mucositis) is rarely associated with systemic symptoms.

Box 14.2   Common drug causes of diarrhea

Laxatives
Thiazide diuretics
Antibiotic-related diarrhea
Allopurinol
Non-steroidal antiinflammatory drugs
Erythromycin
Theophylline
Misoprostil

Diarrhea may also result from intolerance to the excipient ingredients of the medications, such as lactose, to which the patient may be intolerant.

Conversely, patients will often try over-the-counter medications to relieve the symptoms of diarrhea. Some commonly used antidiarrheal agents either alter intestinal motility or transit or decrease secretion. Some antidiarrheal agents also act by solidifying the stools or by absorbing toxins in the stool. While these agents may be very effective in the treatment of acute mild diarrheal illnesses their use in chronic diarrhea should not delay appropriate evaluation.

Medical/surgical history

Inquiry into the previous medical history of a patient may reveal prior gastrointestinal surgery or cholecystectomy, a history of radiation therapy or previous episodes of gastrointestinal disease. A history of autoimmune disease might suggest chronic inflammatory disease of the intestine. Sacroileitis may be associated with ulcerative colitis (Dekker-Saeys et al 1978, Moll 1985). A history of long-standing diabetes suggests a specific differential diagnosis.

Family history

Recent occurrences of acute diarrheal illness in family members or close contacts suggests an infectious cause. Similarly, a detailed family history may reveal a genetic predisposition to inflammatory bowel disease, celiac disease and lactose intolerance.

Ethnic background

Some ethnic groups have an increased risk of specific diseases (Box 14.3). Some diseases once thought not to affect certain ethnic groups may be more related to environment. As Western culture spreads, so also does inflammatory bowel disease (Fellows et al 1990, Sung et al 1994).

Box 14.3 Ethnic predispositions to causes of diarrhea	
Jew	IBD, celiac disease
Near East Africans Orientals	Lactose intolerance
Irish/Western European	Celiac disease
Near East	Immune proliferative small intestinal disease
Tropical regions	Tropical sprue

Social history

A social history may also reveal excessive alcohol intake which can result in osmotic diarrhea. High-risk sexual activity or intravenous drug abuse confers a risk, particularly of HIV infection, and opens a wider vista of potential causes for diarrhea. Anal intercourse preceding an acute attack of proctitis might suggest venereal disease of the rectum as a possibility and needs to be specifically inquired about. A history of recent travel, particularly to a poorly developed area or wilderness, should be inquired for. One should ask about the water supply and animal exposure and close contacts who may have had recent diarrheal illnesses.

PHYSICAL EXAMINATION

The physical examination may be helpful not only in determining the cause of diarrhea but also in evaluating the effects of the diarrhea.

General examination

Initial evaluation should include the general assessment of hydration (Box 14.4). The assessment should not be based solely on such features of the appearance of the individual as lethargy, sunken eyes and decreased skin turgor but also on the measurement of supine and erect blood pressure and pulse.

An orthostatic fall in systolic blood pressure of >10 mmHg or a drop in body weight of 10 pounds or more in an adult suggests significant dehydration. The occurrence of supine hypotension, tachycardia or lethargy suggests severe dehydration calling for immediate and vigorous intervention.

The presence of fever in an acute setting suggests a bacterial or invasive enteric infection. Fever may also occur in severe inflammatory bowel disease. Intermittent or recurring fever over a long period of time suggests Crohn's disease or Whipple's disease.

Box 14.4   Symptoms and signs of dehydration

Symptoms	**Signs**
Thirst	Dry mucous membranes
Dry mouth	Sunken eyes
Fatigue	Orthostasis
Lightheadedness	Tachycardia
Dizziness	Hypothermia
Oliguria	Concentrated urine
Acute weight loss	

The examiner should look for such features of thyrotoxicosis as lid retraction, lid lag, tremor, tachycardia, goiter and a thyroid bruit. The flushed facies of a patient with carcinoid syndrome is apparent during or shortly following an attack. The presence of or history of dermatitis herpetiformis suggests celiac disease. Erythema nodosum and pyoderma gangrenosum occur in association with inflammatory bowel disease. Hyperpigmentation of the skin may result from excess circulating bile salts, as in bile duct obstruction, or from severe malnutrition relating to malabsorption. The presence of an arthropathy affecting the weight-bearing joints or the spinal column suggests ankylosing spondylitis associated with inflammatory bowel disease. The occurrence of iritis, uveitis or chronic conjunctivitis suggests either inflammatory bowel disease or celiac disease. Rarely, tetany may be demonstrable either by the induction of carpopedal spasm (Trousseau's sign) or spasm of the facial muscles (Chvostek's sign). Clubbing of the fingers suggests inflammatory bowel disease, celiac disease or intestinal lymphoma. Scleroderma, most apparent in the face and hands, may be associated with jejunal diverticulosis and consequent malabsorption.

Abdominal examination

The abdominal examination may reveal scars of operations or discoloration from the long-term application of heat for chronic pain. Generalized acute abdominal distension may be the result of excessive gas production due to maldigestion, fecal loading related to severe constipation, toxic megacolon or intestinal ischemia. Chronic abdominal distension may represent chronic partial small bowel obstruction or the distension associated with malnutrition from malabsorption or starvation. Loops of dilated small intestine may be apparent. Palpation of the abdomen may reveal the indentable masses of stool in fecal impaction, a tender palpable left colon in diverticulitis, a palpable colonic cancer or a tender mass in the right lower quadrant from Crohn's disease.

Anorectal examination

The perianal skin may show erythema and excoriation related to severe diarrhea or the excessive use of toilet tissue. Purplish discoloration with possible fissuring or fistulization related to perianal Crohn's disease may occasionally be apparent. A patulous anus suggests fecal incontinence.

The rectal examination must be performed gently because many patients with severe diarrhea have a very sensitive anal canal. The use of a topical anesthetic gel to lubricate the external anal canal reduces the discomfort. The discovery of a large amount of solid stool in the rectum suggests impaction with spurious diarrhea. The finding of normal solid stool in the rectum of a patient complaining of severe diarrhea should also raise the suspicion of a false report. Fissuring of the anal canal suggests Crohn's disease. Similarly, the finding of gross blood on the examiner's finger suggests a colonic process. A soft, fleshy, lobulated rectal mass suggests a villous adenoma or villous adenocarcinoma. The rectal exam also gives a fresh specimen of stool for further evaluation.

Evaluation of stool

The clinician should directly examine the stool. Preferably the patient passes this into a graduated plastic receptacle without contamination with urine. The opportunity to examine the stool directly may confirm the patient's own assessment of the volume, consistency, color and odor.

Color

Stool color is helpful in only a small number of patients with diarrhea. A black and tarry consistency constitutes melena. A dark but solid stool results from the ingestion of bismuth and iron-containing preparations. Pale yellow or gray stools suggest the lack of bile pigment. If such stools are bulky and malodorous, that suggests steatorrhea due to pancreatic insufficiency or small bowel mucosal disease. Silver stools reflect a rare combination of the lack of bile pigment and the presence of altered blood, as can occur in ampullary carcinoma. Gross red or maroon blood in the stool suggests diseases of the colon.

Consistency of stool

Stool consistency is watery in cholera, hormonal diarrheas and other toxin-induced diarrheas. A semiformed stool, one that only partially holds its shape, may be described as bulky or mushy. If the patient has also described it as floating or difficult to flush away, that suggests the presence of fat.

Odor

The fatty stool of malabsorption has a particularly foul odor and that should prompt the consideration of intestinal mucosal or pancreatic disease. Melenic stool is also quite malodorous. While all stools, both normal and diarrheal, may be malodorous to a certain extent, an odor that is sufficiently foul to result in complaints from family members suggests a maldigestive or malabsorptive pathology.

> **Box 14.5** Initial non-specific investigation
>
> Stool examination
>   Occult blood
>   Fecal leukocytes or lactoferrin
>   Culture and sensitivity
>   Ova and parasite exam
>   *Giardia* antigen
> CBC and differential
> Serum chemistries
> Sedimentation rate or C-reactive protein
> Flexible sigmoidoscopy with biopsy

LABORATORY EVALUATION OF DIARRHEA

An extensive range of diagnostic tests can be performed in evaluating patients with diarrhea. However, it is neither safe nor cost effective to apply a broad range of diagnostic tests blindly to patients presenting with diarrhea. The data gleaned from a careful history and physical examination should direct the initial investigative strategy.

Several basic tests that may be useful in initially evaluating patients with either acute severe diarrhea or chronic diarrhea are shown in Box 14.5. In most cases, however, the diagnostic approach can be tailored to the specific clinical situation. To aid this, diarrheal illnesses can be categorized partly by pathophysiologic definition and partly by the clinical presentation.

ACUTE DIARRHEA

Most people will experience at least one episode of acute diarrhea per year, usually lasting less than 2–3 days and not associated with systemic upset. It is often treated empirically with over-the-counter medications and rarely comes to medical attention. This is appropriate and cost-effective self-management. Most of these episodes relate to the ingestion of toxins related to food spoilage, the ingestion of naturally occurring laxative substances in foods, dietary indiscretions, or microbial infections (Box 14.6). A much smaller proportion may represent diseases that usually cause chronic or relapsing diarrhea such as inflammatory bowel disease.

The non-inflammatory causes of diarrhea usually result in a watery diarrhea without systemic features whereas the inflammatory causes frequently show mucosal invasion by infective agents with fever, abdominal pain, tachycardia, abdominal distension, blood in the stools, tenesmus and urgency. Thus, the clinical presentation and the condition of the patient guide investigation. Patients who are elderly, immunocompromised, chronically ill or septic frequently require further diagnostic

---

Box 14.6 Microbial causes of diarrhea

Non-inflammatory	**Inflammatory**
Staphylococcus aureus	*Shigella*
Bacillus cereus	*Salmonella*
E. coli	*Campylobacter jejuni*
Giardia lamblia	Enteroinvasive *E. coli*
Cryptosporidium	*Clostridium difficile*
Clostridium perfringens	*Entamoeba histolytica*
Rotavirus	*Strongyloides*
Norwalk virus	*Microsporidium*
Vibrio cholerae	

---

evaluation. The presence of leukocytes or blood in stool also warrants further investigation.

If gross blood is not present, the stool should be evaluated for the presence of occult blood and the presence either of fecal leukocytes or lactoferrin, a surrogate marker for leukocytes. The latter test has some advantages over the direct examination for white blood cells in the stool in that lactoferrin is stable whereas white blood cells degrade rapidly (Guerrant et al 1992). Box 14.7 outlines a scheme for the investigation of such patients with acute diarrhea.

In an immunocompetent patient, culture of the stools to look for the bacterial causes of enteritis is useful. The stool tests for antigens are much more sensitive than direct stool examinations for giardiasis and Cryptosporidium. A *Clostridium difficile* toxin test should be performed in patients with a current or recent history of antibiotic use. Specific latex agglutination tests should be considered for the cytoverotoxin-producing strain of *E. coli*, 0157-H7.

Box 14.7 Laboratory evaluation of acute infectious diarrhea

Inflammatory	**Non-inflammatory**
Stools:	*Stools:*
Fecal leukocytes present	Fecal leukocytes absent
Routine culture: *Salmonella, Shigella*	No further investigation
and *Campylobacter*	warranted unless patient
O&P exam	condition necessitates
Special cultures: *E. coli* 0157-H7	(fever, abdominal pain,
Yersinia, Clostridium difficile toxin	dehydration)
(if hx of antibiotic treatment)	
Labs:	
CBC	
Electrolytes	
ESR, albumin, total protein	
Sigmoidoscopy *and* biopsy	

TRAVELER'S DIARRHEA

Traveler's diarrhea is the most common kind of acute infectious diarrhea, affecting 10 million travelers each year. Traveler's diarrhea consists of 3–4 unformed stools per 24 hours, usually starts on the third day of travel and lasts 2–3 days. Associated symptoms include anorexia, nausea, vomiting, abdominal cramps, abdominal bloating and flatulence.

The investigation of a returned traveler with persistent diarrhea should take into account the prevalent diarrheogenic pathogens in the area in which the patient traveled. Among travelers to Asia, the most commonly reported pathogens are *E. coli* (33%), *Salmonella* (15%), *Shigella* (4–7%) and *Campylobacter* (2–5%). Enterotoxin-producing strains of *E. coli* are also the most common cause of traveler's diarrhea in Africa and Latin America (Black 1986). Diarrhea after travel to Russia or on domestic camping trips in North America is associated especially with giardiasis (Chester et al 1985). Rotavirus and Norwalk virus often cause traveler's diarrhea (Taylor & Escheverria 1986). Parasitic causes of diarrhea, including *Giardia*, *Entamoeba* and *Cryptosporidium*, while accounting for less than 1% of cases, frequently lead to medical attention because of the long duration of the diarrhea they can cause.

Risk factors for the acquisition of traveler's diarrhea include the location of travel, the hygienic standards of the visited country, the eating practices of the traveler, the immunologic status of the patient and the use of drugs that suppress gastric acid secretion (Black 1986).

ACUTE DIARRHEA LEADING TO CHRONIC DIARRHEA

Persistent bloody diarrhea in a returned traveler more likely reflects inflammatory bowel disease than persistent infectious dysentery. There have been reported instances in which the onset of inflammatory bowel disease has been precipitated by an acute enteric infection, including cytomegalovirus infection (Orvar et al 1993). Some unusual bacterial entities can cause persistent diarrhea, such as *Aeromonas* (Blackstone & Kirsner 1991).

Tropical sprue is a clinical entity characterized by malabsorptive diarrhea in a person returning from a long sojourn in Southeast Asia or in Central or South America. It may be difficult to distinguish from celiac disease clinically but the prompt response to antibiotics with resolution of the intestinal lesion differentiates these entities. In patients with atherosclerosis, dehydration due to the acute diarrhea may precipitate ischemic colitis.

NOSOCOMIAL DIARRHEA

When evaluating patients who develop diarrhea in the hospital, the clinician needs to consider a specific differential diagnosis (Box 14.8). The

Box 14.8   Nosocomial diarrhea

Antibiotic-related diarrheas
Drug-induced diarrheas
Postoperative ileus-associated diarrhea
Stool impaction with overflow
Nutritional (excessively concentrated enteral feedings)
Epidemic infections
Ischemic colitis
Recrudescence of prior condition
Immunosuppressed patients

possibilities include antibiotic-related diarrhea, drug-induced laxative effects, the effects of enteral nutrition and stool impaction with overflow diarrhea. Occasionally, epidemic infections occur in the hospital from spread of the cytoverotoxin-producing 0157-H7 strain of *E. coli* (Carter et al 1987). The possibility of acute ischemia of the colon should be considered in patients with vascular disease and after abdominal aortic aneurysm repair.

Patients who develop acute diarrhea should be promptly evaluated. If the patient has had antibiotics the stool should be tested for *C. difficile* as described below. If the stool is negative the test should be repeated and if it is still negative the patient should have prompt sigmoidoscopy with biopsy. The sigmoidoscopy may reveal characteristic pseudomembranes (Fig. 14.1). A positive test should be followed by appropriate treatment. Examination for ova and parasites is unhelpful in the investigation of nosocomial diarrhea and should not be performed routinely unless there is a history of immunosuppression or if symptoms were present before admission (Morris et al 1992).

ANTIBIOTIC ASSOCIATED DIARRHEA

Antibiotic treatment may result in diarrhea by a variety of mechanisms. The antibiotic may suppress the normal colonic flora. This suppression can result in a decrease in bacterial fermentation of carbohydrate in the colon. This results in a greater osmotic load leading to diarrhea. The diarrhea due to the osmotic effect usually begins shortly after the start of the antibiotics.

Alternatively there may be overgrowth of the toxin-producing *Clostridium difficile*. The illness may range from a mild illness to life-threatening pseudomembranous colitis. Almost all antibiotics can cause pseudomembranous colitis, notably ampicillin, the cephalosporins and clindamycin. Pseudomembranous colitis is almost always associated with the overgrowth of *Clostridium difficile*. Patients with the milder form of antibiotic-

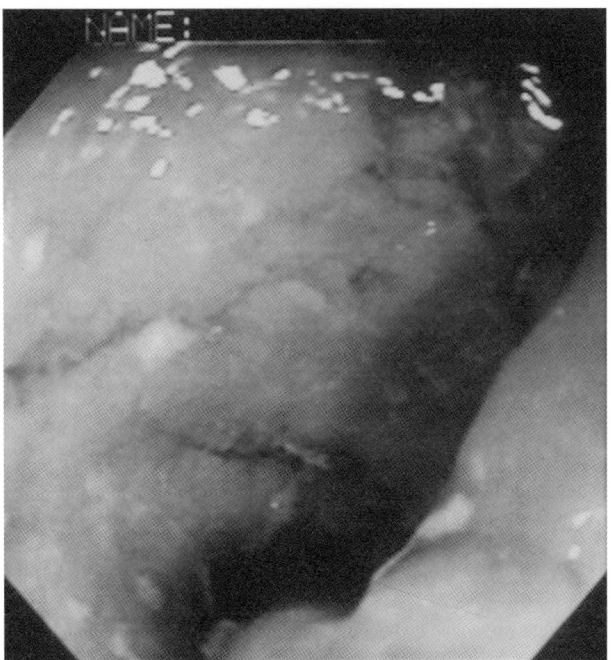

Figure 14.1 Characteristic white plaques adherent to the colonic mucosa of *C. difficile-*associated pseudomembranous colitis (courtesy of D. Hillebrand).

associated diarrhea do not usually appear to be so ill as those with pseudomembranous colitis, who may have high fevers, cramping, severe watery diarrhea and leukocytosis. The disease is often associated with nosocomial or institutional outbreaks.

Sigmoidoscopy usually reveals moderate to severe colitis which may be associated with pseudomembranes. Biopsies may reveal specific changes (Fig. 14.2). *C. difficile* diarrhea is highly infectious. The elderly and those who are fasting are especially at risk. Rarely, the condition may be so severe that perforation can occur rapidly.

Stool tests for *C. difficile*-associated diarrhea vary in sensitivity, specificity and convenience (Box 14.9). Culture of the stool is sometimes difficult and does not identify toxin-producing isolates. Fibroblast cultures are more sensitive but also more expensive to perform and often take 24–48 hours. The ELISA's combined simplicity, rapid result and specificity make it the single most useful stool test (Kelly et al 1987).

DIARRHEA IN IMMUNOCOMPROMISED PATIENTS

Immunocompromised patients are at risk of acquiring opportunistic infections (Chui & Owen 1994). Protozoans are a common cause of

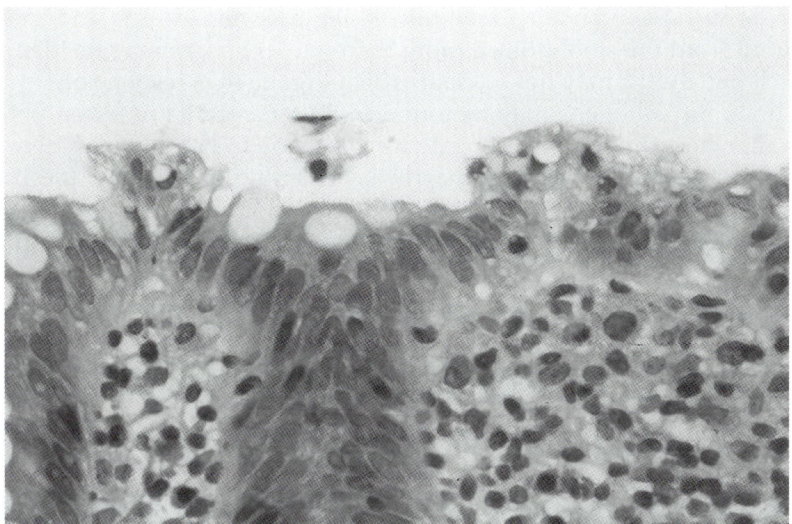

Figure 14.2 Mucosal biopsy demonstrating the summit lesions of pseudomembranous enterocolitis. Summit lesions may also be seen in verotoxin-producing *E. coli* 0157-H7 (courtesy of F. Mitros).

Box 14.9 Comparison of tests for *Clostridium difficile* diarrhea

Lab test	Target	Sensitivity	Specificity	Time required
Culture organism	Culture media	High	Moderate*	48 hours, selective
Tissue culture cytotoxicity	Toxin B	High	High	24–48 hours, tedious
Latex agglutination	gluconate dehydrogenase	moderate	moderate	30 min, simple
ELISA	Toxin A or toxin A & B	High	High	1 hour, rapid

* Does not identify toxin-producing strains
(Adapted from Kelly et al 1987)

infectious diarrhea in HIV-infected patients. *Cryptosporidium, Microsporidium, Isospora belli, Giardia lamblia, Enterocytozoon bieneusi, Strongyloides stercoralis, Septata intestinalis* and *Entamoeba histolytica* are the most common parasites causing diarrhea in such cases. Viruses which commonly cause diarrhea in HIV-infected patients include cytomegalovirus, herpes simplex virus and Epstein–Barr virus (Cello 1993, Jacobson 1988). In addition to the usual bacterial causes of diarrhea, *Mycobacterium avium-intracellulare* and *M. tuberculosis* are common causes and may be cultured from the stools. Since more than one organism may be identified in such patients, it may not be clear which organism is responsible.

Although pathogens may be found in 50–85% of HIV-infected patients with diarrhea, the high carrier rate for protozoa in homosexual men with AIDS, even in those without diarrhea, raises the question of the pathogenic nature of the organism. Those without identifiable pathogens probably have HIV enteropathy or an unrelated diarrheal illness (Dworkin & Rosenthal 1993). The syndrome of chronic diarrhea and wasting often associated with established AIDS may be the result of HIV infection of the intestine with alteration of mucosal function and immune dysregulation (Kotler et al 1993). Such patients may respond temporarily to nutritional supplementation. Lymphoma of the small intestine may also occur in immunocompromised patients. Rarely there may be the coincidental occurrence of inflammatory bowel disease (Bernstein et al 1994, Sturgess et al 1992).

Patients with iatrogenic immunosuppression can have any of the infections that affect patients with AIDS but they are also subject to certain non-bacterial diarrhea. Patients who have had a bone marrow transplant are likely to develop graft vs host disease, typically 30–90 days after allogenic bone marrow transplant. It also can occur after blood transfusions (Ryo et al 1994, Hara et al 1993) or liver transplantation (Roberts et al 1991).

CHRONIC DIARRHEA

Chronic diarrhea can be divided into six pathophysiologic categories:

1. secretory;
2. osmotic;
3. exudative or bloody;
4. malabsorptive (steatorrhea);
5. due to dysmotility;
6. functional.

The function of the normal intestine is to absorb fluid, nutrients and electrolytes and to secrete waste products. *Secretory diarrhea* is a disequilibrium between the absorptive and secretory functions. It occurs as a result of increased intestinal cell secretion secondary to the action of toxins or hormonal hypersecretion as in thyrotoxicosis and the carcinoid syndrome. *Osmotic diarrhea* results from the presence of poorly absorbed solutes in the gut lumen and the ensuing net loss of water. *Exudative diarrhea* results from the discharge of mucus, blood and serum proteins into the intestinal lumen. It occurs primarily as a result of inflammation, as in ulcerative colitis, Crohn's disease and ischemic colitis. *Steatorrhea* results from fat malabsorption. *Dysmotility* may contribute to diarrhea by accelerating transit to such an extent that the intestine may not have time to complete absorption. *Functional diarrhea* is a diagnosis of exclusion when no organic cause can be found and may be associated with psychological stress.

Clinical groupings

While these pathophysiological groupings help to understand the theory of diarrhea they have little utility in practice. This is because most intestinal diseases cause diarrhea by more than one mechanism. Celiac disease causes osmotic diarrhea from the maldigestion of carbohydrates, hypersecretion due to the crypt hyperplasia and dysmotility due to the inflammatory reaction. There are some specific clinical categories (Box 14.10) that should be considered in parallel with the pathophysiologic classification given above.

Laboratory tests in chronic diarrhea

Frequently the history and physical examination do not provide a specific diagnosis and an initial laboratory evaluation (see Box 14.5) may be helpful in distinguishing the different categories of chronic diarrhea as listed above.

Stool tests

The laboratory evaluation of chronic diarrhea should begin with the stool. The simplest test is the identification of occult blood in the stool. This simple test is performed by the application of a dilute hydrogen peroxide solution to a sample of stool smeared on a test card which contains another reagent. A positive reaction produces a deep blue color which can be compared with the positive control spot. Care must be taken with this test in a patient who is taking iron because the greenish discoloration of stool produced by the iron may be confused with a positive test. Rehydration of samples that have dried increases the accuracy of the test.

Box 14.10 Clinical categories

Chronic watery diarrhea (osmotic or secretory)
Diabetes mellitus
Immunosuppression
Stomal diarrhea
Factitious diarrhea

The presence of occult blood suggests an inflammatory or neoplastic process of the gastrointestinal tract.

Fecal leukocytes, while more commonly seen in acute inflammatory diarrheas, may also be seen in chronic inflammatory conditions such as ulcerative colitis. The careful study of multiple samples of stools for ova or parasites may reveal the etiologic agent for diarrhea such as *Giardia*. The detection rate for *Giardia* may be increased by the use of an antigen detection test in stool. Stools can be stored for several days in a refrigerator prior to such testing. Antigen tests are also available for *Cryptosporidium*. Of course, more extensive examination for parasites needs to be performed on immunocompromised patients. The Sudan stain is a simple test to detect excessive fat in the stool. Stool tests for *C. difficile* should be carried out if there is any history of prior antibiotic therapy.

Complete blood count

A complete blood count may be helpful in revealing anemia. Microcytic anemia indicates iron deficiency from chronic blood loss from inflammatory bowel disease, neoplasia, acute dysentery or malabsorption. Normochromic anemia suggests the anemia of chronic disease which also can be seen in inflammatory bowel disease. Macrocytic anemia suggests folic acid or vitamin B_{12} deficiency, usually a manifestation of malabsorption or malnutrition. Combined iron and folate deficiency suggests proximal small bowel disease, celiac disease and tropical sprue (Frisancho et al 1994). An elevated white blood cell count suggests an inflammatory process. Particularly high levels may be seen in pseudomembranous colitis.

Leukopenia may occasionally occur in severe malnutrition. The differential white cell count may reveal eosinophilia, suggestive of infection with metazoan parasites such as hookworm or strongyloides. Lymphopenia may suggest the acquired immunodeficiency syndrome or severe malnutrition. The total platelet count is often increased in patients presenting with Crohn's disease and may be diminished in patients with the cytoverotoxin-producing strain of *E. coli*, 0157-H7.

Serum biochemistry

An elevated blood urea nitrogen indicates significant dehydration. It may be low in severely malnourished patients due to loss of muscle mass. Hypokalemia may result from vomiting and/or diarrhea. In watery diarrhea, hypokalemia suggests a hormonal cause such as Verner–Morrison syndrome or a potassium-secreting villous adenoma of the colon. Hypoproteinemia often indicates inflammatory bowel disease, malabsorption or protein-losing enteropathy. A low globulin fraction suggests protein-losing enteropathy or, in the absence of hypoalbuminemia, suggests a rare immunodeficiency state such as common variable hypogammaglobulinemia. A low serum calcium level, particularly one out of proportion to the serum albumin and confirmed by a diminished serum ionized calcium level, suggests malabsorption of vitamin D, usually associated with small bowel mucosal disease. An elevated alkaline phosphatase with otherwise normal liver function tests may be of bone origin in malabsorption or of intestinal origin in inflammation. An elevated alkaline phosphatase with abnormal tests of hepatocellular function suggests cholestatic liver disease producing steatorrhea due to bile salt deficiency. Elevated serum transaminases can occur in patients with sepsis or celiac disease.

Abnormal non-specific indicators of inflammation, such as the erythrocyte sedimentation rate or the C-reactive protein level, suggest an inflammatory condition but lack sensitivity and specificity. The finding of an elevated sedimentation rate or C-reactive protein level in a patient suspected of having functional bowel disease should prompt a diligent search for organic disease.

CHRONIC WATERY DIARRHEA

A case of chronic watery diarrhea where all the basic tests are negative presents a significant diagnostic challenge. In this situation, identifying the diarrhea as being primarily secretory or osmotic may be quite helpful.

Calculating the fecal osmolar gap may be helpful in distinguishing between secretory and osmotic diarrhea:

[fecal osm–2(sodium + potassium)] = calculated fecal osmolar gap (sodium and potassium are fecal measured values)

In secretory diarrhea, the sodium and potassium and other cations account for the entire osmotic load (fecal osmolar gap <40). In osmotic diarrhea, an osmotic load increases the osmolality of the stool above that of the plasma. Sodium passes into the blood to equilibrate the fecal plasma osmolalities, increasing the gap between the total osmolality and the major cations present (>40). The estimation of the osmolar gap is of limited diagnostic use due to the difficulty in collection and the wide variation in the results. The plasma osmolality may be substituted in most cases for the measured fecal values (Duncan et al 1992).

Many diseases can also cause more than one type of diarrhea. Celiac disease causes both a secretory diarrhea due to the inflammation and an osmotic diarrhea due to maldigested carbohydrates. The finding of a very high stool osmolality relative to plasma osmolality usually indicates contamination of the stool with urine. Conversely a low osmolality probably results from the dilution of the stool with water – factitious diarrhea.

Osmotic diarrhea

If the diarrhea can be characterized as osmotic on the basis of a fecal osmolar gap, the following tests may be useful in determining the etiology (Box 14.11).

The measurement of excreted hydrogen in the breath may be useful to define the cause of maldigestion (King & Toskes 1984). Hydrogen, produced by bacterial degradation of carbohydrates in the colon and small intestine, is rapidly assimilated and excreted in the breath. The patient provides samples of expired breath into sealed containers. The samples are analyzed for the concentration of hydrogen at intervals before and after the ingestion of a substrate carbohydrate. An elevated baseline or an early rise in breath hydrogen within 2 hours of ingestion of glucose, lactulose or lactose suggests bacterial overgrowth. Intolerance to lactose or other disaccharides produces a delayed peak that may coincide with the reproduction of symptoms (Corazza et al 1990). False negative results occur due to colonic resection and prior antibiotic therapy. False positives reflect the lack of compliance with dietary restrictions and smoking. Patients with pancreatic insufficiency or previous gastric surgery may also show false early peaks due to rapid transit.

Serologic tests for celiac disease

Two classes of serologic tests are available for celiac disease. One class identifies deficiencies due to malabsorption by measuring serum concentrations of, for example, carotene, folate, vitamin B_{12} and iron. The second class are antibody tests. These can be autoantibodies, such as reticulin or endomysial antibodies directed against connective tissue, or antigliadin antibodies (Chorzelski et al 1984). The reticulin antibody,

---

Box 14.11   Evaluation of osmotic diarrhea

Hydrogen breath test – lactose/fructose/sucrose
Serologic screening for celiac disease
Trial of antibiotics
72–hour fecal fat
Stool pH (useful in children)
Stool magnesium
Small bowel biopsy and quantitative culture

present in the serum of untreated patients with celiac disease, reacts with reticulin derived from rodent liver or kidney. The endomysial antibodies (usually IgA) recognize the extracellular connective tissue in smooth muscle bundles. Antigliadin antibodies are directed against gliadin, the fraction of gluten thought to be most harmful in gluten-sensitive entero-pathy. The IgA antibodies are more specific but the frequency of selective IgA deficiency in patients with celiac disease means that some false negatives occur. In this situation the IgG antibodies are usually positive. Some reports suggest that these serologic tests have sensitivities and specificities that approach 99%, but these are based on retrospective serologic surveys performed in research laboratories.

The serologic tests cannot yet substitute for intestinal biopsy in the diagnosis of celiac disease (Ferreira et al 1992). They represent a signifi-cant advance in screening patients at risk for celiac disease and probably should replace the more non-specific screening tests that depend upon the demonstration of a deficiency syndrome or a radiographic abnormality.

Occasionally, particularly in elderly patients, bacterial overgrowth syndromes are particularly common and may justify the use of an empiric course of antibiotics as an initial diagnostic trial (Haboubi & Montgomery 1992).

Secretory diarrhea (Box 14.12)

If patients clearly have secretory diarrhea and tests for parasitic, protozoal or common endocrine abnormalities are negative, an evaluation of the colon, both endoscopically and histologically, should be carried out. If this examination is negative, small intestinal biopsies should be obtained. If these are non-diagnostic, then a small bowel contrast study may detect intestinal Crohn's disease or other structural lesions associated with diarrhea such as jejunal diverticulosis, blind loop syndrome, intestinal lymphoma or intestinal carcinoid syndrome.

If the above tests are all negative or unrevealing and the patient continues to produce more than 300 cc of liquid stool output despite fasting, then rarer hormonal causes for diarrhea should be considered

---

Box 14.12 Secretory diarrhea

Giardia antigen, *Entamoeba histolytica* antibody titers and *Yersinia* culture
Fasting serum glucose and thyroid function tests
Colonoscopy with right-sided biopsies
Small bowel biopsy
Small bowel contrast study
Cholestyramine trial for bile acid diarrhea
Fasting gastrin, VIP

Box 14.13 Hormonal diarrheas

Hormone	**Disease/syndrome**
Vasoactive intestinal polypeptide	Severe diarrhea, hypokalemia, hypochlorhydria, acidosis
Calcitonin	Medullary cell carcinoma, associated with MEN 1
Gastrin	Zollinger–Ellison syndrome
Histamine	Systemic mastocytosis, gastric hypersecretion, enlarged liver and spleen
Serotonin	Carcinoid, flushing, wheezing

(Box 14.13). The most common and well described is that of a small tumor producing vasoactive intestinal polypeptide, the Verner–Morrison syndrome; carcinoid syndrome is suggested by the presence of flushing and wheezing and confirmed by 24-hour collection for 5-hydroxy-indole acetic acid, a product of serotonin. Diarrhea as a part of the Zollinger–Ellison syndrome can be checked by measuring fasting serum gastrin levels.

These hormonal causes of diarrhea are rare. Indeed, in one large series of patients investigated for obscure chronic watery diarrhea, 86 out of 193 patients had one or more abnormally elevated peptide levels. On follow-up, none of these patients proved to have a hormone peptide-producing tumor (Schiller et al 1994).

STEATORRHEA

When the presentation strongly suggests steatorrhea rather than diarrhea, or if measurements of fecal fat confirm the presence of excessive fat in the stool, then a specific series of investigations will usually identify the cause of the fat malabsorption (Box 14.14). The utility of a 72-hour fecal fat collection in identifying fat malabsorption is limited by practical concerns relating to the difficulty of adequate collection, the appropriate dietary challenge of at least 100 g of fat per day, the unpleasantness of quantitative analysis and the significant delay in carrying out the test and

---

Box 14.14 Steatorrhea investigations

Giardia antigen on stool
Liver blood tests to screen for cholestatic liver disease
Plain abdominal film for pancreatic calcification
Multiple duodenal or small bowel biopsies
Duodenal or jejunal aspirate for quantitative culture, *Giardia* examination

If above negative:
   Dedicated small bowel contrast study
   Tests of pancreatic function

obtaining the results. In patients with the abrupt onset of steatorrhea, especially if there is a history of foreign travel, exposure to young children or the use of well water, examination of the stool for *Giardia* antigen may be the only test required.

Small intestinal biopsy is the most important diagnostic test for identifying celiac disease, tropical sprue, Whipple's disease and protein-losing enteropathy. Endoscopy is preferred because it allows visual evaluation, directed biopsies and aspiration of fluid for culture and examination for *Giardia*. Pancreatic insufficiency should be considered in patients with chronic alcoholism or diabetes. The finding of a fat secretion of greater than 30 g/day indicates pancreatic insufficiency, especially if the stool water content is not particularly high.

Radiographic contrast studies are useful when the above investigations are negative. A small intestinal series or enteroclysis allows identification of such abnormalities as blind loops, Crohn's disease, jejunal diverticulosis, lymphoma and, rarely, pseudoobstruction syndromes. In older patients or patients with known extensive atherosclerosis, mesenteric arteriography should be considered to investigate ischemia. Other rare conditions, such as lymphoma or immunoproliferative small intestinal disease, are often identified by an abnormal IgA on electrophoresis. Occasionally CT scanning may demonstrate the thickened small intestinal wall or lymphadenopathy suggestive of lymphoma. Some drugs, including cholestyramine, neomycin and colchicine, occasionally precipitate steatorrhea.

The finding of significant steatorrhea without evidence for liver disease or small intestinal disease should prompt evaluation of pancreatic function. A pancreatogram or a CT scan may reveal anatomic abnorm-alities. Tests of pancreatic function are cumbersome and require duodenal intubation to measure the pancreatic secretion of bicarbonate enzymes following stimulation with intravenous CCK. In the bentiramide test (a non-invasive and non-specific measure of pancreatic function), bentir-amide is enzymatically hydrolized by pancreatic chymotrypsin and releases paraaminobenzoic acid (PABA) which is rapidly absorbed by an intact intestinal mucosa and excreted in the urine. This test is a reliable marker for chronic pancreatic exocrine insufficiency. The causes of steatorrhea are listed in Box 14.15.

Box 14.15   Causes of steatorrhea

Giardiasis
Celiac disease
HIV enteropathy
Cholestatic liver disease
Pancreatic exocrine failure
Bacterial overgrowth syndrome

> **Box 14.16** Investigation of chronic exudative diarrhea
>
> CBC
> Serum albumin, total protein
> Sedimentation rate
> Electrolytes
> *Entamoeba histolytica* titer
> Stool culture, *Clostridium difficile*, latex
> agglutination, O&P
> Flexible sigmoidoscopy and biopsies

BLOODY EXUDATIVE COLITIS

The presence of gross blood mixed with the stool implies an inflammatory or neoplastic process affecting the colon.

Exudative diarrhea is nearly always due to colonic inflammation, neoplasia or infection. Grossly bloody diarrhea is always due to a colonic disease. Direct stool tests may occasionally show amebic cysts, bacterial pathogens or the toxin of *C. difficile*. Chronic exudative diarrhea is most often due to inflammatory bowel disease characterized by the presence of anemia, hypoalbuminemia and an increased sedimentation rate. The initial tests that are helpful in assessing exudative diarrhea are listed in Box 14.16.

The endoscopic examination of the colon is essential in differentiating the various forms of colonic inflammation or neoplasia responsible for the diarrhea. Complete colonoscopic examination may be unnecessary or unwise if there is severe or obvious inflammation in the rectosigmoid on initial flexible sigmoidoscopy. However, in older patients or when the cause of the diarrhea is not obvious from history or initial investigation, then a complete colonoscopic examination should be carried out. If the endoscopy is macroscopically normal, biopsies from the right and left side of the colonic mucosa should be obtained. The endoscopic findings and histology should allow discrimination of the various types of colitis (Box 14.17) (Fig. 14.3).

MOTILITY DISORDERS

Motor abnormalities are the primary cause of diarrhea in hormonal disorders (hyperthyroidism, carcinoid syndrome), neuronal disorders (diabetic autonomic neuropathy, dysautonomia) and drug effects (erythromycin, misoprostol, and possibly cisapride). In many of these conditions there is also stimulation of intestinal secretion which aggravates the diarrhea.

Hypomotility of the intestine may also cause diarrhea. The poorly

Box 14.17 Features of chronic colitis

Disease	Endoscopic appearance	Histology
Ulcerative colitis	Continuous inflammation, friability, loss of vascular pattern, superficial ulcers, pseudopolyps	Continuous inflammation, crypt abscesses, inflamtion limited to mucosa
Crohn's disease	Skip lesions, aphthous ulcers, strictures, perianal fissures/fistulae	Transluminal inflammation, granulomas, fibrosis
Lymphocytic/collagenous* colitis	Normal-looking mucosa or erythematous patches	Increased lymphocytes in intercryptal epithelium (Fig. 14.3), *increased thickness in subepithelial collagen (>7 mM). May be associated with celiac disease
Ischemic colitis	Well-demarcated areas, ulcers, strictures, watershed areas, rectum spared	Hemorrhage, fading of entire crypts (ghosts)
Brainerd diarrhea	Normal macroscopic appearance	Clusters of subepithelial inflammatory cells/normal
Radiation colitis	Loss of vascular pattern, telangiectasia, erythema, stricturing	Vasculitis, foamy macrophages, atrophic mucosa, eosinophilic crypt adhesions
Diversion colitis	Similar to ulcerative colitis, occurs in distal colon when fecal stream is diverted via stoma	Continuous inflammation, crypt abscesses, inflammation limited to mucosa

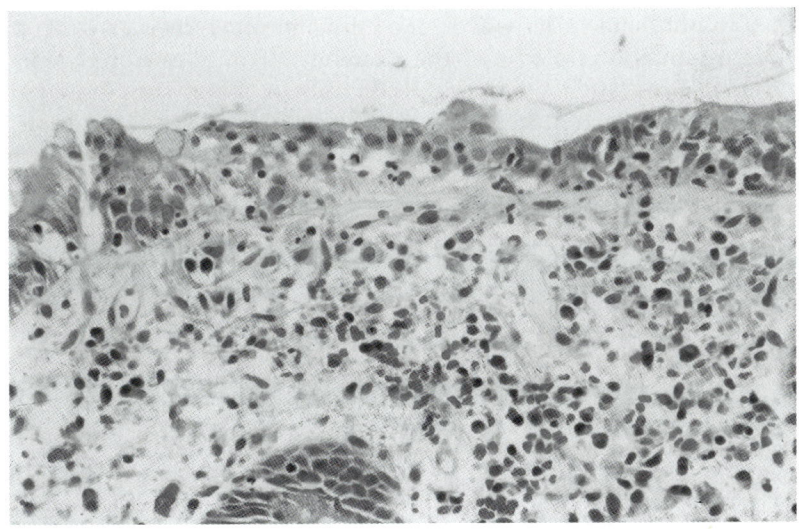

Figure 14.3 This photomicrograph of the colonic mucosa demonstrates the intraepithelial lymphocytosis affecting the intercryptal epithelium that is characteristic of lymphocytic colitis (courtesy of F. Mitros).

contracting gut suffers from stasis and consequent bacterial overgrowth. This is especially common in scleroderma, hypothyroidism, diabetes and in the very old. Colonic hypomotility may lead to severe constipation and fecal impaction with resultant overflow diarrhea. The investigation of primary motor abnormalities relies on anatomic studies demonstrating bowel dilatation or stasis in the absence of mechanical obstruction.

FUNCTIONAL DIARRHEA

In many patients with a disordered bowel habit, careful evaluation fails to reveal an organic cause. Many blame these problems on a presumed irritability of the intestine. The term 'functional' diarrhea suggests anxiety-induced diarrhea. This is likely to represent an exaggeration of a normal physiologic response to stress as exemplified by the medical students' rush to toilet prior to examination.

As a clinical entity, the irritable bowel syndrome or spastic colon defies scientific definition. If one defines such patients as having a syndrome consisting of the onset of GI disturbances at an early age, habitual early morning rush to stool, the frequent passage of small volume and semi-formed or hard stools associated with lower abdominal cramping, and an excitable temperament, it seems highly unlikely that such a syndrome will evolve into an organic disease provided that no features suggestive of organic disease are present (Box 14.18). If none of these features are present and the basic laboratory tests outlined in Box 14.5 are negative, a provisional diagnosis of functional diarrhea may be made. However, the clinician must keep an open mind with regard to the etiology of the diarrhea. If it does not respond to simple measures such as stress reduction or fiber supplementation, further evaluation is required.

Many patients with functional diarrhea have their symptoms aggravated by certain foods. It would be logical to ascribe such symptoms to food intolerance rather than label them as irritable bowel syndrome.

Box 14.18   Features suggesting organic rather than functional diarrhea

Nocturnal diarrhea
Blood in the stool
Weight loss
Late (greater than 40 years)/recent onset
Fever or systemic symptoms
Predominantly watery stools
Abnormality on basic lab tests

Box 14.19 Differential diagnosis of chronic diabetic diarrhea

Idiopathic autonomic diabetic diarrhea
Bacterial overgrowth
Celiac disease
Pancreatic exocrine insufficiency
Ingestion of diabetic foods high in fructose/sorbitol

DIABETES MELLITUS

Diarrhea in diabetes mellitus is associated with a specific differential diagnosis (Box 14.19) (Valdovinos et al 1993). The dietary withdrawal of diabetic foods high in fructose or sorbitol may dramatically improve diarrhea. A trial of antibiotics (metronidazole or tetracycline) can be used if there is a suspicion of intestinal bacterial overgrowth. A plain abdominal X-ray will reveal pancreatic calcification in many cases of pancreatic exocrine insufficiency. Serological tests for the antiendomysial antibody, the antigliadin antibody and the antireticulin antibody may reveal celiac disease (Talal et al 1993). Confirmation requires the demonstration of villous damage and a subsequent clinical improvement on a gluten-free diet. Finally, the diagnosis of idiopathic diabetic diarrhea is suggested by the presence of symptoms of autonomic neuropathy or gastroparesis (Ogbonnaya & Arem 1990).

STOMAL DIARRHEA

The reduced absorptive surface after resection of the intestine increases the likelihood of fluid and electrolyte imbalance. The location of the stoma in the intestine is a major factor in determining the volume of stool. Stomas in the terminal ileum can produce volumes of 1–2 liters per day.

OBSCURE DIARRHEA

In some patients the cause of chronic diarrhea cannot be found (Afzalpurkar et al 1992). In such patients a detailed history without prior reference to any previous record and review of previous test results may reveal something that was overlooked or misinterpreted. The most common causes that have been ultimately found in such cases are listed in Box 14.20.

Brainerd diarrhea

In some patients with abrupt onset of secretory diarrhea where no organic cause can be found, the symptoms resolve spontaneously after 7–31

Box 14.20 Obscure causes of diarrhea

Bile salt diarrhea
Brainerd diarrhea
Factitious diarrhea
Food allergies
Microscopic colitis

---

months (Afzalpurkar et al 1992). This probably represents an enteric infectious process, as exemplified by an epidemic of chronic diarrhea of abrupt onset in Brainerd County, Minnesota (Osterholm et al 1986). Occasionally, careful histologic examination of right-sided colonic biopsies may reveal collections of inflammatory cells in the lamina propria (Janda et al 1991).

Bile salt diarrhea

Malabsorption of bile salts may result from many disease processes, including small bowel resection, Crohn's disease, bacterial overgrowth and small bowel mucosal disease. The delivery of significant amounts of bile salts to the colon incites the colonic enterocytes to secrete. This kind of diarrhea does not always respond to bile acid binding with cholestyramine (Eusufzai 1993).

Malabsorption of bile salts due to ileal resection may deplete the bile salt pool. This depletion can then lead to steatorrhea. In a patient who has distal small bowel disease or has had a resection, a raised fecal fat output suggests depletion of the bile salt pool. Cholestyramine may further deplete the bile salt pool and exacerbate the malabsorption.

Factitious diarrhea

Factitious diarrhea deserves special mention as it is the cause in a significant number of patients with diarrhea of obscure origin. Specific indicators suggesting factitious diarrhea are often present but not recognized by unsuspecting physicians. There may be a history of medical attention-seeking behavior in the past. This occurs classically in a young female patient working in the healthcare field. Features that should raise suspicion include a vague but dramatic history, the lack of visitors, vagueness about the locations and names of physicians who rendered treatments in the past and ignoring hospital rules or dietary restrictions. Physical examination may reveal multiple scars from prior medical/surgical procedures. Such patients are often prepared to be subjected to multiple investigations.

Stool osmolality may be very high if urine has been added to the stool after its passage. A very low stool osmolality indicates the addition of water. Stool magnesium levels are usually elevated in magnesium salt-induced osmotic diarrhea (Fine et al 1991). Sulfate may be detected in the stool of patients taking sodium sulfate. Various laxatives or derivatives that can be detected in the stool (or urine) include phenolphthalein, danthron and bisacodyl. Lactulose use can be inferred from the presence of a high osmotic gap. Such measures as room searches are fraught with legal implications and best avoided unless there is an imminent risk of self-harm or death. These patients should not be immediately confronted with evidence but should be referred for a psychiatric consultation.

REFERENCES

Afzalpurkar R G, Schiller L R, Little K H, Santangelo W C, Fortran J S 1992 The self-limited nature of chronic idiopathic diarrhea. New England Journal of Medicine 327: 1849

Bernstein B B, Gelb A, Tabanda-Lichauco R 1994 Crohn's ileitis in a patient with longstanding HIV infection. American Journal of Gastroenterology 89: 937–939

Black R E 1986 Pathogens that cause travelers' diarrhea in Latin American and Africa. Review of Infectious Diseases 8: S131–S135

Blackstone M O, Kirsner J B 1991 Clinical application of diagnostic tests in selected colonic disorders. In: Phillips S F, Pemberton J H, Shorter R G (eds) The large intestine, physiology, pathophysiology and disease. Raven Press, New York

Carter A O, Borczyk A A, Carlson J A et al 1987 A severe outbreak of Escherichia coli 0157:H7-associated hemorrhagic colitis in a nursing home. New England Journal of Medicine 317: 1496–1500

Cello J P 1993 Evaluation of AIDS-related diarrhea. Hospital Practice 28: 95–102

Chester A C, MacMurray F G, Restifo M D, Mann O 1985 Giardiasis as a chronic disease. Digestive Diseases and Sciences 30: 215–218

Chorzelski T P, Buetner E H, Sulej J, Tchorzewska H, Jablonska S, Kumar V, Kapuscinska A 1984 IgA antiendomysium antibody. A new immunological marker of dermatitis herpitiformis and celiac disease. British Journal of Dermatology 111: 395–402

Chui D W, Owen R L 1994 AIDS and the gut. Journal of Gastroenterology and Hepatology 9: 291–303

Corazza G R, Sorge M, Strocchi A, Lattanzi M C, Benati G, Gasbarrini G 1990 Methodology of the H_2 breath test. II. Importance of the test duration in the diagnosis of carbohydrate malabsorption. Italian Journal of Gastroenterology 22: 303–305

Crowe S E, Perdue M H 1992 Gastrointestinal food hypersensitivity: basic mechanisms of pathophysiology. Gastroenterology 103: 1075–1095

Dekker-Saeys B J, Meuwissen S G, Van Den Berg-Loonen E M, De Haas W H, Agenant D, Tytgat G N 1978 Ankylosing spondylitis and inflammatory bowel disease. II. Prevalence of peripheral arthritis, sacroiliitis, and ankylosing spondylitis in patients suffering from inflammatory bowel disease. Annals of the Rheumatic Diseases 37: 33–35

Duncan A, Robertson C, Russell R I 1992 The fecal osmotic gap: technical aspects regarding its calculation. Journal of Laboratory and Clinical Medicine 119: 359–363

Dworkin B M, Rosenthal W S 1993 Diarrhea in patients with acquired immunodeficiency syndrome. Practical Gastroenterology 17: 9–17

Eusufzai S 1993 Bile acid malabsorption in patients with chronic diarrhoea. Scandinavian Journal of Gastroenterology 28: 865–868

Fellows I W, Freeman J G, Holmes G K 1990 Crohn's disease in the city of Derby, 1951–85. Gut 31: 1262–1265

Ferreira M, Davies S L, Butler M, Scott D, Clark M, Kumar P 1992 Endomysial antibody – is it the best screening test for celiac disease? Gut 33: 1633–1637

Fine K D, Santa Ana C A, Fordtran J S 1991 Diagnosis of magnesium-induced diarrhea. New England Journal of Medicine 324: 1012–1017

Frisancho O, Ulloa V, Ruiz W et al 1994 Megaloblastic anemia associated with chronic diarrhea. A prospective and multicenter study in Lima. Rivista de Gastroenterologia del Peru 14: 189–195

Guerrant R L, Araujo V, Soares E, Kotloff K, Lima A A, Cooper W H, Lee A G 1992 Measurement of fecal lactoferrin as a marker of fecal leukocytes. Journal of Clinical Microbiology 30: 1238–1242

Haboubi N Y, Montgomery R D 1992 Small-bowel bacterial overgrowth in elderly people: clinical significance and response to treatment. Age and Ageing 21: 13–19

Hara Y, Morimoto K, Nakamura Y et al 1993 A case report of graft-versus-host disease caused by using stored blood after aortic valve replacement. Kyobu Geka (Japanese Journal of Thoracic Surgery) 46: 438–441

Jacobson M A, O'Donnell J J, Porteous D et al 1988 Retinal and gastrointestinal disease due to cytomegalovirus in patients with the acquired immune deficiency syndrome: prevalence, natural history and response to gancyclovir therapy. Quarterly Journal of Medicine 67: 473–486

Janda R C, Conklin J L, Mitros F A, Parsonnet J 1991 Multifocal colitis associated with an epidemic of chronic diarrhea. Gastroenterology 100: 458–464

Kelly M T, Champagne S G, Sherlock C H et al 1987 Commercial latex agglutination test for detection of Clostridium difficile-associated diarrhea. Journal of Clinical Microbiology 25: 1244–1247

King C E, Toskes P P 1984 The use of breath tests in the study of malabsorption (review). Clinics in Gastroenterology 12: 591–610

Kotler D P, Reka S, Clayton F 1993 Intestinal mucosal inflammation associated with human immunodeficiency virus infection. Digestive Diseases and Sciences 38: 1119–1127

Moll J M 1985 Inflammatory bowel disease. Clinics in Rheumatic Diseases 11: 87–111

Morris A J, Wilson M L, Reller L B 1992 Application of rejection criteria for stool ovum and parasite examinations. Journal of Clinical Microbiology 30: 3213–3216

Ogbonnaya K I, Arem R 1990 Diabetic diarrhea. Archives of Internal Medicine 150: 262–267

Orvar K, Murray J, Carmen G, Conklin J L 1993 Cytomegalovirus infection associated with onset of inflammatory bowel disease. Digestive Diseases and Sciences 38: 2307–2310

Osterholm M T, MacDonald K L, White K E et al 1986 An outbreak of a newly recognized chronic diarrheal syndrome associated with raw milk consumption. Journal of the American Medical Association 256: 848–849

Roberts J P, Ascher N L, Lake J et al 1991 Graft vs. host disease after liver transplantation in humans: a report of four cases. Hepatology 14: 274–281

Ryo R, Goto M, Takada M et al 1994 Diagnosis of post-transfusion graft-versus-host disease after formalin-fixation. International Journal of Hematology 59: 297–302

Schiller L R, Rivera L M, Santangelo W C, Little K H, Fordtran J S 1994 Diagnostic value of fasting plasma peptide concentrations in patients with chronic diarrhea. Digestive Diseases and Sciences 39: 2216–2222

Sturgess I, Greenfield S M, Teare J, O'Doherty M J 1992 Ulcerative colitis developing after amoebic dysentery, in a haemophiliac patient with AIDS. Gut 33: 408–410

Sung J J, Hsu R K, Chan F K, Liew C T, Lau J W, Li A K 1994 Crohn's disease in the Chinese population. An experience from Hong Kong. Diseases of the Colon and Rectum 37: 1307–1309

Talal A H, Murray J A, Goeken J A, Sivitz W I 1993 Celiac disease in American type I diabetics. American Journal of Gastroenterology 88: 1564

Taylor D N, Escheverria P 1986 Etiology and epidemiology of travelersí diarrhea in Asia. Review of Infectious Disease 8: S136–S141

Tjandra J J, Cuthbertson A M, Penfold C 1990 Sessile adenomas of the rectum: a personal series 1974–1984. Australian and New Zealand Journal of Surgery 60: 883–886.

Valdovinos M A, Camilleri M, Zimmerman B R 1993 Chronic diarrhea in diabetes mellitus: mechanisms and an approach to diagnosis and treatment. Mayo Clinic Proceedings 68: 691–702

15

Assessment of the constipated patient

R. Hutchinson   D. Kumar

Constipation is a symptom and not a disease. It is the patient's subjective impression of an abnormal evacuatory function. Constipation may be due to organic, structural or metabolic disease, abnormal gastrointestinal or pelvic floor function or abnormal perception of normal evacuation. Rational management of the constipated patient depends on determining the cause of symptoms, the site or sites of abnormality and quantification of the severity of the physiological disturbance (Pemberton et al 1991, Wexner et al 1991).

As is routine with the evaluation of other symptoms, the assessment of constipation begins with taking a history and performing a physical examination. This is followed by the logical application of special investigations.

HISTORY

General causes for constipation should be sought with a history of medical illnesses, dietary habits and drug treatments. A detailed history of the bowel habit should be elicited including bowel frequency, consistency of stools, straining, pain on defecation, incomplete evacuation and the use of manual evacuation. Patients should be asked specifically about associated features such as abdominal pain, distension, weight loss and rectal bleeding. The duration of symptoms and whether or not the onset was related to a pelvic procedure should be determined. In women, the relationship of symptoms to the menstrual cycle, obstetric events and gynecological operations should be established. In patients who give an equivocal history, a diary of their bowel habit may be instructive, especially as the correlation between symptoms and objective abnormalities is poor (Probert et al 1994).

There are several definitions of constipation based upon the analysis of symptoms (Drossman et al 1982, Kumar 1992, Probert et al 1994). Some definitions refer to the infrequency of defecation, others to the nature of the stool and others to the patient's subjective feelings of straining, pain, incomplete evacuation or abdominal distension. A consensus definition of constipation is less than three bowel actions per week and/or straining at more than 25% of bowel actions (Drossman et al 1982, Whitehead et al 1991). However, it is important to establish the nature of an individual patient's complaint and to determine which features of constipation are particularly troublesome. Although correlation with objective functional abnormalities is poor, the nature of symptoms may occasionally point to the likely cause of constipation. For example, patients with chronic idiopathic constipation are typically female with little or no urge to evacuate and bowel actions less than once per week with associated abdominal distension (Preston & Lennard-Jones 1986). Symptoms typically begin in adolescence or following a gynecological procedure such as hysterectomy (Smith et al 1990). This type of constipation is usually unresponsive to laxatives.

Constipated patients who also suffer from colicky abdominal pain and abdominal distension related to the phase of the menstrual cycle may have the constipation-predominant type of irritable bowel syndrome (Trotman & Price 1986). Certain 'alarm' symptoms such as weight loss and rectal bleeding in a patient with a relatively short history of constipation should raise the possibility of colorectal malignancy. Anal canal bleeding and pain on defecation suggest a local anorectal cause for constipation such as perianal sepsis or anal fissure.

PHYSICAL EXAMINATION

Physical examination may suggest general medical causes of constipation by revealing features of hypothyroidism, diabetes mellitus or a connective tissue disorder. A thorough neurological examination should be performed. Abdominal examination, perineal inspection, rectal examination and proctosigmoidoscopy are mandatory and may reveal local causes of constipation such as perianal sepsis, an anal fissure or rectal carcinoma.

On perineal inspection, pelvic floor descent should be assessed. Mucosal or full-thickness rectal prolapses may become apparent on straining. Rectal examination should include an assessment of anal sphincter resting tone and squeeze pressures, sphincter defects and rectoceles. Digital evaluation of sphincter function correlates with anal canal manometry (Hallan et al 1989). Fecoliths and megarectum are apparent on digital examination of the rectum. As well as showing specific causes of constipation such as rectal carcinoma, proctosigmoidoscopy may reveal associated features of constipation such as hemorrhoids, solitary rectal ulcer syndrome or melanosis coli. The solitary rectal ulcer syndrome is characterized by distinct histological changes and so biopsies may be diagnostic. Air insufflation may reproduce the typical abdominal pain and this may support a diagnosis of irritable bowel syndrome. (Ritchie 1973).

Features of subacute intestinal obstruction with abdominal distension as a prominent symptom raise the possibility of chronic idiopathic intestinal pseudoobstruction as well as the more common causes of mechanical intestinal obstruction.

INVESTIGATIONS

Hematological and biochemical tests

Abnormalities of blood glucose, calcium or thyroid function may indicate a medical cause for constipation. Anemia may be associated with a colorectal neoplasm. However, blood tests are usually unhelpful in cases of chronic idiopathic constipation.

Imaging tests

Plain abdominal radiographs provide a qualitative assessment of the degree of fecal loading. Fecal impaction and intestinal obstruction may be diagnosed (Mezwa et al 1993). Barium enema examination of the colon is one of the most important investigations in the assessment of the constipated patient to find mechanical causes of symptoms. In addition to mechanical problems, such physiological disorders as adult Hirschsprung's disease, megacolon and solitary rectal ulcer syndrome may also be diagnosed by barium enema (Feczko et al 1980, Goei et al 1988, Levine et al 1986, Ponka et al 1972). Contrast radiology is essential also to differentiate mechanical from acute or chronic intestinal pseudoobstruction (Koruth et al 1985).

Barium enema examination may be safely omitted in constipated patients with a long history of symptoms who fulfill diagnostic criteria for the irritable bowel syndrome (Manning et al 1978). The diagnosis is reliable and the risk of missing other pathology is negligible for patients meeting these criteria (Holmes & Salter 1982). Nevertheless, in practice, a barium enema is usually performed in all patients complaining of chronic constipation. A normal finding is of value in reassuring the patient that mechanical pathology is excluded and that the complaint is being taken seriously by the investigating clinician.

Upper gastrointestinal contrast studies may be considered if the history and physical examination suggest a panenteric motor disorder. However, these conditions are better evaluated with transit studies.

Endoscopy

Rigid proctosigmoidoscopy should be performed on all patients presenting with constipation as part of the initial physical examination. Flexible sigmoidoscopy or colonoscopy is indicated in the assessment of the constipated patient who has a short history of altered bowel habit, especially if 'alarm' symptoms such as rectal bleeding or weight loss raise the suspicion of colorectal malignancy. Colonoscopy is complementary to barium enema examination. The choice of which investigation should come first in the management strategy will usually be influenced by local logistical considerations such as availability of and waiting times for the investigations (Lindsay et al 1988).

FUNCTIONAL ASSESSMENT

If the history, physical examination, imaging investigations and endoscopic procedures discussed above do not reveal a mechanical cause for symptoms, the patient's constipation may be due to a functional gastrointestinal disorder and functional assessment is necessary to guide rational treatment. Recent advances in the evaluation of patients with chronic constipation have enabled more precise definition of the various physiological abnormalities and improved the classification of patients according to their functional defect. Constipated patients may have abnormalities of colonic transit, pelvic floor dysfunction, impaired rectal evacuation, panenteric neuropathies or combinations of these functional abnormalities (Devroede 1988, Kumar 1992, Roe et al 1986).

Colonic transit tests

Techniques of measuring colonic transit that involve the ingestion of non-absorbable markers (Alvarez & Freedlander 1924), colored powders or chemically detectable markers such as chromium oxide (Whitby & Lang 1960) and copper thiocyanate (Dick 1969) are obsolete because they are inconvenient, necessitating the collection and examination of stools for several days. Furthermore, these tests reflect whole gut transit and not colonic transit.

Radiological techniques involving ingestion of radioopaque markers of different shapes or sizes have been devised for the measurement of colonic transit. These tests may require several abdominal radiographs taken up to 7 days following marker ingestion. They can be time consuming and subject the patients to excessive radiation. It may be difficult to determine the positions of the markers within the colon because of gross colonic movements and overlap of bowel loops. Nevertheless, segmental colonic transit can be assessed (Chaussade et al 1989, Hinton et al 1969). The test can be simplified by taking a single radiograph at 5 days from marker ingestion (Evans et al 1992, Metcalf et al 1987). These modifications improve safety and convenience but the radiographs remain difficult to interpret.

Colonic scintigraphy has become the method of choice for assessment of colonic transit (Van der Sijp et al 1993). It has superseded other techniques because it is relatively quick, convenient and non-invasive. Previously, problems with delivery of radionuclide to the colon prevented the widespread use of scintigraphy. Ingestion of the radionuclide resulted in scintigraphic activity distributed throughout the stomach and small intestine as well as the colon (McLean et al 1990). Direct instillation of radionuclide via a fine nasocecal tube (Kamm et al 1988, Krevsky et al 1986) or via a tube placed at colonoscopy (Moreno-Osset et al 1989) is invasive and of doubtful physiological validity. Bowel preparation and colonoscopy may alter colonic transit.

These problems have been overcome with a delivery system which was originally used for the deposition of drugs in the proximal colon (Hardy et al 1985). Briefly, [111]Indium is adsorbed onto resin particles and incorporated into a gelatine capsule coated with a methacrylate polymer. The capsule is ingested and remains intact on passage through the stomach and small bowel. The capsule dissolves at distal ileal pH and releases a bolus of radionuclide into the cecum. The start time of colonic transit measurement can be accurately determined (Proano et al 1990).

We favor a modification of this technique for the measurement of colonic transit. We modified the number of capsule coatings to achieve reliable release of radioisotope in the ileocecal region (Hesslewood et al 1992). Colonic scintigraphy is performed on outpatients without bowel preparation. In our protocol, the subject ingests a capsule at 05.00 and image acquisition starts within 4 hours. Image acquisition is continued hourly between 09.00 and 17.00 on the first day and the subject returns home overnight. Normal activity is encouraged. Imaging is continued for 2 further days between 09.00 and 17.00 with image acquisition at 3–4-hourly intervals. Subjects are asked to collect fecal samples and record the time of evacuation. A mean of 14 images are acquired per subject. Digital images as well as analog pictures are acquired and stored on computer.

From the computerized data, dynamic images are generated and the position of the colon determined. Corrections are made for distance from the gamma camera and for isotope decay. To evaluate segmental colonic transit, regions of interest (ROIs) are defined and transit through each region separately determined. We use five ROIs: ROI 1 = cecum, ascending colon and hepatic flexure; ROI 2 = transverse colon; ROI 3 = splenic flexure; ROI 4 = descending colon, sigmoid colon and rectum; ROI 5 = fecal sample. The proportion of the scintigraphic counts in each region on each image is calculated. These percentages are converted to color- or gray-scale images called condensed parametric images (Notghi et al 1991). These depict the distribution of scintigraphic activity throughout the colon with time.

The advantages of scintigraphy over other methods of measuring colonic transit are that repeated or continuous observations can be obtained without additional radiation hazard. The estimated dose equivalent is less than one abdominal radiograph. Scintigraphy is non-invasive and does not require bowel preparation. Segmental colonic transit can be assessed. It is possible to distinguish sites of normal from abnormal transit, rather than only obtaining an overall impression of delayed colonic transit. It is possible to examine retrograde as well as antegrade movements of colonic contents.

We advocate the condensed parametric image as a method of data presentation because a large amount of data can be summarized on one chart. Each chart contains data of scintigraphic activity in five colonic ROIs at a mean of 14 time points and it provides a visual representation of colonic transit for each subject. The methodology of parametric image production has been described in detail (Notghi et al 1993). Classification of subjects with normal colonic transit, rapid colonic transit, generalized colonic delay, right-sided colonic delay or left-sided colonic delay is straightforward. The protocol can be simplified so that convenience is improved and costs reduced by restricting image acquisition to three occasions without losing diagnostic accuracy (Notghi et al 1994).

Rectal emptying tests

The assessment of rectal evacuation is an important component of the evaluation of the constipated patient because chronic constipation may be attributed to impaired rectal evacuation as well as to slow colonic transit or to a combination of both functional abnormalities. The variety of methods of assessing rectal evacuation testifies to the difficulties and the lack of consensus about the optimum method.

Defecation may be quantified by balloon expulsion tests (Fleshman et al 1992, Preston et al 1984a). However, the tests are of doubtful clinical relevance as patients do not evacuate balloon-shaped boluses of feces and there is considerable variability depending on the contents and compliance of the balloons.

Barium defecating proctography involves the evacuation of a barium-labeled artificial stool (Mahieu et al 1984a). It provides anatomical information on the anorectal angle, pelvic floor descent, rectoceles and mucosal prolapses (Bartolo et al 1985, Mahieu et al 1984b, Turnbull et al 1988). Scintigraphic defecography involves the evacuation of a radio-labeled artificial stool (Barkel et al 1988, O'Connell et al 1986, Papachrysostomou et al 1992). As in conventional proctography, anorectal angle, pelvic floor descent and rectoceles can be measured with reference to markers and the anal canal (Hutchinson et al 1993). However, the scintigraphic technique has several advantages over conventional defecating proctography (Hutchinson et al 1995a). Scintigraphic defecography is a test of function rather than anatomy. Evacuation rate as well as the percentage of rectal emptying can be calculated. The functional significance of anatomical variants such as pelvic floor descent and rectoceles can be assessed. Rectal evacuation is only estimated with barium proctography. Furthermore, the radiation dose associated with the scintigraphic method (1 mSv) is significantly less than it is with conventional barium proctography (Hutchinson et al 1995a). A barium proctogram study typically involves 1–2 minutes of fluoroscopy and two or three radiographs. The effective dose equivalent (EDE) of fluoroscopy is 1 mSv/min (Padovani et al 1987) and the EDE of pelvic radiography is 1.2 mSv/film (Shrimpton 1988). This high radiation dose contraindicates prolonged or repeated testing. Prolonged or repeated investigation of anorectal function is feasible using scintigraphic defecography.

The clinical significance of several of the parameters measured at barium proctography remains controversial and is hotly debated (Felt-Bersma et al 1990). For example, the small anatomical variants present in a high proportion of normal subjects are of no functional significance (Shorvon et al 1989). Similarly, the routine measurement of anorectal angle is not helpful as it is similar among constipated patients and controls and there is no relationship between symptoms and the anorectal angle (Goei 1990). Therefore, it appears that the assessment of anorectal function is more helpful than the assessment of anorectal anatomy in the management of the constipated patient. For these reasons, we favor scintigraphic defecography as the investigation of choice for measuring rectal emptying.

Small bowel transit tests

A small proportion of patients with chronic constipation have delayed gastric emptying or delayed small bowel transit as well as slow colonic transit. Nevertheless, it is important to distinguish this group of patients with a panenteric disorder from those with isolated colonic inertia.

Breath hydrogen analysis can be used to measure orocecal transit (Bond & Levitt 1975). Briefly, the subject ingests a test meal containing non-absorbable carbohydrate under standardized conditions after an overnight fast. Colonic bacteria ferment the non-absorbable carbohydrate to produce hydrogen, which is absorbed into the circulation and excreted via the lungs. Breath samples are analyzed and the time of appearance of hydrogen in the exhaled air corresponds with arrival of the test meal in the cecum.

There are a number of problems with breath hydrogen analysis. There is considerable intra- and intersubject variation in orocecal transit times, depending on the composition of the test meal (Korth et al 1984, Read et al 1980) and the subjects' physical activity and smoking habits (Thompson et al 1985). A misleading early rise in breath hydrogen may occur in patients with bacterial overgrowth in the stomach or small intestine. This may occur in patients with chronic intestinal pseudoobstruction, in achlorhydria and following proximal gastrointestinal surgery. The test can also be affected by the oropharyngeal bacterial flora (Thompson et al 1986).

Sulfasalazine can be used for the measurement of orocecal transit (Kellow et al 1986). Following oral administration, it is hydrolyzed by colonic bacteria into mesalazine and sulfapyridine which is absorbed and can be detected in the blood. The time of detection of sulfapyridine corresponds with orocecal transit.

Gastric emptying and small bowel transit can be studied with a radio-labeled test meal. The subject ingests the test meal after an overnight fast. Images of the abdomen are acquired until gastric emptying is complete and the meal arrives in the cecum. The analysis of data can be difficult and there are several ways of measuring small bowel transit (Kamm 1992). Small bowel transit can be calculated by subtracting gastric half-emptying time from colonic half-filling time (Camilleri et al 1989) or from the time of 10% gastric emptying to 10% colonic filling (Greydanus et al 1990, Stivland et al 1991). Small bowel residence can be determined but the analysis is complex (Read et al 1986). Overlap of small bowel with colon may make identification of cecal filling difficult. Another problem is the interpretation of the significance of prolonged transit times. Transit times vary widely within individuals and between normal subjects (Cummings et al 1976, Wyman et al 1978). This variability appears to depend on test meal composition, psychological stress and the phase of the menstrual cycle (Read 1991).

Despite these limitations, scintigraphy is the preferred method for measuring small bowel transit and there is reasonable correlation between radioisotope arrival in the cecum and the rise in breath hydrogen (Read et al 1986). Minor prolongations of transit should be disregarded, but grossly delayed small bowel transit is a useful indicator of a panenteric motor dysfunction as the cause for constipation.

Tests of anorectal and pelvic floor physiology

'Anorectal physiology' tests refer to a group of investigations which individually may be difficult to interpret but when considered together, may provide an integrated assessment of the mechanisms of continence and defecation. Anorectal physiology tests usually comprise anorectal manometry, electromyography (EMG) and sensory testing. Simultaneous anorectal manometry and measurement of internal anal sphincter (IAS) and external anal sphincter (EAS) electrical activity with the patient at rest, during voluntary sphincter contraction, during straining and during rectal distension may yield interesting results in chronically constipated patients. Occasionally, the findings are diagnostic. For example, anorectal testing may show the absence of the anorectal inhibitory reflex which is characteristic of adult Hirschsprung's disease (Crocker & Messmer 1991). Obstructed defecation due to anismus may be suggested by increased electrical activity in the EAS and puborectalis muscle on attempted defecation (Preston & Lennard-Jones 1985). Abnormalities of rectal sensation following distension or electrical stimulation have been demonstrated in patients with chronic idiopathic constipation (Kamm & Lennard-Jones 1990).

The exact role of anorectal physiology tests in the assessment of the constipated patient remains debatable (Carty et al 1994, Kuijpers 1990, Parks 1992, Rasmussen 1994). The tests are invasive and non-physiological and only rarely do they contribute to the diagnosis or management of the constipated patient. Scintigraphic defecography provides the quantitative information on rectal evacuation necessary for classification of the constipated patient. At present, the general application of anorectal physiological tests cannot be advocated outside specialist units with research interests in chronic constipation.

Functional assessment – other tests

Abnormalities of esophageal, gastric and small intestinal motility (Kumar et al 1989) and of ileocecal transit (Hutchinson et al 1995b) have been demonstrated in some patients with chronic idiopathic constipation. This supports the notion that constipation may occasionally be the manifestation of a panenteric functional disorder of the gastrointestinal tract. Techniques have been devised for the ambulatory measurement of motility in these regions. However, the value of these complex investigations in the management of chronically constipated patients is limited. The measurement of small intestinal or colonic motility is, at present, of research interest only (Bassotti et al 1993, Camilleri 1993, Quigley 1992).

MANAGEMENT STRATEGY (Box 15.1)

A rational approach to the management of the chronically constipated patient depends upon the identification of the cause or causes of symptoms. Metabolic and mechanical causes of constipation are usually apparent following assessment by history, physical examination, barium enema examination or colonoscopy. A small but significant proportion of patients without a metabolic or mechanical explanation for their constipation will have a functional disorder of the gastrointestinal tract. These patients require specialized investigations to identify the site, nature and severity of functional abnormalities. Several functional abnormalities may coexist so quantification is helpful to assess the relative contributions of these abnormalities to the patient's symptoms.

We believe that measurements of colonic transit and rectal evacuation are the minimum requirements for the assessment of a patient with functional constipation. A combination of scintigraphic defecography and colonic scintigraphy permits classification of constipated patients into

---

Box 15.1 Diagnostic and management strategy for the constipated patient

History	**Physical examination**
Duration of symptoms	General
Bowel frequency	Neurological
Consistency of stools	Abdominal
Straining	Perineal inspection
Urge to evacuate	pelvic floor movements
Pain on defecation	mucosal/rectal prolapse
Incomplete evacuation	Rectal examination including
Manual evacuation	assessment of resting anal
Abdominal pain	sphincter tone and squeeze
Abdominal distension	pressures, sphincter defects,
Weight loss	fecaliths, megarectum, rectoceles
Rectal bleeding	Proctoscopy including
Relation to pelvic procedures	hemorrhoids, SRUS
Relation to menstrual cycle	Sigmoidoscopy
Medical illnesses	
Family history	
Diet	
Drugs	
Response to laxatives	

Initial investigations	**Empirical treatment**
Hematological tests	High fiber diet
Biochemical tests	Increased fluid intake
Abdominal radiographs*	Exercise
Barium enema	Avoid constipating drugs
Upper gastrointestinal contrast studies*	
Endoanal ultrasonography*	
Flexible sigmoidoscopy or colonoscopy	

(* optional)

---

those with slow colonic transit, those with impaired rectal evacuation and those with a combination of functional abnormalities (Hutchinson et al 1995c). This guides further investigation and management. The diagnostic and management strategy we advocate is summarized in the flow diagram (Fig. 15.1).

IMPLICATIONS FOR TREATMENT

Patients with functional constipation in whom a panenteric disorder of gut motility has been excluded and in whom slow colonic transit is the only objective abnormality are likely to benefit from colonic resection. Good results have followed colectomy and ileorectal anastomosis in this carefully selected group (Pemberton et al 1991, Roe et al 1986, Wexner et al 1991). It is worth emphasizing that careful selection is the key to success as results from surgery on constipated patients whose functional abnormality is less well defined have been disappointing (Kamm et al 1988b, Preston et al 1984b, Yoshioka & Keighley 1989).

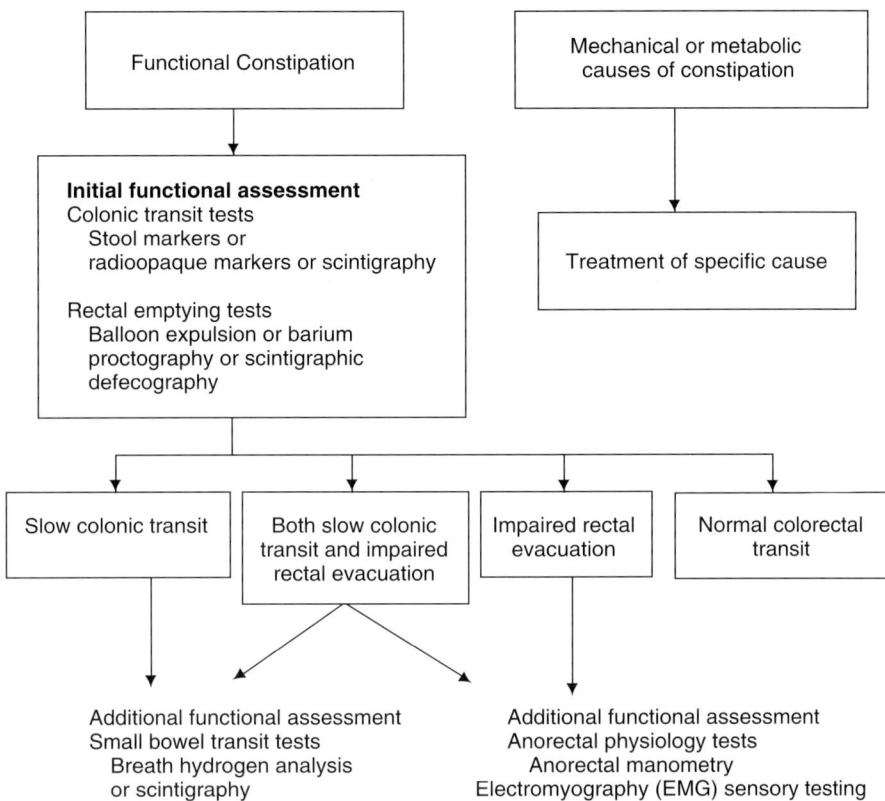

Figure 15.1 Diagnostic and management strategy.

Patients with isolated colonic inertia form only a small proportion of patients with functional constipation. Patients with impaired rectal evacuation and those with a combination of functional abnormalities are more common and more difficult to manage. The results of surgical treatment for functional outlet obstruction are poor (Kamm et al 1988c, Wallace & Madden 1969). The results from biofeedback retraining are encouraging and this is probably now the treatment of choice for obstructed defecation (Bleijenberg & Kuijpers 1987). In patients with both delayed colonic transit and impaired rectal evacuation, initial treatment should address the impaired defecation as disordered defecation may lead to a transit picture that resembles delayed colonic transit.

In summary, the assessment of the constipated patient should follow the usual sequence of history, physical examination and special investigations to distinguish mechanical or metabolic causes of constipation from functional constipation. It is important, in patients with functional constipation, to apply the various functional tests logically in order to identify the small proportion of patients with isolated colonic inertia who might benefit from surgery. More importantly, careful functional assessment ensures that inappropriate surgery is avoided.

FURTHER READING

Alvarez W C, Freedlander B L 1924 The rate of progress of food residues through the bowel. Journal of the American Medical Association 83: 576–580

Barkel D C, Pemberton J H, Pezim M E, Phillips S F, Kelly K A, Brown M L 1988 Scintigraphic assessment of the anorectal angle in health and after ileal pouch–anal anastomosis. Annals of Surgery 208: 42–49

Bartolo D C, Roe A M, Virjee J, Mortensen N J 1985 Evaluation proctography in obstructed defaecation and rectal intussusception. British Journal of Surgery 72: S111–116

Bassotti G, Crowell M D, Whitehead W E 1993 Contractile activity of the human colon: lessons from 24 hours studies. Gut 34: 129–133

Bleijenberg G, Kuijpers H C 1987 Treatment of the spastic pelvic floor syndrome with biofeedback. Diseases of the Colon and Rectum 30: 108–111

Bond J H, Levitt M D 1975 Investigation of small bowel transit time in man utilizing pulmonary hydrogen measurements. Journal of Laboratory and Clinical Medicine 85: 546–555

Camilleri M 1993 Study of human gastroduodenojejunal motility. Applied physiology in clinical practice. Digestive Diseases and Sciences 38: 785–794

Camilleri M, Colemont L J, Phillips S F, Brown M L, Thomforde G M, Chapman N, Zinsmeister A R 1989 Human gastric emptying and colonic filling of solids characterized by a new method. American Journal of Physiology 257: G284–290

Carty N J, Moran B, Johnson C D 1994 Anorectal physiology measurements are of no value in clinical practice. True or false? Annals of the Royal College of Surgeons of England 76: 276–280

Chaussade S, Khyari A, Roche H, Garret M, Gaudric M, Couturier D, Guerre J 1989 Determination of total and segmental colonic transit time in constipated patients. Digestive Diseases and Sciences 34: 1169–1172

Crocker N L, Messmer J M 1991 Adult Hirschsprung's disease. Clinical Radiology 44: 257–259

Cummings J H, Jenkins D J A, Wiggins H S 1976 Measurement of the mean transit time of dietary residue through the human gut. Gut 17: 210–218

Devroede G 1988 Constipation. In: Kumar D, Gustavsson S (eds) An illustrated guide to gastrointestinal motility. John Wiley & Sons, Chichester, pp 411–445

Dick M 1969 Use of cuprous thiocyanate as a short term continuous marker for faeces. Gut 10: 408–412

Drossman D A, Sandler R S, McKee D C, Lovitz A J 1982 Bowel patterns among subjects not seeking health care. Gastroenterology 83: 529–534

Evans R C, Kamm M A, Hinton J M, Lennard-Jones J E 1992 The normal range and a simple diagram for recording whole gut transit time. International Journal of Colorectal Diseases 7: 15–17

Feczko P J, O'Connell D J, Riddell R H, Frank P H 1980 Solitary rectal ulcer syndrome: radiologic manifestations. American Journal of Roentgenology 135: 499–506

Felt-Bersma R J, Luth W J, Janssen J J, Meuwissen S G 1990 Defecography in patients with anorectal disorders: which findings are clinically relevant? Diseases of the Colon and Rectum 33: 277–284

Fleshman J W, Dreznik Z, Cohen E, Fry R D, Kodner I J 1992 Balloon expulsion test facilitates diagnosis of pelvic floor outlet obstruction due to non-relaxing puborectalis muscle. Diseases of the Colon and Rectum 35: 1019–1025

Goei R 1990 Anorectal function in patients with defecation disorders and asymptomatic subjects: evaluation with defecography. Radiology 174: 121–123

Goei R, Baeten C, Arends J W 1988 Solitary rectal ulcer syndrome: findings at barium enema study and defecography. Radiology 168: 303–306

Greydanus M P, Camilleri M, Colemont L J, Phillips S F, Brown M L, Thomforde G M 1990 Ileocolonic transfer of solid chyme in small intestinal neuropathies and myopathies. Gastroenterology 99: 158–164

Hallan R I, Marzouk D E M M, Waldron D J, Womack N R, Williams N S 1989 Comparison of digital and manometric assessment of anal sphincter function. British Journal of Surgery 76: 973–975

Hardy J G, Wilson C G, Wood E 1985 Drug delivery to the proximal colon. Journal of Pharmaceuticals and Pharmacology 37: 874–877

Hesslewood S R, Panagamuwa B, Kumar D, Smith N B, Notghi A, Harding L K 1992 Development of a dosage form for measuring colonic transit. Journal of Pharmaceuticals and Pharmacology 44: S1086

Hinton J M, Lennard-Jones J E, Young A C 1969 A new method for studying gut transit times using radio-opaque markers. Gut 10: 842–847

Holmes R M, Salter R H 1982 Irritable bowel syndrome: a safe diagnosis. British Medical Journal 285: 1533–1534

Hutchinson R, Mostafa A B, Grant E A, Smith N B, Deen K I, Harding L K, Kumar D 1993 Scintigraphic defecography: quantitative and dynamic assessment of anorectal function. Diseases of the Colon and Rectum 36: 1132–1138

Hutchinson R, Deen K I, Mostafa A B, Harding L K, Kumar D 1995a. Scintigraphic defecography: a direct comparison with conventional barium proctography. Diseases of the Colon and Rectum (in press).

Hutchinson R, Notghi A, Smith N B, Harding L K, Kumar D 1995b Scintigraphic measurement of ileocaecal transit in irritable bowel syndrome and chronic idiopathic constipation. Gut (in press).

Hutchinson R, Notghi A, Mostafa A B, Harding L K, Kumar D 1995c. Chronic idiopathic constipation: where is the problem? Gastroenterology (in press).

Kamm M A 1992 The small intestine and colon: scintigraphic quantitation of motility in health and disease. European Journal of Nuclear Medicine 19: 902–912

Kamm M A, Lennard-Jones J E 1990 Rectal mucosal electrosensory testing. Evidence of a sensory neuropathy in severe constipation. Diseases of the Colon and Rectum 33: 419–423

Kamm M A, Lennard-Jones J E, Thompson D G, Sobnack R, Garvie N W, Granowska M 1988a Dynamic scanning defines a colonic defect in severe idiopathic constipation. Gut 29: 1085–1092

Kamm M A, Hawley P R, Lennard-Jones J E 1988b Outcome of colectomy for severe idiopathic constipation. Gut 29: 969–973

Kamm M A, Hawley P R, Lennard-Jones J E 1988c Lateral division of the puborectalis muscle in the management of severe constipation. British Journal of Surgery 75: 661–663

Kellow J E, Borody T J, Phillips S F, Haddad A C, Brown M L 1986 Sulfapyridine appearance in plasma after salicylazosulfapyridine: another simple measure of intestinal transit. Gastroenterology 91: 396–400

Korth H, Muller I, Erckenbrecht J F, Wienbeck M 1984 Breath hydrogen as a test for gastrointestinal transit. Hepatogastroenterology 31: 282–284

Koruth N M, Koruth A, Matheson N A 1985 The place of contrast enema in the management of large bowel obstruction. Journal of the Royal College of Surgeons of Edinburgh 30: 258–260

Krevsky B, Malmud L S, D'Ercole F, Maurer A H, Fisher R S 1986 Colonic transit scintigraphy. A physiologic approach to the measurement of colonic transit in humans. Gastroenterology 91: 1102–1112

Kuijpers H C 1990 Application of the colorectal laboratory in diagnosis and treatment of functional constipation. Diseases of the Colon and Rectum 33: 35–39

Kumar D 1992 Symposium on constipation. International Journal of Colorectal Diseases 7: 47–67

Kumar D, Waldron D, Williams N S, Wingate D L 1989 Slow transit constipation: a panenteric motor disorder. Gastroenterology 96: A277

Levine M S, Piccolello M L, Sollenberger L C, Laufer I, Saul S H 1986 Solitary rectal ulcer syndrome: a radiologic diagnosis? Gastrointestinal Radiology 11: 187–193

Lindsay D C, Freeman J G, Cobden I, Record C O 1988 Should colonoscopy be the first investigation for colonic disease? British Medical Journal 296: 167–169

Mahieu P, Pringot J, Bodart P 1984a Defecography 1. Description of a new procedure and results in normal patients. Gastrointestinal Radiology 9: 247–251

Mahieu P, Pringot J, Bodart P 1984b Defecography 2. Contribution to the diagnosis of defecation disorders. Gastrointestinal Radiology 9: 253–261

Manning A P, Thompson W G, Heaton K W, Morris A F 1978 Towards positive diagnosis of the irritable bowel. British Medical Journal 2: 653–654

McLean R G, Smart R C, Gaston-Parry D et al 1990 Colon transit scintigraphy in health and constipation using oral Iodine-131-cellulose. Journal of Nuclear Medicine 31: 985–989

Metcalf A M, Phillips S F, Zinsmeister A R, MacCarty R L, Beart R W, Wolff B G 1987 Simplified assessment of segmental colonic transit. Gastroenterology 92: 40–47

Mezwa D G, Feczko P J, Bosanko C 1993 Radiologic evaluation of constipation and anorectal disorders. Radiologic Clinics of North America 31: 1375–1393

Moreno-Osset E, Bazzocchi G, Lo S et al 1989 Association between postprandial changes in colonic intraluminal pressure and transit. Gastroenterology 96: 1265–1273

Notghi A, Panagamuwa B, Oya M, Tulley N J, Kumar D, Harding L K 1991 The use of condensed images in colonic motility. Nuclear Medicine Communications 12: 278

Notghi A, Kumar D, Panagamuwa B, Tulley N J, Hesslewood S R, Harding L K 1993 Measurement of colonic transit time using radionuclide imaging: analysis by condensed images. Nuclear Medicine Communications 14: 204–211

Notghi A, Hutchinson R, Kumar D, Smith N B, Harding L K 1994 Simplified method for the measurement of segmental colonic transit time. Gut 35: 976–981

O'Connell P R, Kelly K A, Brown M L 1986 Scintigraphic assessment of neorectal function. Journal of Nuclear Medicine 27: 460–464

Padovani R, Contento G, Fabretto M, Malisan M R, Barbina V, Gozzi G 1987 Patient doses and risks from diagnostic radiology in north-east Italy. British Journal of Radiology 60: 155–165

Papachrysostomou M, Griffin T M J, Ferrington C, Merrick M V, Smith A N 1992 A method of computerized isotope dynamic proctography. European Journal of Nuclear Medicine 19: 431–435

Parks T G 1992 The usefulness of tests in anorectal disease. World Journal of Surgery 16: 804–810

Pemberton J H, Rath D M, Ilstrup D M 1991 Evaluation and surgical treatment of severe chronic constipation. Annals of Surgery 214: 403–413

Ponka J L, Grodsinsky C, Brush B E 1972 Megacolon in teenaged and adult patients. Diseases of the Colon and Rectum 15: 14–22

Preston D M, Lennard-Jones J E 1985 Anismus in chronic constipation. Digestive Diseases and Sciences 30: 413–418

Preston D M, Lennard-Jones J E 1986 Severe chronic constipation in young women: 'idiopathic slow transit constipation'. Gut 27: 41–48

Preston D M, Lennard-Jones J E, Thomas B M 1984a The balloon proctogram. British Journal of Surgery 71: 29–32

Preston D M, Hawley P R, Lennard-Jones J E, Todd I P 1984b Results of colectomy for severe idiopathic constipation in women (Arbuthnot Lane's disease). British Journal of Surgery 71: 547–552

Proano M, Camilleri M, Phillips S F, Brown M L, Thomforde G M 1990 Transit of solids through the human colon: regional quantification in the unprepared bowel. American Journal of Physiology 258: G856–862

Probert C S J, Emmett P M, Cripps H A, Heaton K W 1994 Evidence for the ambiguity of the term constipation: the role of irritable bowel syndrome. Gut 35: 1455–1458

Quigley E M M 1992 Intestinal manometry – technical advances, clinical limitations. Digestive Diseases and Sciences 37: 10–13

Rasmussen O O 1994 Anorectal function. Diseases of the Colon and Rectum 37: 386–403

Read N W 1991 Measurement of small bowel transit in humans. In: Kamm M A, Lennard-Jones J E (eds) 1991 Gastrointestinal transit: pathophysiology and pharmacology. Wrightson Biomedical Publishing Ltd, Petersfield, pp 97–108

Read N W, Miles C A, Fisher D et al 1980 Transit of a meal through the stomach, small intestine and colon in normal subjects and its role in the pathogenesis of diarrhoea. Gastroenterology 79: 1276–1282

Read N W, Al-Janabi M N, Holgate A M, Barber D C, Edwards C A 1986 Simultaneous measurement of gastric emptying, small bowel residence and colonic filling of a solid meal by the use of the gamma camera. Gut 27: 300–308

Ritchie J 1973 Pain from distension of the pelvic floor by inflating a balloon in the irritable colon syndrome. Gut 14: 125–132

Roe A M, Bartolo D C C, Mortensen N J M 1986 Diagnosis and surgical management of intractable constipation. British Journal of Surgery 73: 854–861

Shorvon P J, McHugh S, Diamant N E, Somers S, Stevenson G W 1989 Defecography in normal volunteers: results and implications. Gut 30: 1737–1749

Shrimpton P C 1988 Are X-rays safe enough? In: Faulkner K, Wall B F (eds) Patient doses and the risks in diagnostic radiology. Institute of Physical Sciences in Medicine, York, pp 41–53

Smith A N, Varma J S, Binnie N R, Papachrysostomou M 1990 Disordered colorectal motility in intractable constipation following hysterectomy. British Journal of Surgery 77: 1361–1365

Stivland T, Camilleri M, Vassallo M et al 1991 Scintigraphic measurement of regional gut transit in idiopathic constipation. Gastroenterology 101: 107–115

Thompson D G, Binfield P, DeBelder A, O'Brien J D, Warren S 1985 Extra-intestinal influences on exhaled breath hydrogen measurements during the investigation of gastrointestinal disease. Gut 26: 1349–1352

Thompson D G, O'Brien J D, Hardie J M 1986 Influence of the oropharyngeal microflora on the measurement of exhaled breath hydrogen. Gastroenterology 91: 853–860

Trotman I F, Price C C 1986 Bloated irritable bowel syndrome defined by dynamic ^{99m}Tc bran scan. Lancet ii: 364–366

Turnbull G K, Bartram C I, Lennard-Jones J E 1988 Radiologic studies of rectal evacuation in adults with idiopathic constipation. Diseases of the Colon and Rectum 31: 190–197

Van der Sijp J R M, Kamm M A, Nightingale J M D et al 1993 Radioisotope determination of regional colonic transit in severe constipation: comparison with radio-opaque markers. Gut 34: 402–408

Wallace W C, Madden W M 1969 Experience with partial resection of the puborectalis muscle. Diseases of the Colon and Rectum 12: 196–200

Wexner S D, Daniel N, Jagelman D G 1991 Colectomy for constipation: physiologic investigation is the key to success. Diseases of the Colon and Rectum 34: 851–856

Whitby L G, Lang D 1960 Experience with the chromium oxide method of fecal marking in metabolic balance investigations on humans. Journal of Clinical Investigation 39: 854–863

Whitehead W, Corazziari E, Chaussade S, Kumar D 1991 Management of constipation. Gastroenterology International 4: 99–114

Wyman J B, Heaton K W, Manning A P, Wicks A C B 1978 Variability of colonic function in healthy subjects. Gut 19: 146–150

Yoshioka K, Keighley M R B 1989 Clinical results of colectomy for severe constipation. British Journal of Surgery 76: 600–604

16

Fecal incontinence

D. Kumar

INTRODUCTION

Fecal incontinence is a common and distressing symptom. Due to embarrassment about their symptom, many patients are reluctant to volunteer information about fecal incontinence or do not seek medical help for even moderately severe incontinence. Consequently, many patients suffer social isolation and serious psychological problems. There are no reliable data available on the incidence and prevalence of fecal incontinence in the community (Enck et al 1991). Health surveys in the UK and USA have suggested that between 0.5% and 1.5% of all adults exhibit symptoms of fecal incontinence at least occasionally (Mandelstam 1984, Milne 1976). Drossman et al (1986) reported that more than 5% of healthy subjects experience incontinence, predominantly fecal soiling, but only approximately 20% of these people consult a physician. In another study (Leigh & Turnberg 1982), 51% of women who complained of diarrhea were incontinent but less than half of these patients admitted to the symptom of incontinence when they consulted their doctor. Enck et al (1991) prospectively evaluated the presence of fecal incontinence in selected patient groups and compared it to the incidence in healthy controls. As expected, the incidence of fecal incontinence was higher in the patient groups as compared to controls, but regardless of the mechanism only 5% of the patients had fecal incontinence documented in their medical charts.

Improved understanding of the pathophysiology of fecal incontinence offers more targeted treatment, conservative as well as surgical. Some patients will improve with antidiarrheal agents, suppositories or enemas. Others will improve with pelvic floor exercises, biofeedback training or electrical stimulation of the sphincter. In those where conservative measures fail, operations such as sphincter repair, postanal repair or sphincter reconstruction may restore continence.

MECHANISM OF CONTINENCE

It is important to understand that continence is not maintained just by normal function of the anal sphincter complex, but also by other factors such as normal rectal and colonic function (Fig. 16.1). Factors such as the

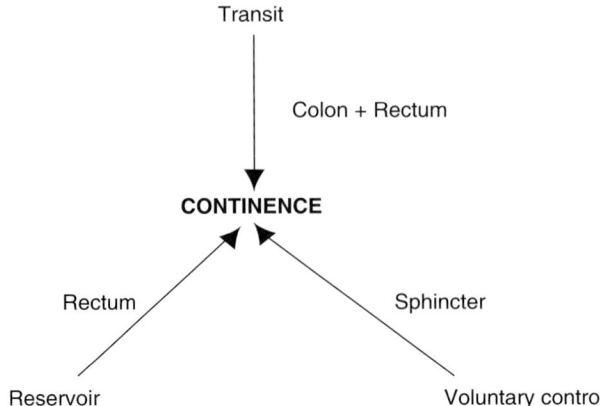

Figure 16.1 Normal rectal and colonic function.

consistency of the stool, motor function of the colon, the capacity of the rectum and the compliance of the rectum are just as important in maintaining continence as integrity of the internal and external anal sphincter muscles, preservation of the sampling reflex and anal sensation. In many patients the challenge of liquid stool entering the rectum at speed is too great and this results in a feeling of intense urgency followed by incontinence. In such patients objective and physiological testing reveals a normal rectum and anal sphincter complex. However, measurement of colonic motor activity will reveal hyperactivity in the colon. In some patients there may be hyperactivity of the small bowel giving rise to intestinal hurry.

In patients with a low capacity rectum, such as seen in those with inflammatory bowel disease, the colonic function may be normal but even a small amount of fecal matter in the rectum produces a strong desire to defecate which, even in the presence of a normal sphincter complex, may result in fecal incontinence.

Thus, normal continence is maintained by an interaction of several factors:

1. normal transit of a normal consistency stool;
2. normal capacity rectum to provide an adequate reservoir;
3. a normal voluntary control and reflex function provided by the anal sphincter complex.

ETIOLOGY

The most common cause of fecal incontinence in adult healthy women is obstetric trauma. Other causes include pudendal nerve neuropathy and iatrogenic causes such as surgical operations on the anal canal. Neurological causes of fecal incontinence include upper motor neuron lesions, lower motor neuron lesions or peripheral nerve lesions from the sacral outflow or pudendal nerve. There may be associated cerebral causes as well. In patients with diabetes mellitus, mixed motor and sensory loss may result in fecal incontinence. Direct trauma to the sphincter can also cause fecal incontinence. Fecal incontinence may be the presenting symptom in patients with fecal impaction and idiopathic constipation. Patients with rectal prolapse, descending perineum syndrome and proctitis may also have associated incontinence. In children, meningocele, Hirschsprung's disease and anorectal malformations can all result in incontinence.

Obstetric Damage

In healthy adult women the most common cause of fecal incontinence is sphincter damage during childbirth. Often there is a history of a difficult vaginal delivery, forceps delivery, perineal tear or cephalopelvic disproportion (MacArthur et al 1991). Several studies have examined pelvic floor neurophysiological changes at childbirth and suggested that incontinence results from damage to the innervation of pelvic floor muscles and not from direct muscle damage (Bartolo et al 1983, Snooks et al 1984a). Sultan et al (1994) studied 128 women during pregnancy and after delivery and found that pudendal nerve latencies were significantly prolonged after vaginal delivery. Only a third of those who had a prolonged pudendal nerve latency were still affected after 6 months, suggesting that the majority of women who sustain sphincter trauma during childbirth appear to recover normal nerve function. With the availability of superior imaging technology, we now know that sphincter disruption is the most common form of obstetric damage (Deen et al 1993). Approximately a third of all primiparous women who deliver vaginally develop a sphincter defect involving one or both muscles (Sultan et al 1993). Patients who sustain a division of the external anal sphincter at delivery also have impaired sensation which persists in the upper anal canal at 6 months (Cornes et al 1991).

Sphincter trauma

This is usually the result of operations on the anal canal for fissures, fistulae-in-ano and hemorrhoids. Anal dilatation has also been shown to damage the anal sphincters. Fecal soiling is a prominent feature in patients after fistula operations. In patients with anal fissure or hemorrhoids, forceful dilatation of the anal sphincter complex (Lord 1968, MacDonald et al 1992) results in a persistent fall in anal canal pressures (Snooks et al

1984b). Repeated anal dilatation in these patients results in a significant risk of fecal incontinence (Henry 1983). Third degree tears during childbirth causing disruption of the anal sphincter complex also result in incontinence. Forceps delivery, primiparous delivery, birth weight greater than 4 kg and occipitoposterior position at delivery predispose to the development of a tear (Kamm 1994).

Fecal impaction

This is usually seen as a cause of fecal incontinence in geriatric patients (Barratt 1992). In younger patients, it is often associated with a mega-rectum or congenital anorectal malformations. Incontinence results from the development of bolus obstruction in the rectum. It is also seen in patients who are on drug therapy for psychiatric illness.

Incontinence secondary to fecal impaction is made worse on treatment with laxatives. Liquid fecal material simply leaks out from an open anal canal while the fecal bolus remains unaffected. However, the symptoms of incontinence can be prevented by using mild laxatives after the fecal impaction has been removed from the rectum.

EVALUATION OF PATIENTS WITH FECAL INCONTINENCE

History

All patients attending gastroenterology clinics should be asked directly about fecal incontinence as many will hide this symptom and will complain of diarrhea when they are suffering from urgency and fecal incontinence. If the patient admits to incontinence then the frequency of occurrence and the nature of the leakage should be recorded. The use of questionnaires may be helpful in obtaining an accurate history. Careful attention should be paid to the stool consistency, history of straining and a previous history of difficult vaginal delivery with or without the use of forceps. Neurological symptoms must always be documented. Attention should always be paid to symptoms suggestive of colonic or rectal disease such as the presence of diarrhea and the leakage of mucus or blood in patients with inflammatory bowel disease. Any previous pelvic or anal operations, especially anal dilatation, fistula surgery and prolapse repair, should be noted. Any associated history of urinary incontinence and uterovaginal prolapse should also be recorded.

Physical examination

The perineum, anus and rectum are best examined with the patient in the left lateral decubitus position. Prior to examination of the perineum and the anorectum, the patient should be examined as a whole because incontinence can be a manifestation of disease outside the anorectum. The anus and the perineum should be inspected for the nature of perianal skin, scarring, signs of fecal leakage, external openings of a fistula, a patulous anus and a mucosal or full-thickness rectal prolapse. Abnormal perianal descent relative to the ischial tuberosities, both at rest and on straining, is associated with pudendal neuropathy. Gaping of the anal canal at rest or on traction of the perianal skin suggests reduced resting tone. The integrity of perineal innervation is tested by pinprick sensation and the anocutaneous reflex which is evoked by stroking the perianal skin. This causes a transient contraction of the external anal sphincter. It tests the integrity of the pudendal nerve and sacral plexus and may be absent in fecal incontinence.

Digital examination of the anorectum allows qualitative assessment of the resting anal tone and changes which occur on voluntary contraction and coughing. The presence of fecal impaction, palpable tumors or masses and tenderness in the rectum should be recorded. All patients should undergo proctosigmoidoscopy to exclude inflammatory bowel disease, neoplasia, fistulae, mucosal prolapse and hemorrhoids. History and examination alone will often identify the nature of any sphincter weakness and other rectal and colonic factors which can be quantified by more sophisticated physiological tests.

Clinical grading of continence

It is useful to have a simple clinical classification of continence. This provides a helpful guide to the severity of symptoms. We grade continence according to the following four categories:

- **Grade 1:** continent to solid and liquid stool and gas.
- **Grade 2:** continent to solid and liquid stool only, but incontinent to gas.
- **Grade 3:** continent to solid stool, but incontinent to liquid stool and gas.
- **Grade 4:** incontinent to solid and liquid stool as well as gas.

INVESTIGATIONS

In a significant number of patients the cause of fecal incontinence will be found on a careful history and clinical examination. However, in the remaining patients specialist investigations will be required to find a cause.

Anal manometry

The function of both internal and external anal sphincters is assessed using anal canal pressures. A variety of pressure measuring equipment is available which utilizes perfused tubes, air or water-filled balloons or microtransducer-tipped catheters. These are inserted into the rectum and then gradually withdrawn. When the high pressure zone is reached, the distance from the anal verge is recorded and the pressure in the anal canal measured at 1 cm intervals as the catheter is withdrawn. This measures the resting pressure produced by the internal anal sphincter as well as the resting sphincter length. Manometry is the only method of measuring resting tone in the anal canal. The internal sphincter is responsible for approximately 70–80% of the resting tone (Frenckner & von Euler 1975). Measurement of the resting tone therefore provides an assessment of the internal anal sphincter.

The procedure is repeated, but this time the patient is asked to close the anal canal as tightly as possible so that the maximum squeeze pressure produced by the external anal sphincter can be recorded. Voluntary squeeze pressure is the greatest pressure achieved above resting pressure during a maximal voluntary contraction. It is mainly an expression of anal sphincter muscle function. The patient should not use the gluteal muscles during voluntary squeeze as this will result in an erroneous recording of the squeeze pressure. In almost all patients with incontinence the resting and squeeze pressures are significantly lower than in normal subjects (Delechenaut et al 1992, Read et al 1979, 1983). Also, patients who are incontinent to liquids and solids have lower squeeze pressures than those who are incontinent to liquids alone. The length of the high pressure zone is shorter in patients with incontinence than in normal subjects (Nivatvongs et al 1981).

Reflexes

The integrity of the rectoanal inhibitory reflex can be assessed by measuring anal pressures during incremental inflation of a rectal balloon. There should be a significant fall in anal canal pressure after the introduction of 50 mL of air in the balloon (Aaronson & Nixon 1972). The anocutaneous reflex is elicited by stroking the perianal skin and recording contraction of the external sphincter muscle (Bartolo et al 1983b). Absence of the anocutaneous reflex is suggestive of neuropathy. The sampling reflex can be detected as spontaneous episodes of internal sphincter relaxations during ambulatory manometry. In patients with incontinence the episodes of spontaneous relaxation may be of longer duration than those seen in healthy controls (Fig. 16.2) (Kumar et al 1989). In some patients the sampling reflex may be absent (Binnie et al 1990).

Rectal volume sensation

This can be measured using an ordinary balloon tied to a catheter (Fig. 16.3). The assembly is inserted into the rectum and known aliquots of air

Control

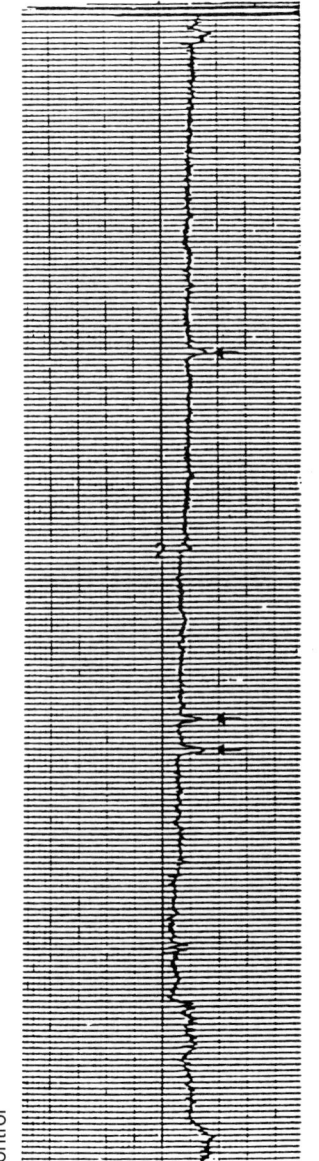

Incontinence

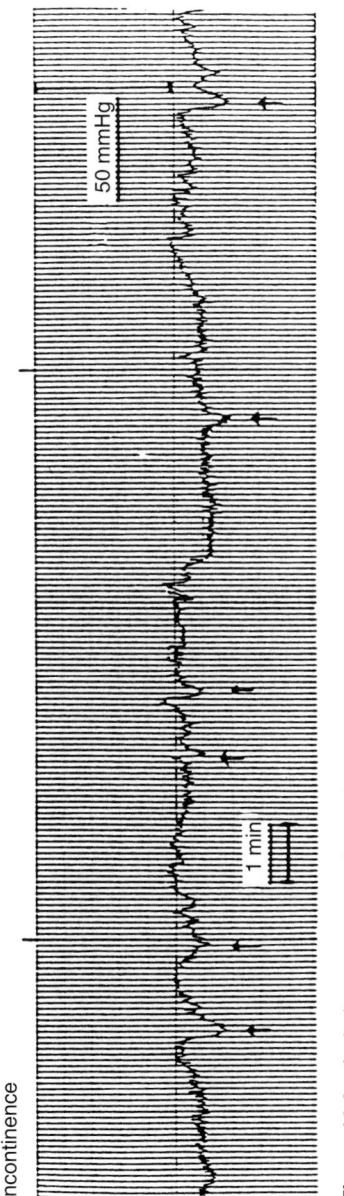

Figure 16.2 Ambulant manometry from a healthy subject (top trace) and a patient with fecal incontinence (lower trace). Note that the episodes of sampling reflex (arrows) are more frequent in fecal incontinence.

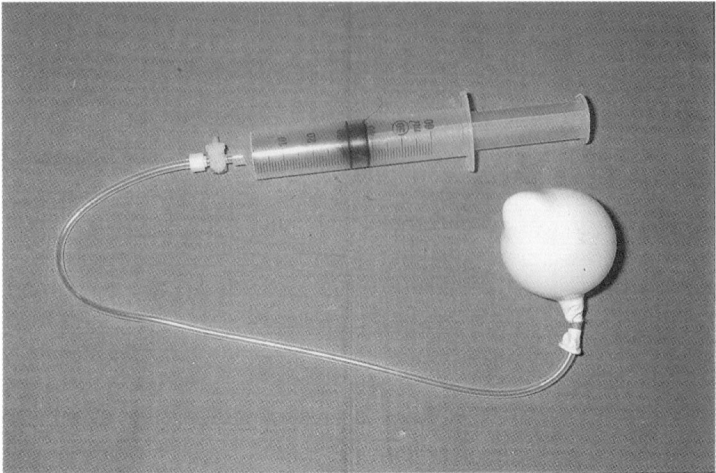

Figure 16.3 Assembly used to test rectal sensation.

are pumped into the balloon. The volume of air at first perception is the threshold volume. The volume at which the patient is constantly aware of the balloon is the volume at constant sensation and the volume at which the patient has a constant urge to defecate is the maximum tolerated volume. In patients with fecal incontinence due to rectal factors, the volume at constant sensation is often lower than normal. The maximum tolerated rectal volume may also be impaired in patients with fecal incontinence. In some patients constant sensation or maximum tolerability at a low volume may be the only abnormality. These patients often have symptoms of severe urgency associated with fecal incontinence.

Anal sensation

In addition to measuring rectal sensation, it is useful to quantify anal sensation as well. This is achieved by measuring anal mucosal electro-sensitivity (Roe et al 1986). A constant current of increasing strength is applied between two electrodes mounted on a catheter placed within the anal canal (Fig. 16.4). The level at which a tingling sensation is first perceived is recorded. Separate measurements are made for the upper, middle and lower anal canal. Anal sensation is impaired in most patients with fecal incontinence.

Electromyography

Electromyography is used to assess denervation/reinnervation in patients

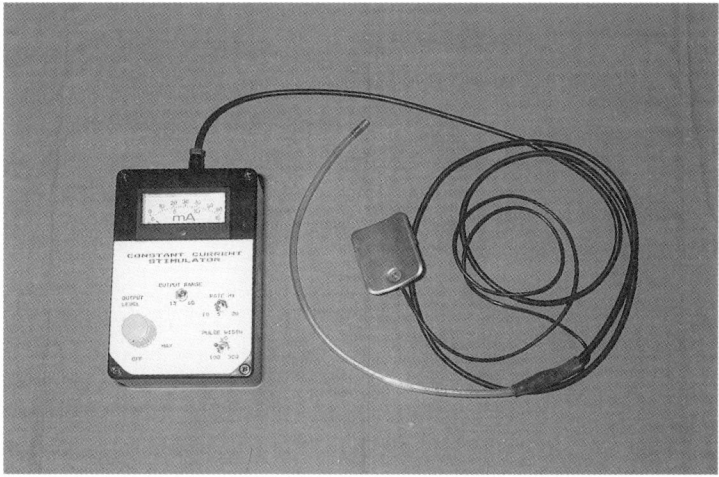

Figure 16.4 Assembly to test anal mucosal electrosensitivity.

with fecal incontinence. It is performed using either a concentric or single fiber needle electrode. The concentric needle electrode has a relatively large uptake area and records the activity of several motor units. It allows quantification of the activity in different muscles and within different parts of a muscle. The EMG activity will be reduced where the number of functioning fibers is reduced. This is seen when there has been denervation of muscle fibers due to neuropathy or in the presence of fibrosis due to direct muscle trauma. Patients with neuropathic fecal incontinence have reduced activity in both puborectalis and external anal sphincter muscles.

EMG can be used for sphincter mapping in patients who are suspected of having a sphincter defect (Kiff 1983). It is said to be particularly helpful in cases of suspected direct sphincter injury where the damaged muscle area is electrically silent. As the name implies, single fiber EMG allows analysis of changes in single muscle fibers. It demonstrates reinnervation of previously denervated muscle fibers by surviving neurons and is expressed as fiber density. It is increased in patients with neurogenic fecal incontinence and is said to be a sensitive index of neuropathy (Neil & Swash 1980).

Pudendal nerve terminal motor latency

Pudendal nerve terminal motor latency measures conduction in the terminal part of the pudendal nerve. The pudendal nerve is stimulated as it crosses the ischial spine whilst recording the evoked potential in the external anal sphincter (Fig. 16.5). This is studied using a specially designed glove (Lubowski et al 1988). Recordings are made from both

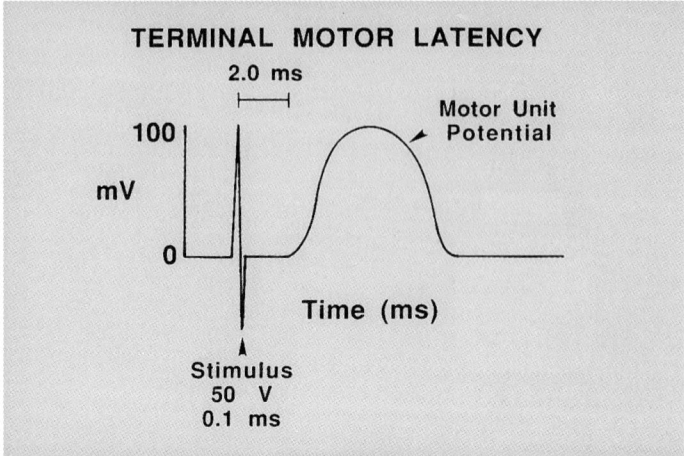

Figure 16.5 Schematic diagram showing pudendal terminal motor latency—time between the application of the stimulus and motor unit potential.

sides of the pelvis as pudendal nerve damage may be asymmetrical in some patients. Pudendal nerve terminal motor latency is prolonged in patients with idiopathic fecal incontinence. However, it must be remembered that pudendal nerve terminal motor latency and fiber density increase with age and this should be considered when interpreting the data (Vernava et al 1992).

Radiology

A contrast outline of the anorectum is obtained using barium proctography. Radiological images are obtained at rest, during straining and during defecation. Measurements of anorectal angle and pelvic floor descent and movement are subsequently made. The presence of anatomical abnormalities such as rectoceles and intussusceptions is also documented. In patients with fecal incontinence the anorectal angle may be obtuse and there may be associated abnormalities such as rectoceles and occult rectal intussusceptions (Womack et al 1985). The efficiency of rectal emptying is also assessed by measuring percentage evacuation and the rate of emptying. In some patients with incontinence there may be evidence of anal funneling and a rectocele.

Endoanal ultrasonography

Endoanal ultrasound provides high resolution images of both the internal and external anal sphincter and the puborectalis muscle. The examination is performed with the patient in the left lateral position and serial images

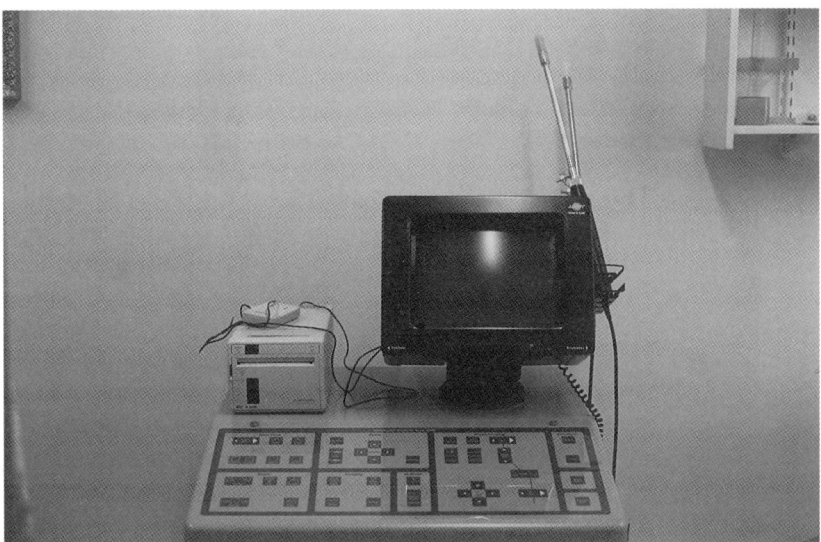

Figure 16.6 Ultrasound machine with the rotating probe used to perform endoanal ultrasonography.

are obtained at rest and during squeeze in the lower, mid and upper anal canal. The equipment used to perform endoanal ultrasonography is shown in Figure 16.6. The normal ultrasound (Fig. 16.7) consists of a

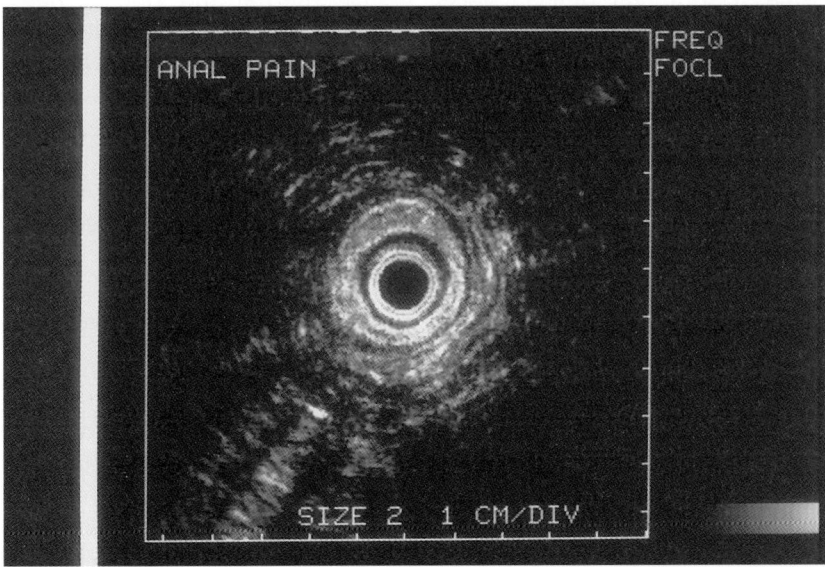

Figure 16.7 Example of a normal anal ultrasound showing a complete internal and external sphincter complex.

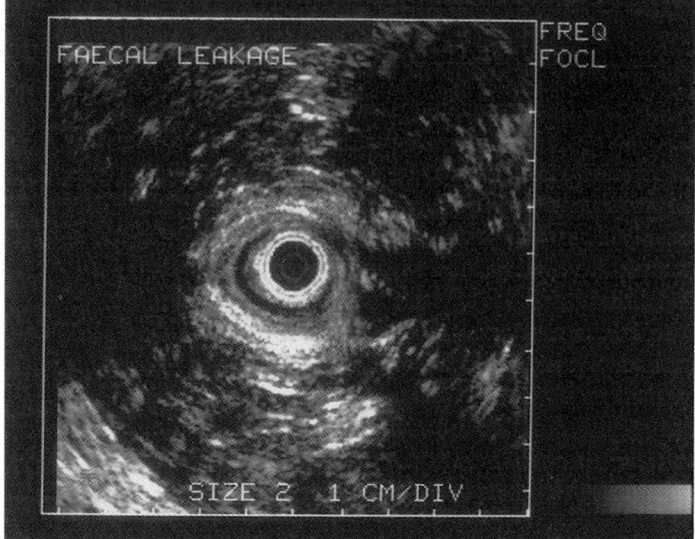

Figure 16.8 Anal ultrasound scan showing an internal and external sphincter defect anteriorly.

complete ring of the internal sphincter surrounded by the uninterrupted external sphincter. In patients with a direct sphincter injury or obstetric trauma, a sphincter defect is seen in the internal and/or external anal sphincter (Fig. 16.8). This method also provides a dynamic assessment of the sphincter muscles on voluntary contraction. We have found an excellent correlation between anal ultrasonography and defects in the internal and external anal sphincters as displayed during surgical dissection (Deen et al 1993). This is one of the most useful investigations in the assessment of fecal incontinence. It is relatively non-invasive and delineates sphincter defects and other anatomical abnormalities, such as prolapses and rectoceles, with precision.

TREATMENT
Conservative treatment

A significant proportion of patients with fecal incontinence can be managed successfully on conservative treatment which should be tried in all patients except those with inflammatory bowel disease, carcinoma or rectal prolapse. Figure 16.9 summarizes our approach to the management of fecal incontinence. The aim of conservative management is to produce a solid stool once each day.

First-line treatment in patients with diarrhea should be the use of

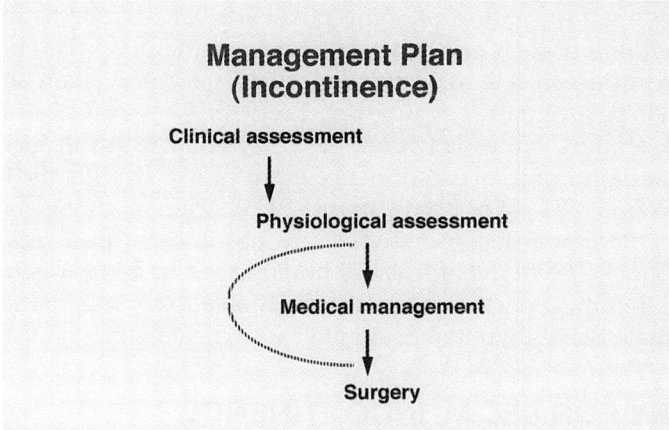

Figure 16.9

simple constipating agents such as codeine phosphate or loperamide. Loperamide may be particularly helpful in those with diarrhea due to excessive small intestinal motility. It acts by slowing transit and also improves resting anal sphincter tone (Goke et al 1992, Ruppin 1987). Dietary manipulation in the form of fiber-rich food and fiber supplementation with methyl cellulose or ispaghula may improve the consistency of a liquid stool. Miller et al (1988) reported a successful outcome in 40% of patients treated by diet and drugs alone, whereas Keighley & Fielding (1983) reported improvement in only 15% of patients.

Another conservative measure commonly employed is the use of suppositories or disposable enemas to ensure that the rectum is empty and contains no fecal material. The main problem with these measures is patient compliance because of dislike of the use of suppositories and enemas.

Other conservative measures include pelvic floor exercises, biofeedback and electrical stimulation. Pelvic floor physiotherapy is useful in patients who have occasional incontinence of liquids. The aim is to reeducate patients in the use of their pelvic floor muscles. However, these techniques are time consuming and have not yet been shown to be of long-term benefit.

Biofeedback training

Biofeedback utilizes the patient's self-control over bodily functions. The patient is provided instantly with information on the current function of the external anal sphincter by using visual or auditory information through an electronic device. This procedure is based on the assumption that the involuntary nature of some physiological responses, and hence the impossibility of their self-control, stem from the poor afferent information from the anorectal continence mechanisms rather than irremedial defects in efferent signals (Loening-Baucke 1990).

In some studies, biofeedback has been reported to result in improvement in symptoms of fecal incontinence in up to 80% of patients (Cerulli et al 1979, Wald 1981, Whitehead et al 1985). The mechanisms for the improved continence in these studies are not known. In a recent study (Loening-Baucke 1990) the efficacy of biofeedback training was compared to medical therapy alone in eight patients. Biofeedback was found to have no additional benefit than that provided by medical therapy alone.

SURGERY FOR FECAL INCONTINENCE

In patients where conservative measures fail to improve the problem or those in whom there is a demonstrable sphincter defect, surgical intervention should be considered. The plan of surgical management for fecal incontinence is outlined in Figure 16.10. A permanent stoma should only be considered when all other measures have failed.

Direct sphincter repair is performed in patients who have experienced sphincter trauma where the defect has been delineated on endoanal ultrasonography. The ends of the external anal sphincter are isolated and an overlap repair is performed using non-absorbable sutures. Following this type of repair, up to 90% of patients can hope to have continence restored (Browning & Motson 1983). In patients with neurogenic fecal incontinence, postanal repair is the most commonly performed operation. The levators

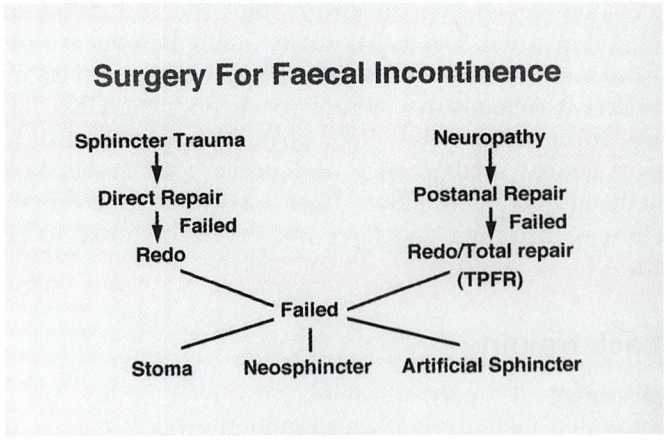

Figure 16.10

are approximated using non-absorbable sutures and the external anal sphincter is also plicated using a similar suture. It must be ensured that the muscles are not opposed under tension as this may result in necrosis.

The quality of continence achieved after a postanal repair is often imperfect (O'Kelly & Mortensen 1992). It was previously thought that postanal repair works by restoring the anorectal angle but it has now been shown that continence is improved by increasing sphincter pressures and improving anal canal sensation (Miller et al 1988).

Patients who fail to benefit from either a direct repair or postanal repair are faced with a difficult choice about a permanent stoma. In these patients the repair can be repeated or a newer option such as gracilis neosphincter reconstruction or an artificial sphincter can be considered.

REFERENCES

Aaronson I, Nixon H H 1972 A clinical evaluation of anorectal pressure studies in the diagnosis of Hirschsprung's disease. Gut 13: 138–146

Barratt J A 1992 Colorectal disorders in elderly people. British Medical Journal 305: 764–766

Bartolo D C C, Jarratt J A, Read M G, Donnelly T C, Read N W 1983a The role of partial denervation of the puborectalis in idiopathic faecal incontinence. British Journal of Surgery 70: 664–667

Bartolo D C C, Jarrat J A, Read N W 1983b The cutaneoanal reflex: a useful index of neuropathy. British Journal of Surgery 70: 660–663

Binnie N R, Kawimbe B M, Papachrysostomou M, Smith A N 1990 Use of the pudendoanal reflex in the treatment of neurogenic faecal incontinence. Gut 31: 1051–1055

Browning G G P, Motson R W 1983 Results of Parks operation for faecal incontinence after anal sphincter injury. British Medical Journal 286: 1873–1875

Cerulli M A, Nikoomannesh P, Shuster M M 1979 Progress in biofeedback conditioning for faecal incontinence. Gastroenterology 76: 742–746

Cornes H, Bartolo D C C, Stirrat G M 1991 Changes in anal canal sensation after childbirth. British Journal of Surgery 78: 74–77

Deen K I, Kumar D, Keighley M R B 1993 Correlation between anal ultrasound and surgery. Annals of Surgery 218: 201–205

Deen K I, Kumar D, Williams J G, Oliff J, Keighley M R B 1993 The prevalence of anal sphincter defects in faecal incontinence: a prospective endosonic study. Gut 34: 685–688

Delechenaut P, Leroi A M, Weber J, Touchais J Y, Czernichow P, Denis P H 1992 Relationship between clinical symptoms of anal incontinence and the results of anorectal manometry. Diseases of the Colon and Rectum 35: 847–849

Drossman D A, Sandler R S, Broom C M, McKee D C 1986 Urgency and faecal soiling in people with bowel dysfunction. Digestive Diseases and Sciences 31: 1221–1225

Enck P, Bielefeldt K, Rathmann W, Purrmann J, Tschope D, Erckenbrecht J F 1991 Epidemiology of faecal incontinence in selected patient groups. International Journal of Colorectal Disease 6: 143–146

Frenckner B, von Euler C 1975 Influence of pudendal nerve block on the function of the anal sphincters. Gut 16: 482–489

Goke M, Ewe K, Donner K, Meyer zum Buschenfelde 1992 Influence of loperamide and loperamide oxide on the anal sphincter. Diseases of the Colon and Rectum 35: 857–861

Henry M M 1983 The descending perineum syndrome. Sir Alan Parks memorial symposium. Annals of the Royal College of Surgeons of England 65 (Suppl): 24–25

Kamm M A 1994 Obstetric damage and faecal incontinence. Lancet 344: 730–733

Keighley M R B, Fielding J W L 1983 Management of faecal incontinence and results of surgical treatment. British Journal of Surgery 70: 463–468

Kiff E S 1983 The clinical use of anorectal physiology studies. Sir Alan Parks memorial symposium. Annals of the Royal College of Surgeons of England 158: 498–512

Kumar D, Waldron W J, Williams N S, Wingate D L 1989 Home assessment of anorectal motility and external sphincter EMG in idiopathic faecal incontinence. British Journal of Surgery 76: 635–636

Leigh R J, Turnberg L A 1982 Faecal incontinence: the unvoiced symptom. Lancet i: 1349–1351

Loening-Baucke V 1990 Efficacy of biofeedback training in improving faecal incontinence and anorectal physiologic function. Gut 31: 1395–1402

Lord P H 1968 A new regime for the treatment of haemorrhoids. Proceedings of the Royal Society of Medicine 61: 935

Lubowski D Z, Swash M, Nicholls R J, Henry M M 1988 Increase in pudendal nerve terminal motor latency with defecation straining. British Journal of Surgery 75: 1095–1097

MacArthur C, Lewis M, Knox E G 1991 Health and childbirth. British Journal of Obstetrics and Gynaecology 98: 1193–1204

MacDonald A, Smith A, McNeill A D, Finlay I G 1992 Manual dilatation of the anus. British Journal of Surgery 79: 1381–1382

Mandelstam D A 1984 Faecal incontinence. Social and economic factors. In: Henry M M, Swash M (eds) Coloproctology and the pelvic floor. Pathophysiology and management. Butterworth, London, pp 217–222

Miller R, Bartolo D C C, Locke-Edmunds J C, Mortensen N J McC 1988 Prospective study of conservative and operative treatment for faecal incontinence. British Journal of Surgery 75: 101–105

Milne J S 1976 Prevalence of incontinence in the elderly age group. In: Wallington E L (ed) Incontinence in the elderly. Academic Press, London, pp 9–31

Neil M E, Swash M 1980 Increased motor unit fiber density in the external anal sphincter muscle in ano-rectal incontinence: a single fibre EMG study. J Neurol Neurosurg Psychiatry 43: 343–347

Nivatvongs S, Stern H S, Fryd D S 1981 The length of the anal canal. Diseases of the Colon and Rectum 67: 216–220

O'Kelly T J, Mortensen N J McC 1992 Investigation and management of anorectal incontinence. Current Practice in Surgery 4: 49–55

Read N W, Harford W V, Schmulen A C, Read M G, Santa Ana C, Fordtran J S 1979 A clinical study of patients with faecal incontinence and diarrhoea. Gastroenterology 76: 747–756

Read N W, Haynes W G, Bartolo D C C 1983 Use of anorectal manometry during rectal infusion of saline to investigate sphincter function in incontinent patients. Gastroenterology 85: 105–113

Roe A M, Bartolo D C C, Mortensen N J 1986 New method of assessment of anal sensation in various anorectal disorders. British Journal of Surgery 73: 310–312

Ruppin H 1987 Loperamide — a potential antidiarrhoeal with actions along the alimentary tract. Alimentary Pharmacological Therapy 1: 179–190

Snooks S J, Swash M, Setchell M, Henry M M 1984a Injury to innervation of pelvic floor sphincter masculature in childbirth. Lancet ii: 546–550

Snooks S, Henry M M, Swash M 1984b Faecal incontinence after anal dilatation. British Journal of Surgery 71: 617–618

Sultan A H, Kamm M A, Hudson C N, Bartram C I 1993 Anal sphincter disruption during vaginal delivery. New England Journal of Medicine 329: 1905–1911

Sultan A H, Kamm M A, Hudson C N 1994 Pudendal nerve damage during labour: prospective study before and after childbirth. British Journal of Obstetrics and Gynaecology 101: 22–28

Vernava A M III, Longo W E, Daniel G L 1992 Pudendal neuropathy and the importance of EMG evaluation of faecal incontinence. Diseases of the Colon and Rectum 35: 11

Wald A 1981 Biofeedback therapy for faecal incontinence. Annals of Internal Medicine 95: 146–149

Whitehead W E, Burgio K L, Engel B T 1985 Biofeedback treatment of faecal incontinence in geriatric patients. Journal of the American Geriatric Society 33: 320–324

Womack N R, Williams N S, Holmfield J H, Morrison J F B, Simpkins K D 1985 New method for dynamic assessment of anorectal function in constipation. British Journal of Surgery 72: 994–998

17

The investigation of rectal bleeding

A. M. Gudgeon   R. J. Leicester

CLINICAL FEATURES

Rectal bleeding is a common symptom reported to occur in 6.4% of the population (Chappuis et al 1985). If all were referred for a specialist opinion 300 consultations a week would be required for a hospital serving a population of 250 000. This figure includes all forms of bleeding, however minor. Such numbers of patients would obviously be unmanageable so it is important to investigate patients selectively. Twenty percent of patients referred to a specialist with rectal bleeding have anal disease alone, 25% have a clinically important colorectal lesion such as adenoma, adenocarcinoma, diverticular disease, inflammatory bowel disease or angiodysplasia, another 25% will have combined anal and colorectal disease whilst in the remaining 30% no cause will be found.

Patients with rectal bleeding fall into one of three major groups:

1. chronic intermittent blood loss;
2. major lower gastrointestinal hemorrhage, defined as greater than 30 mL of blood loss per hour;
3. occult hemorrhage.

Which category the patient falls into, together with his age, will influence the type, extent and urgency of investigation.

A detailed history is followed by careful examination and relevant special investigations. The nature of the bleeding must be established to make a crude estimate of the source and thus direct the appropriate investigations. Fresh blood unmixed with stool suggests an anorectal origin. Darker blood, clots and blood mixed with the stool indicate a more proximal lesion. The latter symptom predicts left-sided colonic neoplasia in 8–25% of individuals (Irvine et al 1988, Silman et al 1983). An estimate of the quantity of blood loss and the duration of symptoms helps to establish the urgency of investigation and the need for resuscitation. A coexistent change in bowel habit raises the likelihood of inflammatory bowel disease or malignancy, while abdominal pain, anorectal pain, change in appetite and weight loss will also influence subsequent investigation. Gastrointestinal symptoms may not be a feature in patients with occult bleeding but the whole of the gastrointestinal tract may need to be investigated before the cause is found.

Specific questions concerning the past medical history of the patient should concern previous intestinal neoplasia, colitis, travel abroad and previous radiation therapy. A history of vascular disease raises the possibility of ischemic colitis. Aneurysm repair may be complicated by aortointestinal fistula and aortic or mitral valve disease are related to angiodysplasia. The history must include specific questions regarding past bleeding disorders and details of medication to identify users of aspirin, other non-steroidal antiinflammatory agents or anticoagulants. A family history of a first-degree relative suffering from colonic neoplasia should prompt a more extensive investigation even if the bleeding is thought to be due to hemorrhoids.

Clinical examination should identify clinical signs of anemia, lymphadenopathy, telangiectasia and aortic stenosis while evidence of shock should prompt rapid resuscitation in patients with major rectal bleeding. Abdominal examination will frequently be unhelpful but may provide useful clues such as the presence of scars from previous surgery, tattoos for radiotherapy, organomegaly and abdominal masses. Examination is concluded with inspection of the anal verge and digital anorectal examination.

DIFFERENTIAL DIAGNOSIS

Any lesion, area of ulceration or vascular abnormality in the gastrointestinal tract is capable of causing rectal bleeding. The more common causes are listed in Box 17.1.

Box 17.1 Common causes of rectal bleeding

In children	In adults
Perianal conditions – fissure, sexual child abuse	Perianal conditions – hemorrhoids, fissure, prolapse
Inflammatory – ulcerative colitis, Crohn's disease	Inflammatory – ulcerative colitis, Crohn's disease, ischemic colitis
Intussusception	Infective – infective colitis, amebiasis, CMV colitis, typhoid
Intestinal hemangiomas	Vascular – aortoenteric fistula, angiodysplasia
Meckel's diverticulum	Diverticulosis, jejunal diverticula
Juvenile polyps, hamartomas – Peutz–Jeghers syndrome	Neoplasia – benign/malignant polyps, adenocarcinoma, lymphoma
Bleeding diatheses	Bleeding diatheses Massive upper gastrointestinal hemorrhage

SPECIAL INVESTIGATIONS

All patients with rectal bleeding require clinical examination, rectal examination and proctosigmoidoscopy followed in most cases by either double contrast barium enema or colonoscopy. The choice between radiological and endoscopic investigation will depend upon a number of factors including expertise and local availability. For anorectal bleeding under the age of 40 sigmoidoscopy plus treatment of the hemorrhoids or fissure is usually quite adequate, but it is important to follow these patients to ensure that symptoms resolve and therefore minimize the risk of overlooking a proximal lesion.

Blood tests

A full blood count and hemoglobin estimation must be performed on all patients. In addition it may be indicated to measure liver function, urea, electrolytes and clotting function in patients over 50 or those with major blood loss.

Proctoscopy and rigid sigmoidoscopy

Both instruments should be used routinely in the initial assessment of patients with rectal bleeding, whether mild or severe, unless there is severe pain from an anal fissure. In cases of major hemorrhage, irrigation and suction equipment must be available. It has been stated that the majority of large bowel neoplasms can be diagnosed with a rigid sigmoidoscope since they lie within the range of the instrument (Rubin 1975) but in practice only about 12% are visible (Farrands et al 1983) due to difficulty advancing the instrument beyond the rectosigmoid junction (Nichols & Dube 1982, Nivatvongs & Fryd 1980). The instrument is invaluable as it is quick to use, simple, cheap and easy to clean. Disposable instruments have become available recently. A good view of the rectum is usually achieved, stool consistency and color can be assessed and the site of bleeding distinguished as anorectal or more proximal. In the event of poor mucosal visualization due to feces, glycerine suppositories may be given before repeating the examination. Some prefer to give these routinely before sigmoidoscopy but this precludes stool visualization. In addition, the rigid sigmoidoscope is more accurate than the flexible instrument in measuring the distance of a lesion from the anal verge.

The proctoscope or anoscope is of more limited value but will demonstrate hemorrhoids and facilitate their treatment with rubber band ligation, infrared coagulation or oily phenol injection. Following these initial investigations the clinician should have established a provisional diagnosis and the choice of subsequent tests will depend upon this as well as their local availability and reliability. These include further direct vision using flexible sigmoidoscopy, colonoscopy and upper gastrointestinal endoscopy as well as radiological and radionucleotide imaging.

Flexible sigmoidoscopy

Although the value of the rigid sigmoidoscope must not be under-estimated in the investigation of rectal bleeding, the flexible instrument measuring 60 cm has conclusively been shown to be more superior in identifying left-sided neoplasms (Farrands et al 1983, Leicester et al 1982). The procedure takes 5–8 minutes and can be readily performed in the outpatient department without the need for sedation. It can be done without bowel preparation but a better view is obtained following a single phosphate enema. The majority of large bowel neoplasms will be iden-tified using this technique, as 70% occur in the rectum and left colon. Rigid sigmoidoscopy followed by double contrast barium enema has an appreciable false negative rate, particularly in the presence of diverticular disease (Ott et al 1980). Flexible sigmoidoscopy complements such an investigation (Brewster et al 1994) and considerably improves the diag-nostic sensitivity and specificity (Farrands et al 1983).

If an adenomatous polyp is found, the patient should be referred for colonoscopy to exclude additional neoplasia. Polypectomy can be per-formed using a snare or hot biopsy forceps. It should not be performed at flexible sigmoidoscopy because of inferior bowel preparation and limited maneuverability of the instrument. Polypoid lesions should be removed by snare polypectomy at colonoscopy as biopsy may be misleading.

Colonoscopy

Colonoscopy is indicated for patients with rectal bleeding or anemia following the exclusion of anorectal pathology, following a normal barium enema or when additional risk factors for colorectal cancer exist, such as previous adenomas or cancer, bowel cancer in a first-degree relative or ulcerative colitis for more than 10 years.

It is dangerous to attribute rectal bleeding to diverticular disease without excluding a lesion endoscopically as up to 34% will have a signi-ficant anorectal lesion. Boulos et al (1985) found that the barium enema was inaccurate in 45 of 105 (43%) patients with symptomatic diverticular disease and recommended endoscopy in patients with sigmoid divert-icular disease (Boulos et al 1985).

Colonoscopy is now regarded by many as the 'gold standard' in primary investigation for rectal bleeding even though it is reported to be twice as expensive as barium enema (Cowen & Macrae 1992). The crude cost of the investigation, however, is not representative when those patients referred for colonoscopy following an inadequate or equivocal barium enema are considered or where a polyp has been identified which requires colonoscopic polypectomy. The additional cost of missed polyps and early carcinomas also has to be taken into account. An early report from Swarbrick et al (1978) highlighted this by describing 239 patients undergoing colonoscopy after rectal examination, proctosigmoidoscopy and a negative barium enema. A cause of bleeding was identified in 95 (40%), 23 (10%) of the series had carcinomas and a further 39 (16%) had adenomatous polyps.

Unlike barium enema, colonoscopy has a negligible false positive rate. It has additional advantages over double contrast barium enema as a primary investigation, including:

- detection of angiodysplasia and minimal colitis not visible on barium enema;
- simultaneous therapeutic procedures such as biopsy, coagulation, snare polypectomy, stricture dilatation and laser treatment of inoperable tumors;
- increased sensitivity and specificity over barium enema;
- for elderly patients, a high quality double contrast barium enema is difficult to obtain (Irvine et al 1988).

Other therapeutic options available are the dilatation of benign strictures, the removal of foreign bodies and laser treatment of tumors. It should be remembered that lesions can be missed on colonoscopy and a double contrast barium enema may be done as a complementary investigation.

The advantages of colonoscopy outweigh the disadvantages in most centers but the technique requires expertise, experience and adequate training. An experienced endoscopist should be able to reach the cecum in over 90% of cases but this figure varies enormously with some reports of failure to reach the cecum in 45% of cases (Aldridge & Sim 1986). Despite this, in 27% of those patients colonoscopy revealed neoplastic lesions not detected by double contrast barium enema.

Enteroscopy

Small bowel enteroscopy is less widely available than colonoscopy, is more time consuming and often incomplete (Lewis & Waye 1988). It should therefore be reserved for those patients where other investigations have been unhelpful.

Upper gastrointestinal endoscopy

Upper gastrointestinal endoscopy must be performed within 12 hours of hospital admission in all cases of major rectal bleeding in order to exclude an upper gastrointestinal source. A complete examination must visualize the fourth part of the duodenum in order to exclude an aortoduodenal fistula which can cause intermittent bleeding. By using a pediatric colonoscope as an upper gastrointestinal endoscope it is frequently possible to examine the proximal jejunum for diverticular and vascular malformations. Bleeding lesions may then be treated by injection sclerotherapy or laser or localized for resection by injection with Indian ink.

Angiography

The patient with massive rectal bleeding warrants angiography once an upper gastrointestinal cause has been excluded by endoscopy. Angiography should also be considered in patients with continuous subacute blood loss where other investigations are negative (Whitaker & Gregson 1993). In order to detect a bleeding lesion, the rate of blood loss must be at least 1–1.5 mL/minute (Zuckerman et al 1993). Angiography requires trained personnel to be available 24 hours a day and hence its ready availability may be limited in some centers. The main advantage of the technique is that it requires minimal patient preparation, needing only urethral catheterization to avoid the accumulation of contrast medium in the bladder and to monitor urine output.

Bleeding most commonly arises from the middle or right colic arteries (Baum et al 1974), therefore selective angiography of the superior mesenteric artery is usually performed preferentially. If this fails to locate a source of bleeding, the inferior mesenteric artery is studied. Finally, the celiac artery is cannulated to exclude anatomical aberrations and to identify upper gastrointestinal causes not identified at endoscopy such as a hepatic artery aneurysm. The ability of angiography to show upper gastrointestinal hemorrhage is limited because the nature of the usual lesions there is such that the bleeding is usually intermittent and of a variable rate (Sos et al 1980). However, in the absence of active bleeding it may still be possible to show anatomical abnormalities of the vasculature (Fig. 17.1). Radiological signs of hemorrhage include extravasation of contrast medium which may fill a diverticulum in diverticular hemorrhage (Fig. 17.2), irregular vessels and aneurysms (Welch et al 1978). Extravasation of the contrast medium in angiodysplasia is less common but such lesions have a characteristic appearance, a vascular tuft accompanied by an early and persistent prominent draining vein. Angiodysplasias are commonly located in the cecum and ascending colon where magnification techniques may be required to confirm their presence (Zuckerman et al 1993).

Digital subtraction angiography is of limited use in the examination of the lower gastrointestinal tract because of artefact related to bowel peristalsis, a limited field of view and poor spatial resolution (Rees et al

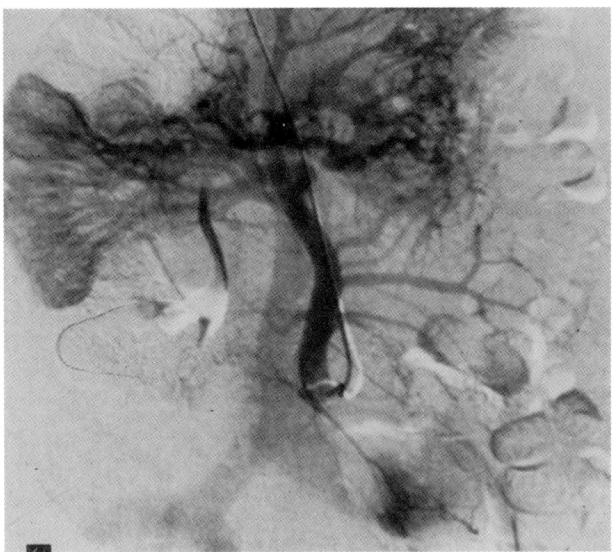

Figure 17.1 Angiograph showing anatomical abnormalities of the vasculature.

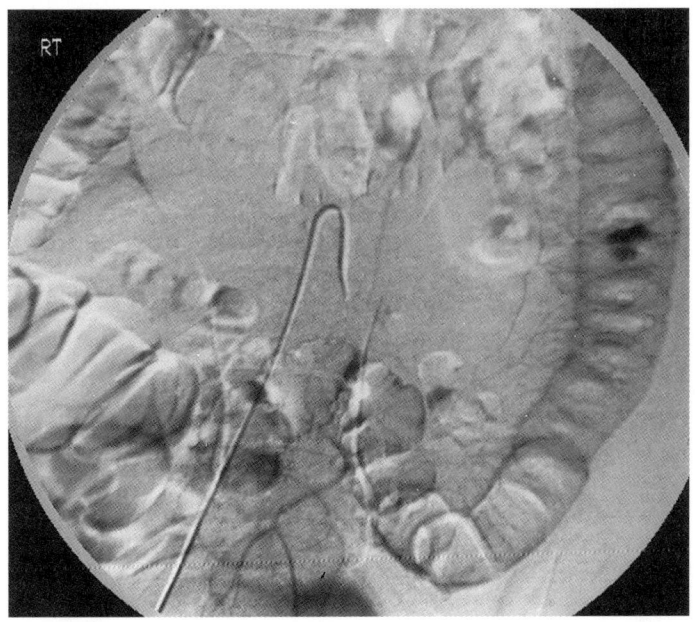

Figure 17.2 Angiograph showing diverticular hemorrhage.

1988). These disadvantages are not compensated for by such advantages as decreased examination time, decreased contrast requirements and improved contrast resolution.

In patients with HIV-related disease and profuse gastrointestinal hemorrhage, angiography often enables identification of a specific site of hemorrhage which can be stopped with transcatheter embolization and/ or vasopressin infusion (Sharma et al 1992). Embolization requires super-selective localization of the feeding vessels prior to infusion of embolic agents as mistakes can cause irreversible ischemia, leading to bowel infarction or stricture formation. Vasopressin infusion does not require these techniques and may be used to help stabilize the patient prior to surgery.

Scintigraphy

The site of massive rectal bleeding is often difficult to establish even when disease has been demonstrated by colonoscopy or barium enema. When selective angiography has failed to demonstrate the site of bleeding, nuclear medicine techniques can be used. There are essentially three types of scan available:

1. [99]technetium pertechnetate scintigraphy to identify gastric mucosa in Meckel's diverticula (Jewett et al 1970);
2. [99]technetium sulfur colloid scintigraphy (Alavi 1982);
3. [99]technetium-labeled red blood cell scintigraphy.

[99]Technetium pertechnetate scintigraphy ('Meckel's scan')

This investigation is particularly important in children and adolescents with rectal bleeding of obscure origin as it is sensitive in the demon-stration of a Meckel's diverticulum, one of the common causes of bleeding in this age group. The Meckel's scan should be performed before a Tc-labeled red cell scan because of interference (Yen & Lanoie 1992). It may be necessary to perform a repeat scan in negative or equivocal cases as 50–91% of bleeding Meckel's diverticula in this age group contain gastric mucosa (Imaeda et al 1990). The simultaneous use of an H_2 antagonist reduces acid secretion and the intraluminal release of pertechnate without impairing its uptake, thereby improving the accuracy of the technique (Baum 1981). Scintigraphy is more accurate than any other currently available non-surgical technique in detection of a Meckel's diverticulum.

[99]Technetium sulfur colloid and [99]technetium-labeled red blood cell scintigraphy

These techniques, introduced in the late 1970s (Alavi et al 1977, Pavel et al

1977), involve the radiolabeling of red blood cells or sulfur colloid. The main problem with the ^{99}Tc sulfur colloid is its rapid clearance from the circulation by the reticuloendothelial system and hence a short half-life, 2.5–3.5 minutes in patients with normal liver function (Alavi 1982). The detection of minute amounts of bleeding, in the range of 0.05–0.1 mL/minute, has been demonstrated away from areas of high activity. Because of the short half-life the patient must be actively bleeding at the time of injection (Robinson 1993).

Alternatively ^{99}Tc-labeled rbc scans may be positive even with intermittent bleeding but they may take several hours to produce results, although they tend to be more accurate than the sulfur colloid technique (Chaudhuri 1991). Reports on the sensitivity and specificity of the investigation vary enormously and results therefore have to be interpreted with caution because of the high false positive and false negative rate (Whitaker et al 1993). The most useful application is in patients with recurrent or prolonged bleeding, inconclusive endoscopy studies and a high risk for operation.

The technetium rbc scan is often a reliable tool for the assessment of unexplained lower gastrointestinal bleeding, when the scan is positive in the first 24 hours and an upper gastrointestinal bleeding source of the hemorrhage has been excluded. However, incorrect localization can occur due to the rapid transit of labeled red cells in the small bowel in antegrade or retrograde directions. Localization can be improved by using dynamic scanning. Used in combination with angiography, the technique has been reported to localize the bleeding source in 70% of patients (Ohri et al 1992).

Finally, in the difficult case of major rectal bleeding which has come to surgery, intraoperative scintigraphy may be used to help find the source of a hemorrhage which is difficult to locate (Biener et al 1990).

In conclusion, ^{99}Tc-labeled rbc scintigraphy is a sensitive, non-invasive technique which has problems of misinterpretation and inaccurate localization. It has a role in the investigation of the patient with major gastrointestinal hemorrhage and with increasing experience the results of the techniques are improving.

Barium enema

If colonoscopy has failed to identify the source of bleeding, it is unlikely that a barium enema will do so. However, while colonoscopy is regarded as the 'gold standard' in colonic examination, it is often impractical as a first-line investigation as there is limited availability of colonoscopy in many centers and the entire colon may not be seen in up to 40% of cases. The barium enema remains a valuable investigation, particularly in conjunction with flexible sigmoidoscopy (Brewster et al 1994), but negative results must be viewed with caution and full colonoscopy performed if symptoms persist. An air contrast technique must be used with the colon empty of feces.

Enteroclysis

When other techniques have failed to identify a source of bleeding, contrast imaging of the small intestine may be employed. In recurrent obscure bleeding such imaging may identify such causes as jejunal diverticula, strictures, ulcers or small bowel tumors but it is unreliable for demonstrating vascular anomalies or Meckel's diverticulum. Enteroclysis (contrast delivered to the small bowel via intubation) has an advantage over a small bowel follow-through of barium with a significantly improved diagnostic yield.

The small bowel remains the most difficult area to study reliably (Rex et al 1991). Recently an alternative double contrast small bowel technique has been reported that uses an acid-resistant effervescent agent administered orally (Klein & Gunther 1993). Reports suggest it provides better views of the ileum than enteroclysis but the latter provides superior imaging of the jejunum.

It is important to avoid enteroclysis if angiography or CT scanning is to be employed as the barium may remain in the bowel for several days and so interfere with interpretation in these investigations.

Computed tomography and ultrasound scanning

CT and ultrasound scanning have a very limited role in the primary investigation of gastrointestinal hemorrhage except in selected cases. Very elderly and infirm patients tolerate barium enema and colonoscopy poorly. Computed tomography will not detect mucosal polyps or subtle mucosal abnormalities but this may not be so important in the elderly. Computed tomography following four 300 mL doses of dilute oral contrast medium over the 2 days prior to the examination has now become an accepted method for investigating the colon (Fink et al 1994). The technique can demonstrate carcinomas and diverticular disease as well as lesions in other organs.

New techniques

The transrectal installation of water has recently been described as a technique for improving sonographic imaging of the lumen and wall of the colon. The technique, known as colonic intraluminal sonography, has shown a sensitivity of 91% for the detection of colonic tuberculosis, 89% for ulcerative colitis and 83% for colonic cancers (Walter et al 1993). It appears to be worthy of further evaluation. As a first-line investigation, however, it has a limited role. It is reserved for those patients who are unable to tolerate other procedures that give more accurate results.

SURGERY

Surgery is necessary in cases of massive blood loss where it is not possible to locate a source of continuing bleeding using the described techniques. There is now little place for blind limited resection or subtotal colectomy. In the absence of an easily identifiable lesion, the patient should have on-table bowel irrigation (Radcliffe & Dudley 1983) and intraoperative endoscopy (Batch et al 1981, Campbell et al 1985, Lau et al 1989). In difficult cases, it is quite possible to examine the whole of the gastrointestinal tract peroperatively. The technique is frequently rewarding and quick to perform (Strodel et al 1984).

OVERVIEW

While this chapter outlines many standard diagnostic tests available for the investigation of rectal bleeding, they are all highly observer-dependent

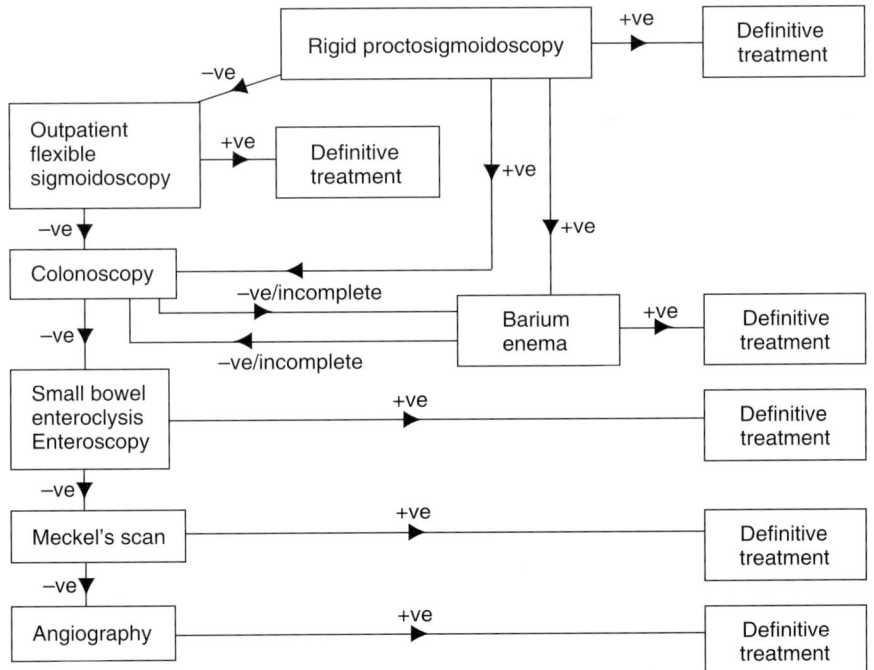

Figure 17.3   Investigation of chronic blood loss.

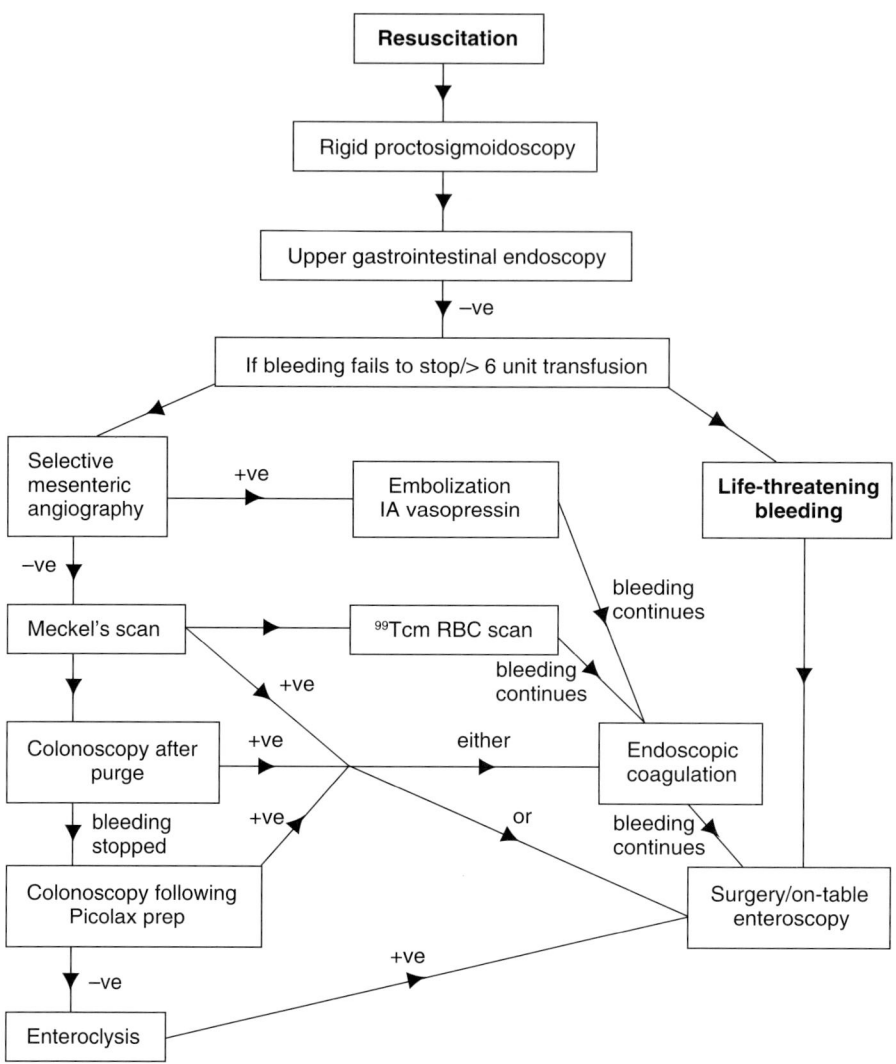

Figure 17.4 Investigation of major blood loss.

with the best results produced by observers with a special interest. No one investigation is universally ideal and the diagnostic techniques employed will depend upon many different factors. It should be remembered that investigations are often complementary and that more than one investigation may be needed to identify a source of bleeding. The algorithms in Figures 17.3, 17.4 and 17.5 demonstrate the preferred order of investigation for the three major categories of rectal bleeding.

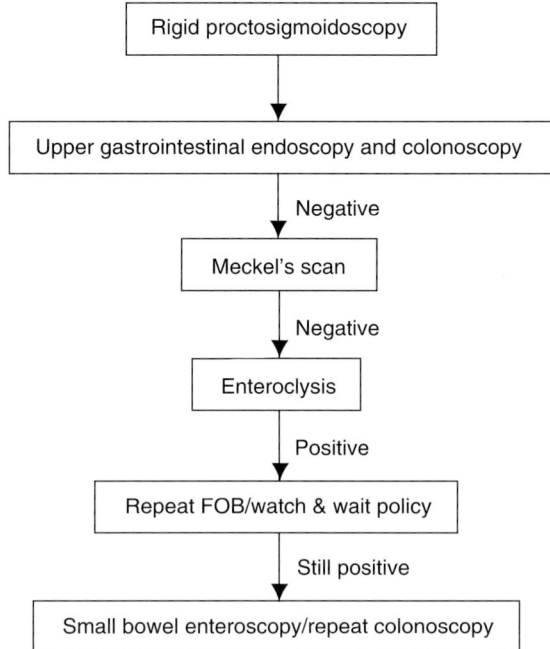

Figure 17.5 Investigation of occult blood loss.

REFERENCES

Alavi A 1982 Detection of gastrointestinal bleeding with ^{99m}Tc-sulphur colloid. Seminars in Nuclear Medicine 12: 126–138

Alavi A, Dann R, Baum S, Biery D N 1977 Scintigraphic detection of acute gastrointestinal bleeding. Radiology 124: 753–756

Aldridge M C, Sim A J W 1986 Colonoscopy findings in symptomatic patients without X-ray evidence of colonic neoplasms. Lancet ii: 833–834

Batch A J G, Pickard R G, DeLacey G 1981 Peroperative colonoscopy in massive rectal bleeding. British Journal of Surgery 68: 64

Baum S 1981 Pertechnetate imaging following cimetidine administration in Meckel's diverticulum of the ileum. American Journal of Gastroenterology 76: 464–465

Baum S, Athanaascoulis C, Waltman A 1974 Angiographic diagnosis and control of large bowel bleeding. Diseases of the Colon and Rectum 17: 447–453

Biener A, Palestro C, Lewis B S, Katz L B 1990 Intraoperative scintigraphy for active small intestinal bleeding. Surgery, Gynecology and Obstetrics 171: 388–392

Boulos P B, Cowin A P, Karamanolis D G, Clark C G 1985 Diverticula, neoplasia or both? Early detection of carcinoma in sigmoid diverticular disease. Annals of Surgery 202: 607–609

Brewster N T, Grieve D C, Saunders J H 1994 Double contrast barium enema and flexible sigmoidoscopy for routine colonic investigation. British Journal of Surgery 81: 445–447

Campbell W B, Rhodes M, Kettlewell M G W 1985 Colonoscopy following intraoperative lavage in the management of severe colonic bleeding. Annals of the Royal College of Surgeons of England 67: 290–292

Chappuis P H, Goulston K J, Tait A D, Dent O F 1985 Predictive value of rectal bleeding in screening for rectal and sigmoid polyps. British Medical Journal 290: 1546–1548

Chaudhuri T K 1991 Radionuclide methods of detecting acute gastrointestinal bleeding. International Journal of Radiation Applications and Instrumentation – Part B, Nuclear Medicine & Biology 18: 655–661

Cowen A E, Macrae F A 1992 Gastrointestinal endoscopy: an accurate and safe primary diagnostic and therapeutic modality. Medical Journal of Australia 157: 52–57

Farrands P A, Vellacott K D, Amar S, Balfour T, Hardcastle J D 1983 Flexible fibreoptic sigmoidoscopy and double-contrast barium enema examination in the identification of adenomas and carcinoma of the colon. Diseases of the Colon and Rectum 26: 725–727

Fink M, Freeman A H, Dixon A K, Coni N K 1994 Computed tomography of the colon in elderly people. British Medical Journal 308: 1018

Imaeda T, Kanematsu M, Sone Y, Iinuma G, Hirose Y, Miya K, Shimokawa K 1990 A case of intermittent bleeding Meckel's diverticulum. Annals of Nuclear Medicine 4: 107–110

Irvine E J, O'Connor J, Frost R A, Shorvon P, Somers S, Stevenson G W, Hunt R H 1988 Prospective comparison of double contrast barium enema plus flexible sigmoidoscopy v colonoscopy in rectal bleeding: barium enema v colonoscopy in rectal bleeding. Gut 29: 1188–1193

Jewett T C, Duszaynski D O, Allen J F 1970 The visualisation of Meckel's diverticulum with 99Tc^m pertechnetate. Surgery 68: 567–570

Klein H M, Gunther R W 1993 Double contrast small bowel follow-through with an acid-resistant effervescent agent. Investigative Radiology 28: 581–585

Lau W Y, Wong S Y, Yuen W K, Wong K K 1989 Intraoperative enteroscopy for bleeding angiodysplasias of the small intestine. Surgery, Gynecology and Obstetrics 168: 341–344

Leicester R J, Pollett W G, Hawley P R, Nicholls R J 1982 Flexible fibreoptic sigmoidoscopy as an outpatient procedure. Lancet i: 34–35

Lewis B S, Waye J D 1988 Chronic gastrointestinal bleeding of obscure origin: role of small bowel enteroscopy. Gastroenterology 94: 1117–1120

Nichols R J, Dube S 1982 The extent of examination by rigid sigmoidoscopy. British Journal of Surgery 69: 438

Nivatvongs S, Fryd D 1980 How far does the proctosigmoidoscope reach? New England Journal of Medicine 303: 380–382

Ohri S K, Desa L A, Lee H, Patel T, Jackson J, Spencer J 1992 Value of scintigraphic localisation of obscure gastrointestinal bleeding. Annals of the Royal College of Surgeons of Edinburgh 37: 328–332

Ott D J, Gelfand D W, Ramquist N A 1980 Causes of error in gastrointestinal radiology. Gastrointestinal Radiology 5: 99–105

Pavel D G, Zimmer A M, Patterson V N 1977 In vivo labelling of red blood cells with ^{99m}Tc: a new approach to blood pool visualisation. Journal of Nuclear Medicine 18: 305–308

Radcliffe A G, Dudley H A F 1983 Intraoperative antegrade irrigation of the large intestine. Surgery, Gynecology and Obstetrics 156: 721–723

Rees C, Palmaz J, Alvarado R, Tyrrel R, Ciaravino V, Register T 1988 DSA in acute gastrointestinal haemorrhage: clinical and in vitro studies. Radiology 169: 499–503

Rex D K, Lappas J C, Maglinte D D 1991 Clinical utility of enteroclysis. Tropical Gastroenterology 12: 15–20

Robinson P 1993 The role of nuclear medicine in acute gastrointestinal bleeding. Nuclear Medicine Communications 14: 849–855

Rubin P 1975 Cancer of the GI tract: colon, rectum and anus. Journal of the American Medical Association 231: 513–516

Sharma V S, Valji K, Bookstein J J 1992 Gastrointestinal haemorrhage in Aids: arteriographic diagnosis and transcatheter treatment. Radiology 185: 447–451

Silman A J, Mitchell P, Nichols R J et al 1983 Self reported dark red bleeding as a marker comparable with occult blood testing in screening for large bowel neoplasms. British Journal of Surgery 70: 721–724

Sos T, Lee J, Wixson D, Sniderman K 1980 Intermittent bleeding from minute to minute in acute massive gastrointestinal haemorrhage: arteriographic demonstration. American Journal of Radiology 131: 1015–1017

Strodel W E, Eckhauser F E, Knol J A, Nostrant T T, Dent T L 1984 Intraoperative fibreoptic endoscopy. American Surgeon 50: 340–344

Swarbrick E T, Fevre D I, Hunt R H, Thomas B M, Williams C B 1978 Colonoscopy for unexplained rectal bleeding. British Medical Journal 2: 1685–1687

Walter D F, Govil S, William R R, Bhargava N, Chandy G 1993 Colonic sonography: preliminary observations. Clinical Radiology 24: 200–204

Welch C E, Athanasoulis C A, Galdabini J J 1978 Haemorrhage from the large bowel with special references to angiodysplasia and diverticular disease. World Journal of Surgery 2: 73–83

Whitaker S C, Gregson R H 1993 The role of angiography in investigation of acute or chronic gastrointestinal haemorrhage. Clinical Radiology 47: 382–388

Whitaker S C, Perkins A C, Wastie M L 1993 The value of scintigraphic studies in the assessment of patients with acute or chronic gastrointestinal haemorrhage. Nuclear Medicine Communications 14: 411–418

Yen C K, Lanoie Y 1992 Effect of stannous pyrophosphate red blood cell gastrointestinal bleeding scan on subsequent Meckel's scan. Clinics in Nuclear Medicine 17: 454–456

Zuckerman D A, Bocchini T P, Birnbaum E H 1993 Massive haemorrhage in the lower gastrointestinal tract in adults: diagnostic imaging and intervention. American Journal of Radiology 161: 704–711

18

Anorectal pain

R. W. Summers

INTRODUCTION

Discomfort and pain in the anorectal region are common and distressing problems affecting most people at one time or another. Discussing the problem is usually uncomfortable and embarrassing for patients and so many physicians neglect or abridge an adequate history or avoid a careful physical examination of the anorectum. The subject of anorectal pathology is not considered to be sufficiently important to deserve educational time in some medical schools' curricula and both our understanding of the pathophysiology of diseases and the development of effective treatments have lagged because of inadequate basic research and insufficient clinical studies. Even in the meetings of professional societies of gastroenterology the topic of anorectal disorders is usually relegated to the last hours of the conference. There is no question that this topic is important and needs more attention than it gets.

There is growing awareness and recognition of anorectal problems. Direct questioning with sensitivity is critical in obtaining a helpful and complete understanding of these diseases. The history can be very helpful in finding the cause of the symptoms and the anorectum is easily accessible to direct examination. New modes of investigation have increased our understanding of the pathophysiology of anorectal disease.

Understanding anorectal symptoms requires a knowledge of anatomy and physiology. In evaluating anorectal pain, the scope of inquiry is the same as with any kind of pain. The onset, character, location, radiation, timing or chronology, associated symptoms and events, severity, aggravating and relieving factors must all be systematically explored in every case. It is essential to inquire how the pain is affected by having a bowel movement. These facts are essential in determining the etiology of the pain and the kind of pathologic process which caused it in order to plan an effective therapeutic strategy. It is worthwhile remembering that most pathologic processes in this region are structural or degenerative, inflammatory (including infections) or neoplastic.

ANATOMY OF THE ANORECTUM

The *anal canal* is approximately 4 cm in length (Fig. 18.1). It originates at

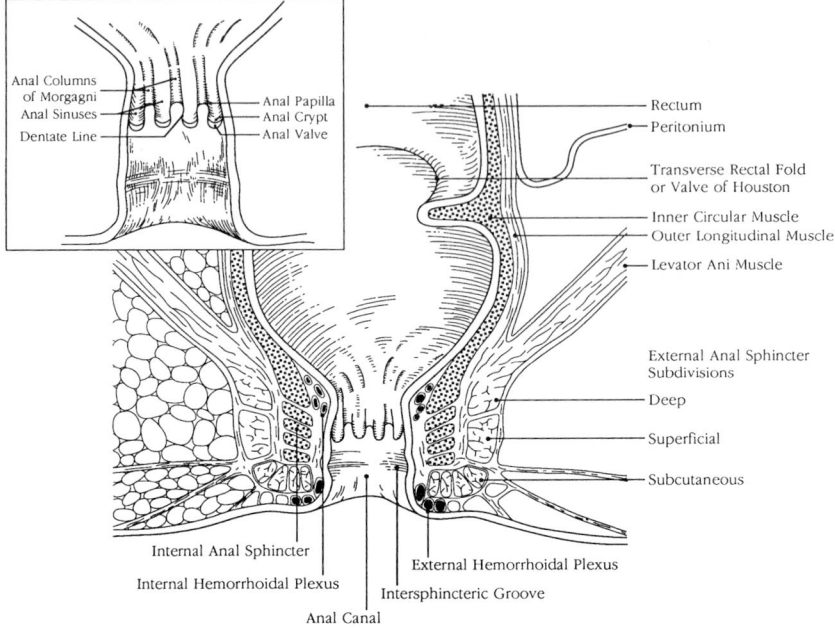

Figure 18.1 Normal anatomy of the anus and rectum.

about the pelvic diaphragm and ends at the anal skin margin. The inner circular smooth muscle layer of the rectum becomes thickened distally and forms the internal anal sphincter. It has a well-defined lower border which can readily be observed on proctoscopic examination and palpated on digital examination as the intersphincteric groove. The external anal sphincter is made up of striated muscle and is composed of three distinct parts: the subcutaneous, superficial and deep. The deep portion is fused with the puborectalis muscle and is essential in maintaining fecal continence. This sling muscle wraps around the lower rectum at the anorectal junction and pulls it forward. It can readily be palpated on digital examination. The puborectalis is the most medial of four parts of the levator ani muscle. Lateral to it is the pubococcygeus (whichs runs from the pubis to the coccyx), next is the iliococcygeus and the most lateral is the ischiococcygeus. Together they make up a continuous sheet of striated muscle which forms a type of pelvic diaphragm supporting the pelvic viscera.

The upper anal canal is lined by rectal mucosa and the lower half by specialized skin (anoderm) devoid of hair follicles and sweat glands. The mucocutaneous junction, called either the dentate or pectinate line, is somewhat scalloped and is bounded by several important structures. Elevated ridges of mucosa are called the columns of Morgagni or rectal papillae; between them are the rectal sinuses. At the inferior margin of the sinuses between the papillae are the anal crypts which are bounded by filmy anal valves. Within the crypts are the anal glands which may become involved in pathologic processes (mostly inflammatory and neoplastic).

The *rectum* is 12.5–15 cm long and it lies against the distal sacrum and the coccyx. It is covered anteriorly and laterally by the peritoneum in its upper third, anteriorly in its middle third, but the lower third has no peritoneum. The peritoneal reflection on the anterior surface of the middle rectum extends to the posterior wall of the bladder in the male and to the uterus in the female, forming the rectovesical or rectouterine pouches respectively. Peritoneal inflammation produces tenderness of the pouch induced by deep digital examination; peritoneal metastatic implants in the pouch produce fixed hard masses which can also be palpated on rectal examination.

There is no distinct transition from the colon to the rectum, but the rectum differs from the colon in that it has no haustra, no tenia coli and no appendices epiploicae. Instead, it has a complete longitudinal coat. The anterior and posterior longitudinal muscles are slightly shorter than the lateral muscle and this arrangement, plus the redundant mucosa and circular muscles, produces three lateral shelves which indent the lumen. These are called the superior, middle and inferior rectal valves or valves of Houston.

Blood vessel and lymphatic anatomy

The major arterial supply of the upper rectum and upper anal canal is the superior rectal (or hemorrhoidal) artery which is the terminal extension of the inferior mesenteric artery (Fig. 18.2). The lower rectum receives several small middle rectal arteries which are branches of the internal iliac arteries, bilaterally. The anus and sphincters receive their blood supply from the inferior rectal arteries which arise from the internal pudendal arteries, also branches of the internal iliac arteries.

The venous return represents a watershed of two separate systems, the portal and systemic circulations. The superior rectal veins drain the proximal rectum into the inferior mesenteric vein and eventually into the portal vein. The middle rectal veins drain the lower rectum and upper anal canal into the internal iliac veins. Similarly, the inferior rectal veins drain the anal canal and the lower rectum into the iliac veins via the internal pudendal veins.

The lymphatic channels from the upper and middle rectum parallel the superior rectal artery and vein and terminate in the inferior mesenteric and paraaortic nodes (Fig. 18.3). Some of the lymphatics from the lower rectum drain lymph in the same direction, but other channels are oriented laterally and terminate in the lateral pelvic walls. Below the dentate line, the lymph channels usually drain into the inguinal nodes, but they may also drain via the superior rectal or middle rectal channels.

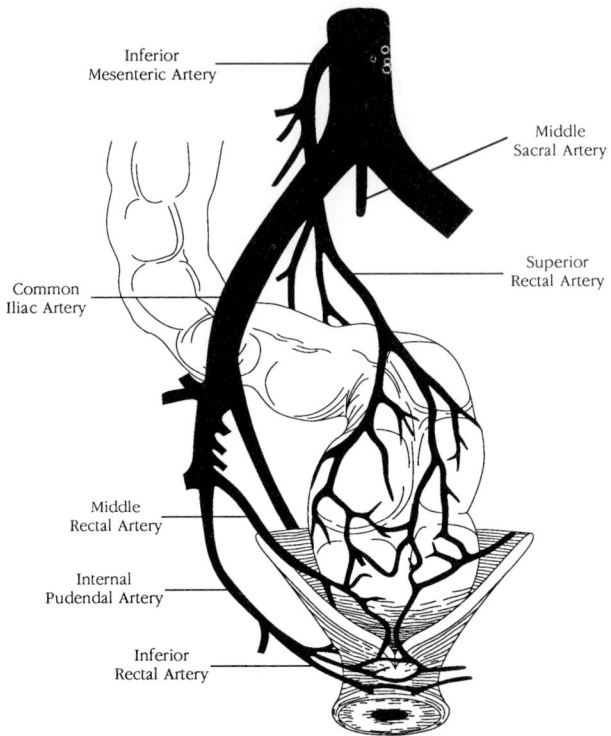

Figure 18.2 Arterial supply to the anus and rectum.

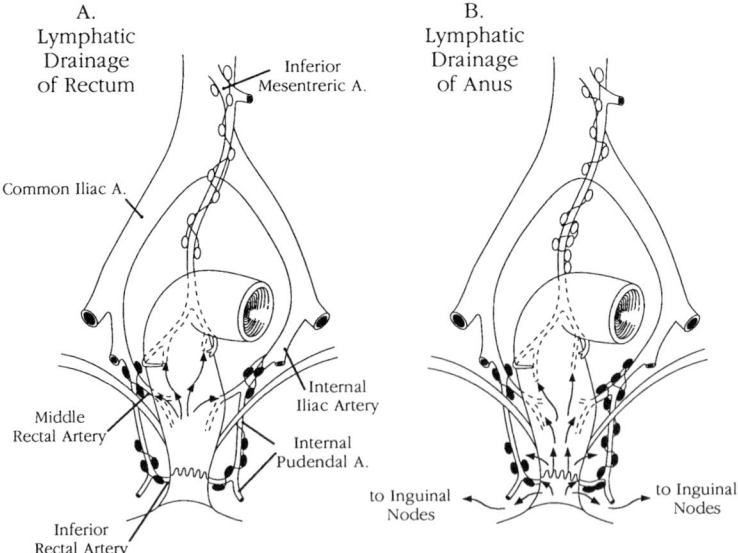

Figure 18.3 Lymphatic drainage of the anus and rectum.

Nerve supply

The rectum and upper half of the anal canal are supplied with both sympathetic and parasympathetic nerve fibers (Fig. 18.4). The preganglionic sympathetic fibers originate from the second to the fourth lumbar splanchnic nerves via the left and right hypogastric nerves and the postganglionic fibers terminate on the sigmoid colon, rectum and upper anal canal via the pelvic plexus. The preganglionic parasympathetic nerves originate in the sacral cord (S2–S4), emerge as the nervi erigentes and become the pelvic splanchnic nerves, terminating on the same viscera supplied by the inferior mesenteric artery, i.e. the sigmoid, rectum and upper anal canal.

The internal anal sphincter is tonically contracted, largely through intrinsic myogenic properties. Stimulation of the parasympathetic nerves relaxes the internal anal sphincter while stimulation of the sympathetic branches of the hypogastric plexus causes contraction. α-adrenergic

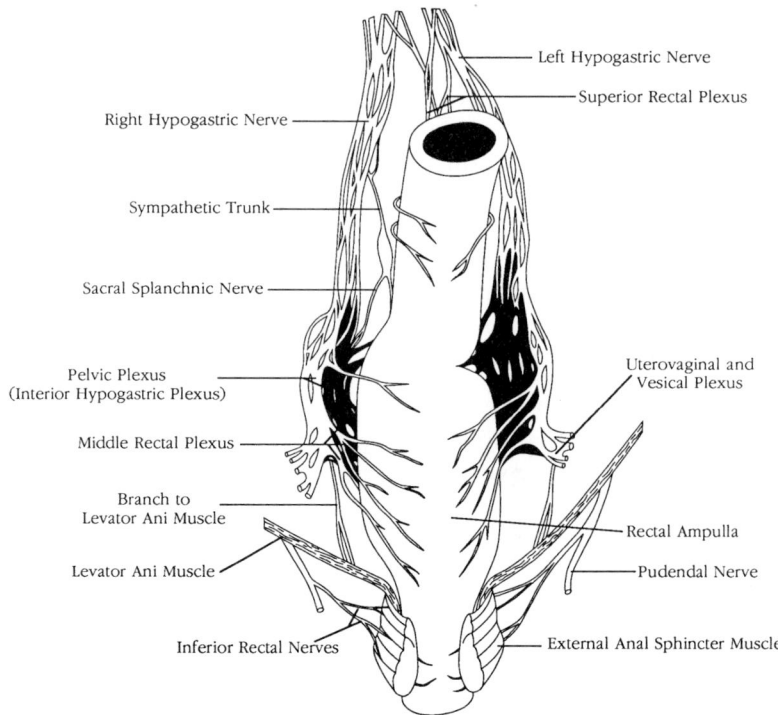

Figure 18.4   Nerve supply of the anus and rectum.

receptors are excitatory while β-adrenergic receptors are inhibitory. Electrical field stimulation produces evidence of inhibition of the sphincter through the release of nitric oxide, the mediator of the non-adrenergic, non-cholinergic nervous system. Control of the external anal sphincter and the striated muscles of the pelvic floor is mediated exclusively through the somatic nervous system (S1–S4).

The sensory fibers of the rectum and upper anal canal are derived from the autonomic nervous system and enter the cord at the Ll, L2, S2, S3 and S4 levels. They are relatively insensitive to painful stimuli but do respond to distension and stretching. Disease processes of the rectum and upper half of the anal canal above the dentate line produce poorly localized visceral pain in the lumbosacral region. Pain may also be referred to the somatic nerve distribution of these same dermatomes. Inflammation of the rectal mucosa heightens the sensitivity to stimuli and lowers the threshold of pain and reflexes. The lower half of the anal canal and the external anal sphincter are supplied by branches of the right and left pudendal nerves called the inferior rectal nerves. The anoderm of the anal canal is richly supplied with spinal somatic nerves and is highly sensitive.

DEFINITIONS

Proctalgia is true anal or anorectal pain. *Urgency* is the uncontrollable desire to have a bowel movement. *Tenesmus* is the ineffectual and painful straining to defecate even after complete evacuation. This complaint in the presence of diarrhea usually indicates the presence of inflammation of the rectum. However, it may occur in constipation as incomplete evacuation of a fecal bolus initiates painful spasms in a distended rectum. *Dyschezia* is painful defecation. The painful passage of stool indicates inflammation or ulceration in the anal canal. *Pruritus ani* is itching around the anus and repeated excoriation or secondary infection may cause burning and soreness of the traumatized skin.

HOW TO ELICIT AND INTERPRET A DETAILED AND SYSTEMATIC HISTORY OF ANORECTAL PAIN

1. **Pain.** *Where* is the pain felt? Is it on the skin around the anal opening, near or at the opening or in the rectum? Does the pain seem to occur in any other place (explore the urogenital tract, the lumbosacral spine or the lower abdomen)?

What is the pain like? Burning or stinging, sharp or knifelike, dull or aching? Burning or stinging pain often indicates inflammation of the anal canal or perianal skin. Sharp or knifelike pain is often caused by an ulcer or fissure in the anal canal and this may also be the description of proctalgia fugax. Dull and continuous pain describes either spasm of the musculature or an inflammatory process or mass in the pelvis.

How severe is the pain? Mildly aggravating to unbearable and preventing other activity or bowel movements? This question indicates the importance of the pain to the patient, but it does not always indicate the importance of the underlying problem.

When does the pain occur? During and/or after the bowel movement or at other times? Is it continuous or does it come and go away? What makes it worse and what makes it better (positions like sitting, lying down, etc. should be explored as well as sitting in hot water)? Pain from anal fissures is increased during and following a bowel movement. Is it getting better, worse or not changing? Pain due to an abscess gradually worsens as it enlarges and is not relieved until it is drained or it drains spontaneously.

2. **Bleeding.** Does the bleeding occur just with bowel movements or at other times? If the bleeding occurs almost continuously, it is probably outside the anal sphincters. If it occurs only with bowel movements, it is coming from within the bowel. Is it seen in the toilet bowl, on the paper, or on the underclothing? External bleeding may be noted only on the paper or underclothes. Is it bright red, dark red or maroon, or black? Bright red blood usually means that active bleeding is occurring from a distal site. Bleeding from the colon is usually maroon in color unless the bleeding from the upper gastrointestinal tract is massive.

Is it just on the surface of the stool in streaks or does it seem to be mixed in with the stool? If the blood is just on the surface, a distal origin is likely. Does it occur with every bowel movement or intermittently? Can you estimate how much there is? Are there clots, does it turn the water pink or red, does it occur in just a few drops, is it about a teaspoon, a cup full or other amounts? Do you feel weak, light-headed or as if you are going to pass out? Are you easily worn out or tired? Significant acute blood loss produces an inadequate circulating blood volume and orthostatic hypotension requiring urgent recognition and treatment. Chronic blood loss allows replacement and maintenance of blood volume, but causes an iron-deficient anemia and chronic fatigue.

3. **Discharge.** Is there discharge from the anus or rectum? If the discharge occurs only with bowel movements, the inflammatory process likely involves the rectum. If it is continuous, a fistula from the bowel to the skin is likely. Is it mucoid, purulent or bloody? Clear or whitish mucus is usually not important, but increased amounts may indicate the presence of a rectal villous adenoma. Pus usually indicates an inflammatory process and blood can occur in a severe inflammatory or malignant process.

4. **Pneumaturia.** Do you pass air in the urine when you void? If pneumaturia is present, it suggests the occurrence of a fistula from the bowel to the urinary tract, often a rectovesical fistula. Such a fistula also

causes frequent urinary tract infections which are manifest by dysuria, increased frequency and passage of malodorous and cloudy urine.

5. **Vaginal discomfort or discharge.** Vaginal infections are often manifest by burning, discharge and dyspareunia. They are usually caused by gynecologic disorders, but can be secondary to a rectovaginal fistula. The latter is especially likely if stool or air are passed spontaneously into the vagina.

6. **Swelling.** Do you notice any swelling or bulging in or around the anal opening? Does the swelling come and go or is it there all of the time? Hemorrhoids and rectal prolapse are both aggravated by straining at stool, but neoplastic and inflammatory masses are usually present all of the time and do not change much with straining.

Is it soft or hard? Is it painful or tender to the touch? A soft painful mass is usually inflammatory (infection, abscess) while a hard, non-painful mass is frequently a neoplasm.

7. **Prolapse.** Does anything (tissue) come out when you push to have a bowel movement? Does it occur with every bowel movement? Does it go in on its own or does it have to be pushed in? Prolapse usually occurs with each bowel movement, but a polyp only comes out intermittently.

8. **Change in bowel habits.** Has there been a change in consistency of your stools recently? Do you have loose or watery stools? How many times during an average 24-hour period do you have a bowel movement? Do you have to get to the bathroom in a hurry when you feel the urge or can you postpone the trip until it is more convenient? Do you have to get up during the night to have a bowel movement? How many times? Are there times when you do not make it to the bathroom in time and you lose stool or soil your underclothes? Urgency, incontinence and nocturnal bowel movements suggest the presence of inflammation of the rectal mucosa.

Has the stool or movement changed in caliber? Smaller or larger? Small caliber bowel movements sometimes suggest the presence of a distal mass or stenosis of the rectum or anus, but more are related to a softer consistency of the stool. Are you constipated? If so, what do you mean by that? How many bowel movements do you have in an average week? Is it difficult to have a bowel movement? Is the stool small, hard and dry?

9. **Other important issues.** How is your general health and sense of well-being? What other medical problems do you have? What is happening with your weight? Are you gaining or losing? How much and over what period of time? Have you ever been physically or sexually abused? What is your sexual preference? How many children have you had and did you sustain any injury or tears during childbirth? Have you had any operations in the rectal area – if so when, what was done and what was the outcome? What have you done or what has been prescribed for your problem and how has it been affected – better, worse or no change?

SPECIFIC ENTITIES CAUSING ANORECTAL PAIN

Hemorrhoids result from a pressure increase in the hemorrhoidal veins and deterioration of the supporting tissues of the anal cushion. It is postulated that these arterial and venous plexuses become engorged with blood during straining with defecation. With repetitive straining and engorgement because of severe diarrhea or difficulty in passing hard, dry pellets of stool, the supporting tissues become stretched and damaged, resulting in a tendency to prolapse downward. The typical low fiber, low residue Western diet is thought to play an important etiologic role in hemorrhoidal disease. In the early stages, the prolapsed tissues may reverse and return to their normal position, but with continued straining, the tissues remain prolapsed and must be replaced manually.

Hemorrhoids are categorized by their origin and relation to the dentate line. *External* hemorrhoids are derived from the inferior hemorrhoidal plexus (see Fig. 18.1). They are found below the dentate line and are covered by stratified squamous epithelium. Their occurrence is painless, but when clots form within these vessels (thrombosed external hemorrhoids), they cause the sudden onset of extreme steady pain for at least 2–4 days. A bluish lump is usually palpable at the anal orifice and the area may be exquisitely tender on examination. Large clots resolve more slowly and may leave a permanent *skin tag* after resolution.

Internal hemorrhoids are derived from the superior hemorrhoidal plexus. They occur proximal to the dentate line and are lined by rectal mucosa. Bleeding can occur with irritation or straining. The bleeding is bright red and may be on the toilet tissue, on the surface of the stool or drip into the water after defecation. The hemorrhoids may protrude below the dentate line with straining (see Box 18.2 for classification). They too are painless, but when more advanced lesions prolapse through the anus, they may induce discharge, perianal irritation and anorectal discomfort. In rare cases, sphincter spasm may prevent reduction of the prolapse and both internal and external hemorrhoids become so engorged that the blood supply is compromised and the vessels become strangulated and

---

Box 18.1   Common conditions associated with anorectal pain

Hemorrhoids, external and internal
Anal fissure, primary and secondary
Anorectal abscesses
Pruritis ani
Proctitis
Solitary ulcer syndrome
Proctalgia fugax
Coccygodynia
Rectal prolapse (procidentia)
Rectal adenocarcinoma

Box 18.2	Classification of internal hemorrhoids
Type	**Description**
First degree	Enlarged hemorrhoidal veins; non-prolapsing, painless, but may bleed
Second degree	Veins outside anal canal which prolapse with defecation but reduce spontaneously
Third degree	Veins prolapse outside anal canal with defecation but can be reduced manually
Fourth degree	Veins continuously prolapsed but cannot be reduced

eventually gangrenous. This situation causes intense pain and requires immediate attention.

An *anal fissure* is a superficial tear which may eventually develop into an infected ulcer in the anal canal. The tear develops because of trauma from either passage of a large hard stool, rectal intercourse or insertion of a foreign body. The vast majority (>90%) of primary fissures (unknown cause) arise in the midline posteriorly. Rarely in men and in about 10% of women, they arise in the anterior midline. Patients describe a sharp, burning, tearing or throbbing pain during and soon after a bowel movement (*dyschezia*).

Acute fissures cause severe incapacitating pain which may last for hours. Bleeding is very common with bright red blood on the toilet paper. The pain may be so severe that the patient will strenuously avoid having a bowel movement and may become severely constipated. This is especially true with children. Healing may be temporary or incomplete and the problem recurs again and again. The patient will experience recurrent spells of bleeding and dyschezia.

If fissures become so deep that they involve the internal sphincter, the pain becomes dull, aching, severe and intractable and spasm leads to anal stenosis. Examination reveals a short rent or ulcer which is best demonstrated by spreading the buttocks and gently opening the anal canal with two fingers. Chronic fissures have a slightly elevated margin, an edematous skin tag at the distal end (sentinal pile) and a hypertrophied anal papilla at the proximal end (Fig. 18.5). These fissures partially heal and frequently recur and usually require surgical repair to achieve permanent healing.

Secondary anal fissures can occur in any quadrant and may be caused by Crohn's disease, leukemia, aplastic anemia, agranulocytosis, tuberculosis, anal trauma or intercourse or AIDS. The ulcers due to Crohn's disease are often larger and deeper than primary fissures, but curiously they are often not as painful. However, the ulcers associated with blood dyscrasias and immunosuppression are more superficial, but necrotic and intensely painful.

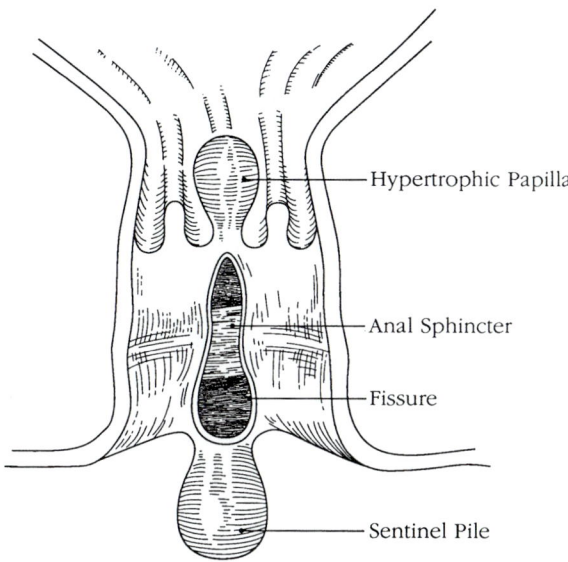

Figure 18.5 Anal fissure.

Anorectal abscesses are infections of the perineal soft tissues in potential pararectal spaces bounded by muscles and pelvic bones (Fig. 18.6). The infections appear to arise from obstructed anal glands of the anal canal at

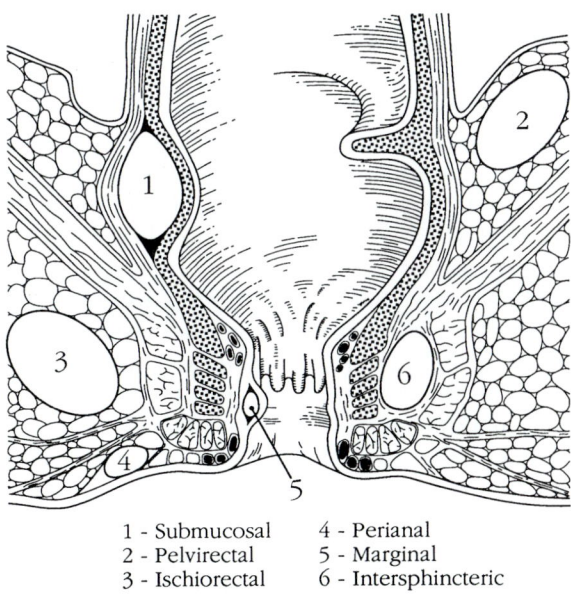

1 - Submucosal   4 - Perianal
2 - Pelvirectal   5 - Marginal
3 - Ischiorectal   6 - Intersphincteric

Figure 18.6 Sites where anorectal abscesses may occur.

the level of the dentate (pectinate) line and then spread to the various anatomic spaces. Most frequent is the perianal abscess which is located under the anal skin and lower rectal mucosa. If it penetrates more deeply through the muscular layers, it becomes an ischiorectal abscess. Rarely, it may penetrate through the levator muscles and is then called a supra-levator abscess. If the abscess occurs anteriorly, it may penetrate and rupture the septum, producing a rectovaginal fistula.

The pain begins in the anal region and becomes progressively more severe as the abscess enlarges. It is described as throbbing or dull and aching and is aggravated by walking, sitting, straining and sneezing or coughing. It may be accompanied by malaise, chills, fever and rigors as sepsis develops.

Perianal and ischiorectal abscesses are located close to the skin surface and tenderness and swelling of the medial buttock usually makes the diagnosis obvious. However, intersphincteric and supralevator abscesses often have minimal, if any, superficial signs or symptoms. The patient notes pain on rectal examination and/or with bowel movements which corresponds to an area of fullness or a mass and tenderness on rectal examination.

Management depends on a thorough knowledge of the anatomy. The patient may note that the pain suddenly disappears and this is often accompanied by the appearance of a large amount of purulent drainage. This suggests that the abscess has ruptured, relieving the expanding lesion and temporarily alleviating the problem. If not treated, the abscess has a high likelihood of recurring at a later time.

A *fistula in ano* is usually the result of a perianal abscess which does not heal completely. It begins in an anal crypt and tracks to an opening in the perianal skin by way of the sphincters. It often follows a surgical drainage procedure or may occur spontaneously. Patients experience drainage from the opening to the skin and recurrent abscesses. Such a fistula becomes painful when the secondary opening in the skin temporarily heals and the abscess begins to expand because there is no place for it to drain. It will continue to recur unless the primary opening in the crypt is closed.

It is important to know that fistulas frequently occur in patients who have Crohn's disease and actually may be the initial manifestation of the disease. If they do not heal or are associated with symptoms such as abdominal pain or intermittent diarrhea, further investigation is indicated to search for other manifestations of the disease.

Pruritus ani has multiple causes, although itching and scratching are the major problems. Skin irritation, soreness and pain result from severe excoriations and secondary inflammation and infection which in turn induces more itching and scratching. The local causes associated with this symptom include hemorrhoids, prolapse, fissures and fistulae, condyloma acuminatum, neoplasms, diarrhea and fecal incontinence. Most of these disorders have fecal and mucoid soilage as a common inciting factor. Dermatologic disorders include eczema, psoriasis, seborrhea, lichen planus, excessive dryness or moisture, chemical irritants including soaps, perfumed toilet tissue, medications and poor personal hygiene. Infectious disorders include fungi (*Candida* and *Epidermophyton* organisms), parasites (pinworms) and secondary mixed bacterial infection of diseased and macerated skin. A number of systemic diseases are sometimes associated with pruritus ani including diabetes mellitus, lymphomas and leukemias and diarrhea of any cause.

Discussion of causes would not be complete without mentioning psychologic disorders. Compulsive and overzealous cleansing of the anus and perineum can be a manifestation of a number of psychiatric disorders, including a variety of psychoneurotic disorders and obsessive–compulsive behavior, and these can be the most difficult problems to diagnose and treat.

Proctitis is inflammation of the rectal mucosa. The causes are multiple including infections, radiation injury, ischemia, foreign body, chemical or idiopathic. Patients are usually bothered by rectal discharge, urgency, tenesmus, rectal cramps and pain and hematachezia. However, the severity of pain varies considerably. Some infections are associated with systemic symptoms such as malaise, fever, rigors or sweats and others are devoid of systemic symptoms.

Patients tend to have frequent and small stools because even small fecal volumes trigger local reflexes which stimulate defecation and occasional fecal and even urinary incontinence. When the extent and severity of the inflammation are limited, diarrhea is unusual. This is true not only with infectious proctitis but also with ulcerative proctitis.

Sexually-related diseases are becoming much more common and can be caused by a multitude of organisms (Box 18.3). Syphilitic chancres and venereal warts are essentially painless, non-LGV and gonococcal proctitis are mildly to moderately painful, but LGV and herpetic infections are intensely painful. HSV proctitis is often associated with severe anorectal pain and a distinctive syndrome consisting of fever, tenesmus, anorectal discharge and inguinal adenopathy. Discharge and bleeding are proportional to and generally parallel the degree of pain. Diarrhea is not constant and patients may even have constipation. Some male patients with HSV have neurologic symptoms in the distribution of the sacral nerves including paresthesias, genital and thigh pain, bladder dysfunction and erectile difficulties.

The diagnoses of these disorders is usually made by appropriate culture, biopsy or serologic testing. It is important to realize that patients with sexually-acquired disease and especially AIDS-related infections may have multiple organisms involved in the disease process. In this situation, it is essential to investigate the inflammatory process completely. Appro-

---

Box 18.3 Incidental and sexually-related inflammatory diseases of the colon and rectum

Non-infectious disorders
  Idiopathic ulcerative colitis
  Crohn's colitis
  Radiation enterocolitis or proctitis
  Chemical proctitis
  Ischemic proctocolitis
Rectal enteric infections +/– sexually-related
  Campylobacter species
  Salmonellosis
  Shigellosis
  Amebiasis
  Giardiasis
Anorectal infections – usually sexually-related
  Chlamydia (lymphogranuloma venereum – LGV or non-LGV serotypes)
  Condylomata acuminata or venereal warts (human papilloma virus – HPV)
  Gonococcal proctitis
  Herpes simplex proctitis (HSV)
  Anorectal syphilis (chancre)
Primarily AIDs-related disorders (HIV)
  Candidiasis
  Cryptosporidiosis
  Cytomegalovirus (CMV)
  Isosporiasis
  Histoplasmosis
  Microsporidiosis
  Mycobacterium avium intracellulare
  Kaposi's sarcoma
  Lymphoma

---

priate therapy for one organism may not be effective because of failure to treat a concurrent infection with another organism.

Solitary rectal ulcer syndrome is usually seen as a single, shallow ulcer of variable size on the anterior wall of the rectum, 6–12 cm from the anal orifice. The term is not optimal because multiple ulcers are present in about 30% of cases and occasionally heaped up and exuberant nodular masses are seen. These polypoid multilobulated nodules grossly resemble adenomas or even carcinomas, but histologically they are made up of hyperplastic mucosa with benign colonic epithelium and cysts deep to the muscularis mucosa. The problem is thought to be associated with obstructed defecation and secondary to prolapse causing ischemia and necrosis of a localized portion of the rectal mucosa (Fig. 18.7). It is often associated with constipation, obstructed defecation and excessive straining during defecation.

In about 10% of cases, rectal prolapse may occur concurrently with the solitary rectal ulcer syndrome. A history of rectal intercourse or foreign body trauma should be sought. Patients commonly complain of rectal

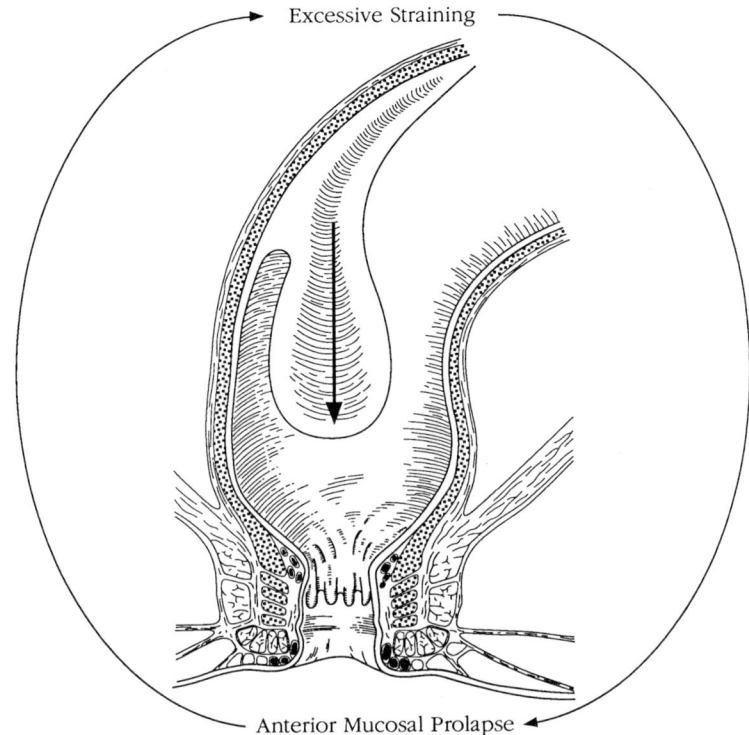

Excessive Straining

Anterior Mucosal Prolapse

Figure 18.7   Mucosal prolapse and solitary rectal ulcer.

bleeding, pelvic pain, a feeling of incomplete evacuation and tenesmus. The pain, if present, is dull, boring and constant and may be aggravated during and after defecation.

The diagnosis is made by the typical history and physical findings, but can be confirmed by biopsies showing proliferation of fibroblasts and extension of smooth muscle into the lamina propria in addition to hemosiderin deposits which are evidence of ischemia.

Rectal prolapse (procidentia) is an intussusception (turning inside out) of the rectal wall. In the early stages of the disease, the patient may experience only mild discomfort during defecation or a feeling of incomplete evacuation. In this first stage, nothing can be seen on physical examination. In stage two, the rectum is visible through the anus during straining (doughnut sign). Eventually in stage three, the rectum protrudes and remains outside the anus. In stage three, the problem is obvious, but in stages one and two, the only way to establish the diagnosis is to observe the patient straining or pushing when lying on their side or preferably while sitting on a toilet or commode.

Proctalgia fugax is a very painful condition of the rectum without a known mechanism or cause. Although variable, the pain is often excruciating, but it usually lasts only a few seconds or minutes. It has been described as a sensation like sitting on a ice-pick. Although unproven, it is thought to be the result of muscle spasm, possibly of the levator ani muscle which can be triggered by a small piece of hard stool in the rectum coincident with a distended bladder. There are no associated symptoms or known aggravating or relieving factors and no pathologic or physical findings. If the pain is long-lasting and recurrent, it is often called the *levator syndrome*. It is described as burning, throbbing or aching in the same region. The muscle in spasm can sometimes be palpated on rectal examination. It may be associated with prolonged sitting or having a bowel movement. No tests are available to establish the diagnosis with either of these distinct but related problems.

Coccygodynia refers to pain and tenderness of the coccyx. Patients describe an aching or sharp pain which may radiate into the rectum or buttocks. It is aggravated by sitting. Coccygeal pain may occur following a fall or childbirth or develop in association with arthritis. The pain may be similar to that occurring in rectal infections and prostatitis. It is confirmed on physical examination by tenderness and reproduction of the pain by manipulation of the coccyx.

Foreign bodies can be the cause of anorectal pain. The anal orifice is a source of sexual gratification and can be used to conceal illegal substances in order to avoid the law. A wide variety of devices and containers have been discovered in the rectum and there they can cause perforation, obstruction and other painful and traumatic problems. Removing them requires imaginative and sometimes quite invasive approaches.

Rectal adenocarcinomas usually do not present with pain but with rectal bleeding, a feeling of incomplete evacuation, obstruction or a mass on digital examination. *Primary anal squamous cell cancers*, on the other hand, usually have multiple symptoms including bleeding, mucous discharge, pain, mass, tenesmus and a change in bowel habits, especially a decrease in stool caliber. A variant is the *cloacogenic carcinoma* which arises from the anal glands.

Malignant melanomas, basal cell carcinomas and *Kaposi's sarcomas* may also originate in this region. Kaposi's sarcoma should be suspected in patients with AIDS and is recognized as a purple nodular lesion. An unusual tumor is *Bowen's disease* or extramammary Paget's disease. These are intraepidermal carcinomas and often appear as reddish plaques. Evidence is growing to support the observation that persons with condylomata acuminata are at increased risk of developing anal malignancy. HPV, the etiologic agent, is frequently present in primary anal cancers and invasive carcinomas are not uncommonly found within condylomata acuminata.

INVESTIGATING ANORECTAL PAIN

Physical examination

Inspection of the perineum must be carried out in good light. First, look for excoriation, hemorrhoids, tags, scars and warts. Excoriation may be associated with skin irritation from rectal discharge or feces secondary to incontinence or poor anal hygiene, from parasites such as pinworms or from skin diseases such as candidiasis or psoriasis. Prominent hemorrhoidal tags, especially if they are edematous, may point to anal fissures or ulcerations. In Crohn's disease, the skin tags are often a dusky purple color. The anus should be examined by pulling apart and separating the skinfolds of the canal with two closely approximated thumbs or fingers. Fistulous tracts from the proximal anal canal appear as small holes at variable distances from the anal orifice. Abscesses cause asymmetric fullness or swelling in the perirectal space and the bulge is exquisitely tender. Rectoceles or prolapse will likely be missed unless the patient is asked to strain and bear down. The best method to detect prolapse is to examine the patient straining in the squatting position or seated on a toilet or commode.

Palpation of the perineum around the rectum is very useful to detect tenderness, especially if there is some asymmetry of the perineal contour. It is important to look for reflexes. Gently scratch or stroke the perineum and look for a 'wink' reflex. There is no reason to perform percussion or auscultation in this region.

The rectal examination is a critical part of the physical examination and it is mandatory when evaluating rectal pain. It is usually conducted with the patient lying in the left lateral decubitus position, but the patient may be asked to bend over the bed or examination table. It may be a very distressing and embarrassing experience for the patient and should be conducted gently with a well-lubricated finger. If patients indicate that they have severe anal soreness or pain, the anal canal should be anesthetized with 2–5% lidocaine for several minutes before the examination.

Insert the finger slowly but with constant pressure in order to avoid spasm and undue pain. If a fissure or thrombosed hemorrhoid is present, pressure should be exerted away from the lesion to reduce pain on insertion. Note the degree of resistance to digital insertion which is an indication of sphincter tone. The anal canal should be smooth and symmetric and one can detect the internal and external sphincters. Sweep around the anal canal to detect induration or tender fissures. Ask the patient to squeeze or pinch as hard as possible, noting the normal increase in sphincter tone.

The puborectalis muscle may be palpated posteriorly and while pressing against it, test its function by asking the patient to pinch or squeeze and alternately relax. If there is little or no increase, this may indicate that a neuromuscular disorder is present. Then ask the patient to bear down and push out the examining finger as if expelling a stool. The sphincters should relax and some force to eliminate should be detectable. The examiner should also note the degree of perineal descent as the patient strains.

As the finger is advanced, the presence or absence of stool in the rectal vault should be determined. The rectum is usually empty in intestinal obstruction. If stool is present, the character (hard, soft or liquid) should be noted. The color of the stool is important and may indicate the nature of the process. The normal color is brown. White, light tan or cream stool may indicate biliary obstruction or recent barium, black stools may indicate digested blood from the upper gastrointestinal tract, maroon stools may indicate massive bleeding from the upper tract or the proximal colon while bright red stools usually indicate brisk bleeding from the left side of the colon or rectum. Bleeding in the absence of bile may produce a silver stool. Unless the stool is grossly bloody, it should always be tested for occult blood.

Palpation should be conducted systematically. It is a good idea to exert pressure posteriorly against the sacrum first because abnormalities here are unusual and one can determine the baseline level of patient discomfort. Again, sweep around the rectal cavity as the finger is advanced to detect masses, indurated areas and tenderness. Anteriorly and superiorly is the pouch of Douglas. Tenderness and fluctuation may indicate the presence of pus and a pelvic abscess or appendicitis. Fullness without tenderness may indicate blood or fluid in the cul de sac. A hard shelflike mass indicates the presence of malignant deposits in the rectouterine or

---

Box 18.4 Checklist for a rectal exam

Anal canal and perianal tissues (hemorrhoids, tags, fistulae, warts, sentinel piles, abnormal contour, tenderness)

Anocutaneous wink reflex elicited in all four quadrants by stroking the perianal skin

Caliber and symmetry of anal canal

Baseline sphincter tone

Squeeze pressure

Sphincter and puborectalis relaxation on bearing down (also note prolapse and perineal descent)

Presence and character of stool (test the stool for occult blood)

Masses and tenderness in rectum

Genital organs (cervix, uterus, fallopian tubes, ovaries and rectovaginal septum in women and prostate and seminal vesicles in men)

rectovesical pouch. Tenderness of the prostate or seminal vesicles indicates acute inflammation and frequently infection of these organs.

Vaginal examination allows the best examination of the uterus, ovaries and fallopian tubes although the uterus and cervix can be palpated through the rectal wall. Be careful not to interpret a vaginal tampon as a rectal mass. Movement of the cervix which causes pain indicates inflammation of the pelvic tissues around the uterus (pelvic inflammatory disease). Finally, the rectovaginal septum should be palpated bidigitally.

Endoscopy of the lower gastrointestinal tract

The indications for an endoscopic examination of the lower gastrointestinal tract include gross or occult bleeding per rectum, suspected polyps or cancer, abdominal or perineal pain of unknown cause, a change in bowel habits (especially diarrhea but also recent onset constipation) and follow-up of inflammatory bowel disease.

The term *proctoscopy* is usually confined to the examination of the anus and lower rectum and the instrument is only a few inches long. It can be performed without preparation in the examining room. One can see and biopsy the rectal mucosa, identify and classify hemorrhoids and detect anal fissures and other inflammatory and neoplastic lesions of the anal canal. In these times of cost containment, this test can be used to diagnose and follow up many disorders with minimal cost.

The instrument has a blunt but pointed tip and should be warmed if it is metal. Always choose an instrument with a slotted or bevelled barrel. This feature is essential in order to see lesions which might touch the anoscope. Carefully look for fissures, hemorrhoids, inflammation or tumors.

Rigid sigmoidoscopy is done less frequently now because of the development of the flexible sigmoidoscope. However, there is still an important place for this examination. Not all physicians are trained in the use of the flexible scope and it is also a much more expensive examination. The equipment for rigid sigmoidoscopy is much less costly and the procedure can be done on the examination table or in the bed in just a few minutes. Specimens of stool or rectal biopsies can be easily taken and the visualization of the rectum and anal canal is excellent. The patient is prepared by a simple tap water or commercial phosphate enema just prior to the procedure. However, if the patient has watery diarrhea or suspected colitis, no preparation should be done in order to examine the mucosa without causing subtle changes in its appearance with the enema.

A rectal exam must be done before the procedure to determine the direction of insertion of the instrument and to detect any masses or tenderness which might be present and to 'prepare' the patient for the examination.

Carefully inspect the anal canal for fissures and masses. Note landmarks such as the pectinate line, the rectal crypts and papillae and look for hemorrhoids and other pathologic findings.

Most of the examination is done on withdrawal of the instrument using a corkscrew motion. Examine behind each fold in order to see 100% of the mucosa. Note the character of the rectal and colonic lining. Look for edema and erythema which can obscure the normal delicate submucosal vascular pattern. Look for granularity, erosions, ulcerations, mucopus, polyps, masses and spontaneous bleeding. Be certain to check for friability at several points. This is done by vigorously rubbing or swabbing the mucosa with a long moistened rectal swab or cotton ball on a grasping forceps. Hold the scope tip at the same point for a minute and look for punctate oozing of blood indicating an inflamed mucosa.

Biopsies may be easily obtained with appropriate forceps with only a small risk of bleeding. Cultures can be obtained directly from the rectal mucosa with brushings or scrapings. It is worthwhile performing a Gram stain on some of the specimen and in some cases a Wright stain.

Flexible sigmoidoscopy is performed after obtaining informed consent. If an anal ulcer, perianal fistula, abscess or fistula in ano is present, additional tests to exclude Crohn's disease should be done including colonoscopy or barium enema and a small bowel series.

Most of the examination is done on withdrawal of the instrument, being careful to look behind all of the folds, valves and bends. Note the appearance of the mucosa, looking for the normal appearance of the delicate submucosal vascular network. If it is not seen, edema and erythema are probably present, indicating the presence of inflammation (see chapter 4, pp. 110–116 for more details).

It is common in elderly patients to see the orifices of multiple diverticula in the sigmoid and descending colon. These are often accompanied by circular muscular hypertrophy which reduces the diameter of the lumen.

Radiography

Plain abdominal/pelvic films are often helpful in evaluating rectal pain in order to determine the amount and distribution of gas within the colon and rectum or to look for gas outside the gastrointestinal tract. Absence of gas in the rectum or distal colon in the presence of clinical obstruction and failure to have a bowel movement constitute strong evidence of a lesion or volvulus of the bowel. Ordinarily, the standard AP (anteroposterior) standing and supine films are adequate to evaluate these features. A left lateral decubitus or crosstable lateral abdominal film can be ordered for especially ill or elderly patients. A prone X-ray of the abdomen may be helpful in determining the presence or absence of rectal gas. Rarely, a coned down lateral film of the rectum is needed.

In addition to the evaluation of gas patterns, plain X-rays may demonstrate wall thickness, soft tissue masses, extraluminal gas collections and calcifications. The wall may become thickened in association with ischemia and severe inflammation of the bowel wall.

Barium enemas are used to better delineate the mucosa and the lumen of the colon. If there is any suggestion of a perforation, barium should not be used because it is extremely inflammatory when it escapes the confines of the colon. For example, it would be unwise to introduce barium if the patient exhibits fever, rigors, a distended abdomen, has free air within the abdominal cavity with rebound tenderness or air outside the bowel on a plain film. If a contrast study is deemed necessary under similar circumstances a water-soluble substance, such as Hypaque, should be used to distend the bowel and to outline its contours.

Defecography is the dynamic radiological study of the process of defecation using barium for radiocontrast. It is indicated to evaluate internal procidentia (occult rectal prolapse) and suspected solitary rectal ulcer syndrome, abnormal pelvic floor descent during straining and rectal prolapse, enterocele, rectocele and obstructed defecation.

It is performed with the patient sitting on a radiolucent commode after the instillation of approximately 300 mL of barium into the rectum. The fluoroscopy is done from the lateral position at rest and during attempted defecation. One can assess the anorectal angle, perineal descent and mucosal prolapse.

This is the best test to demonstrate rectal intussusception, both complete and incomplete. It is important to recognize that mild intussusception occurs in normal persons and that the demonstration of mucosal prolapse of a minor degree is not an indication for surgical intervention to prevent or correct incontinence. The typical findings in patients with outlet obstruction include failure to widen the anorectal angle (or to produce a more acute angle) during straining, an increase in pelvic floor descent greater than 3 cm and a tightening of the external anal sphincter during defecation (anismus). The abnormal straining may result in rectal intussusception, anterior rectal wall prolapse, complete rectal prolapse and a rectocele.

Other imaging studies

Endoscopy or barium contrast studies are the best methods to assess the lumen and mucosa, but techniques to image the pelvic organs in cross-section allow visualization of the thickness of the tubular gut, the extent of invasion of colorectal masses and the spread of inflammatory or neoplastic processes to nearby tissues, organs and lymph nodes.

Ultrasonography

Surface ultrasonography is a relatively inexpensive method of imaging the rectum and pelvis. Although ultrasonography can potentially detect abscesses, hematomas and neoplasms, it does not play a major role in comparisons with other imaging techniques. If there is a large amount of gas in the rectum, reflection of the sound beam interferes with adequate penetration and the quality of the study is greatly compromised. A water enema can be introduced into the rectum to enhance the image and the contrast.

Intrarectal ultrasound is most useful in evaluating the anal sphincters when there is a history of fecal incontinence and rectal carcinomas preoperatively. The probe is inserted into the rectum and scanning is done radially to image the entire circumference of the rectum and the anal canal. This technique can delineate the five layers of the normal rectal wall and determine the symmetry of the anal sphincters. It can help to determine whether a mass seen endoscopically invades any or all of these layers. It may also detect inflammatory or metastatic lymph nodes. The suspected diagnosis can be confirmed using ultrasound-guided needle biopsy.

Preliminary results suggest that intrarectal ultrasound is equal to or greater in accuracy than CT in detecting spread of tumor beyond the bowel wall. This instrument may also be useful in detecting abscesses, but its use has been limited and other imaging modalities are probably more appropriate.

Computed tomography

This can be most helpful in identifying pelvic abscesses and locating their exact position. In doing so, many of them can be treated definitively by CT-directed needle drainage in combination with appropriate antibiotic coverage. In addition, CT can be very helpful in staging pelvic and anorectal carcinomas. Spread of tumor beyond the confines of the bowel wall is often readily seen because the rectum is normally surrounded by fat which provides good radiocontrast. Directed biopsies have the potential to make the diagnosis definitively.

Magnetic resonance imaging

MRI has not been used as widely as CT scans, but promises to be of use in some difficult cases to find occult abscesses and enlarged lymph nodes. Because one can obtain sagittal views, it can be helpful to demonstrate the anatomic relationships of the rectosigmoid with the uterus and vagina in women and the bladder, seminal vesicles and urethra in men.

Anorectal manometry

This is not usually indicated to evaluate acute rectal and perineal pain, but it can be helpful in chronic or refractory pain. In addition to the measurement of intrarectal and anal pressures at rest and during defecation, tests of compliance and sensation can be helpful in evaluating patients with obscure pelvic and anal pain. In many neurologic disorders, rectal sensation is impaired, as measured by distending a rectal balloon. These disorders include spinal cord disorders, Hirschsprung's disease, megarectum and pudendal nerve injury from abnormal perineal descent. However, if the rectal mucosa is inflamed, the threshold sensation is exaggerated and this is responsible for causing tenesmus and rectal pain.

We have also identified patients with unexplained rectal pain who exhibit a hypersensitive rectum and reduced rectal compliance. These patients have no evidence of mucosal inflammation and the underlying reason for the hypersensitivity is unknown. A similar abnormality has been demonstrated in the so-called 'nutcracker esophagus' and, indeed, this abnormality may coexist with the hypersensitive rectum.

Anorectal manometry is also useful in the diagnosis of the solitary rectal ulcer syndrome.

Nuclear scans

Nuclear scans can be used to detect occult pelvic abscesses and tumors in unusual cases. In most situations, these lesions can be demonstrated with routine endoscopy, barium contrast studies and CT scans. Indium-labeled leukocytes are best for identifying infections and inflammatory lesions while ^{99m}Tc-HMDP has been used to localize malignant tumors.

More recently there has been interest in using radiolabeled monoclonal antibodies directed against subcellular tissue-specific tumor antigens such as CEA to localize neoplasms, although the early clinical results are disappointing.

Summary of studies to consider in evaluating anorectal (and pelvic) pain

1. The examination should include a careful rectal (and pelvic) examination in every patient with abdominal or rectal pain.
2. If there is a suggestion of infection, e.g. diarrhea, discharge, tenderness, fluctuance or fever, appropriate stool cultures should be done for bacterial pathogens, fungi and viruses. Gram stains may be helpful in some cases. Guided aspirates should be done when abscesses are suspected.

3. Anoscopy and / or proctoscopy is the next test to be done. It is essential to perform this study in almost all patients who have abdominal and rectal pain. Biopsies should be done to look for viral inclusions, mucosal inflammation, microabscesses, malignant or premalignant changes and evidence of acute or chronic inflammation.

4. Barium contrast studies should be done next, being careful to avoid the test with suspected perforation or complete bowel obstruction. If perforation is suspected, always ask for water-soluble contrast to be used first because of the hazards of barium beyond the mucosal lining.

5. If the diagnosis is not clear at this point, imaging studies may be of value in evaluating patients who have anorectal pain. The choices are quite broad and each test is selected according to its individual merits and deficiencies. They include external or endoscopic ultrasound, nuclear medicine imaging, computed tomography or magnetic resonance imaging. It is often helpful to consult with the radiologist before making a final decision about which test would be more appropriate in each clinical setting.

6. Finally, anorectal manometry may be selected if there is evidence of sphincter dysfunction or a dysmotility syndrome.

FURTHER READING

Bielefeldt K, Enck P, Erkenbrecht J F 1990 Sensory and motor function in the maintenance of anal continence. Diseases of the Colon and Rectum 33: 674–678

Haas P A, Fox T A Jr, Haas G P 1984 The pathogenesis of hemorrhoids. Diseases of the Colon and Rectum 27: 442–450

Hyder J W, MacKeigan J M 1988 Anorectal and colonic disease and the immunocompromised host. Diseases of the Colon and Rectum 31: 971–976

Kaufman J P, Straus E W 1988 Gastrointestinal manifestations of AIDS: endoscopic procedures in the AIDS patient: risks, precautions, indications and obligations. Gastrointestinal Clinics of North America 17: 495–506

Levine D S 1987 'Solitary' rectal ulcer syndrome and 'localized' colitis cystica profunda analogous syndromes caused by rectal prolapse. Gastroenterology 92: 243–253

Metcalf A M, Loening-Baucke V 1988 Anorectal function and defecation dynamics in patients with rectal prolapse. American Journal of Surgery 155: 206–219

Quinn T 1988 AIDS and other medical problems in the male homosexual: clinical approach to intestinal infection in the homosexual male. Medical Clinics of North America 70: 611–634

Smith L E, Henrichs D, McCullah R D 1982 Prospective studies on the etiology and treatment of pruritus ani. Diseases of the Colon and Rectum 25: 358–363

19

Jaundice

E. Elias   A. Mendoza

INTRODUCTION

The initial step when evaluating a jaundiced patient is to determine if the etiology of the disease is likely to be *hemolytic, constitutional, cholestatic* or *hepatitic*. There is an extensive variety of techniques to study jaundiced patients and the initial clinical evaluation is the most important way of reaching an appropriate diagnosis (Frank 1989) (Figure 19.1).

METABOLISM OF BILIRUBIN

Under physiological conditions 70% of daily bilirubin production originates in the extrahepatic reticuloendothelial system via degradation of hemoglobin-heme liberated from senescent erythrocytes. The remaining 30% results from turnover of hepatic heme and hemoproteins, of which cytochrome P-450 is the most important (Crawford et al 1988). The rate-limiting step of hepatocellular transport of bilirubin and bile acids is at the level of the canalicular membrane, in which secretion is carrier mediated (Suchy 1993).

In the gut the bilirubin conjugates are hydrolyzed to an unconjugated form by bacterial β-glucoronidases in the terminal ileum and colon. Bilirubin is reduced by colonic bacteria to a group of colorless tetra-pyrroles known as urobilinogen or stercobilin, which when oxidized produce orange-colored urobilin. Urobilinogen undergoes an entero-hepatic circulation, but less than 20% of the amount produced daily is reabsorbed because it is produced in the colon where the absorption rate is low. About 90% of the urobilinogen that undergoes the enterohepatic circulation is reexcreted by the liver and 10% is lost in urine.

HEMOLYTIC JAUNDICE

In hemolysis hemoglobin is degraded in excessive amounts, consequently increasing serum bilirubin beyond the liver's capacity to excrete it. In mild cases, which constitute the majority, the hyperbilirubinemia is mostly in the form of albumin-bound unconjugated bilirubin and none is detectable in the urine which, however, contains an excess of urobilinogen. In massive hemolysis, conjugated hyperbilirubinemia may produce bili-rubinuria.

Tissue siderosis is a feature of most types of hemolytic anemias. The gallbladder and bile passages contain dark, viscid bile and calcium bilirubinate pigment calculi are found in half to two-thirds of patients. Secondary cholecystitis may complicate formation of multiple, mixed gallstones. When massive, hemolysis may also be accompanied by acute renal failure, e.g. after severe intravascular hemolysis or traumatic myoglobinuria. Anemia with reticulocytosis and jaundice secondary to the accumulation of a blood clot in the peritoneal cavity is often confused with hemolytic anemia. A suspicion of bleeding in such patients will orientate the diagnosis.

Clinical factors

The patient is examined for features of anemia; for splenomegaly which characterizes some hereditary hemolytic disorders and for other stigmata such as leg ulceration. Racial characteristics may suggest a hemoglobin-

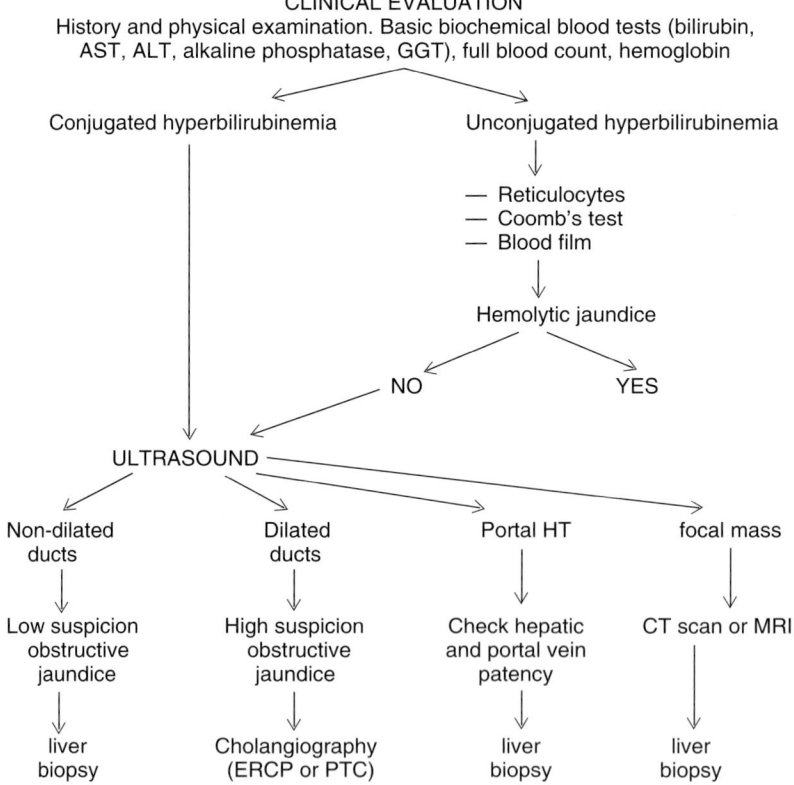

Figure 19.1 Algorithm for clinical evaluation of jaundiced patients.

opathy, e.g. HbS. A family history may establish a pedigree for an inherited hemolytic tendency such as hereditary spherocytosis or pyruvate kinase deficiency. Recent ingestion of a drug may have precipitated massive hemolysis due to glucose-6-phosphatase dehydrogenase (G6PD) deficiency. Intercurrent infection may have heralded a sickling crisis.

Jaundice is usually mild and lemon yellow. Stones in the common bile duct may cause obstructive jaundice and the coexistence of two types of jaundice can confuse the clinical picture.

CONSTITUTIONAL JAUNDICE

Also known as familial non-hemolytic hyperbilirubinemia, this term denotes jaundice caused by defective elimination from the body in the absence of any other evidence of liver abnormality.

Gilbert's syndrome

Defined as a familial, benign, mild unconjugated hyperbilirubinemia (1–5 mg/dL or 17–85 µmol/L), not due to hemolysis and with a normal liver function. It occurs in up to 5% of the population although only a small proportion of the patients present clinically (Okolicsanyi et al 1988).

The hepatic uridine diphosphate (UDP)-glucoronosyl transferase activity is decreased to about 25% of normal. Three types have been differentiated according to bromosulftalein clearance.

The typical history is of mild jaundice without bilirubinuria, usually occurring at a time of reduced calorie intake such as during an intercurrent illness with nausea and anorexia. This combination can easily trap the unwary physician into a false diagnosis of hepatitis which causes unnecessary anxiety for the patient who is intimidated by advice about the need for prolonged convalescence, an uncertain prognosis, avoidance of contagion and restriction on numerous activities including exercise, alcohol ingestion and sex. Diagnosis can usually be performed with biochemical tests (Box 19.1) and rarely is liver biopsy required (Elias 1989).

Crigler–Najjar type 1

UDP-glucuronosyl transferase activity is absent in this disease and cannot be induced. These patients usually develop kernicterus and die and recently have been treated with auxiliary liver transplantation, after involving left segmentectomy of a living related donor.

Box 19.1   Biochemical diagnosis of Gilbert's syndrome

Routine
Normal Hb, MCV, reticulocytes and blood film. Normal AST, GGT, alk. phosp., and all blood chemistries except bilirubin. Predominantly unconjugated bilirubinemia. Absence of bilirubinuria, normal urinary urobilinogen.

Supplementary
- *Nicotinic acid stress test*
  Indomethacin 100 mg by i.m. injection is given 1 hour before nicotinic acid to prevent flushing. Sensitivity and specificity 100% when bilirubin rises by more than 18 µmol/L in the 4 hours after i.v. nicotinic acid (5.9µmol/kg).
- *Calorie restriction*
  Calorie intake is restricted to 400 kcal/day for 48 hours. In Gilbert's the final serum bilirubin is more than double the baseline value. A lesser rise is seen in other forms of hyperbilirubinemia.

Crigler–Najjar type 2 (Arias syndrome)

There is a partial deficiency of the enzyme UDP-glucuronosyl transferase that can be induced by phenobarbital (Arias et al 1969). Serum bilirubin levels are higher than in Gilbert's syndrome, but only of unconjugated bilirubin and usually <20 mg/dL or 340 µmol/L.

Dubin–Johnson and Rotor's syndromes

These diseases are much rarer forms of constitutional hyperbilirubinemia. Dubin–Johnson is a chronic, benign intermittent jaundice with conjugated hyperbilirubinemia. It is probably inherited as an autosomal recessive disorder and may manifest after ingestion of oral contraceptives or during pregnancy when there is reduced hepatic excretory function. Persistence of jaundice is associated with hepatomegaly which may be tender in about half of the patients and vague abdominal pain is a common complaint. The age of onset of jaundice is variable; most appear in childhood or adolescence but some are delayed to adult life when jaundice may be noted for the first time during medical surveillance, especially in pregnancy (Cohen et al 1972).

Diagnostic tests

Prolonged bromosulftalein (BSP) excretion test

In Dubin–Johnson syndrome, BSP retention at 45 minutes may be increased or within the normal range and there is a characteristic secondary rise such that plasma BSP retention at 90 minutes exceeds that at 45 minutes (Abe & Okuda 1975).

Urinary coproporphyrin

In Dubin–Johnson syndrome, more than 80% of urinary coproporphyrin is isomer I compared to less than 30% in normals. In Rotor's syndrome and cholestatic conditions the ratio coproporphyrin I:III is increased, but the proportion of coproporphyrin I is not as high as 80%. In Dubin–Johnson syndrome total urinary coproporphyrin excretion is normal whereas in Rotor's syndrome, as in cholestasis, values increase several fold.

Liver histology

The liver in Dubin–Johnson syndrome is macroscopically dark gray or black as in protoporphyria and on microscopy shows coarsely granular pigment resembling melanin within hepatocytes, with a predominantly centrolobular distribution. In Rotor's syndrome liver histology is normal.

CHOLESTATIC JAUNDICE

The typical triad of cholestatic jaundice is of pale stools, dark urine and pruritus; it is essential to determine whether the lesion is intrahepatic or extrahepatic. Ultrasonography is the initial technique used to identify bile ducts, and when dilated cholangiography should be obtained endoscopically or percutaneously to demonstrate the site and extent of obstruction as well as to establish proof of its nature (Elias 1976).

Extrahepatic cholestasis

Calculi in major bile ducts

Calculi are found in the common bile duct in 10% of patients with calculous disease (Johnson et al 1992). Many remain asymptomatic for many months but eventually complications progress, such as hepatocellular function impairment and cholangitis. Obstructive jaundice occurs most frequently when the calculi are impacted in the lower end of the common bile duct above the ampulla; jaundice may fluctuate if the calculus is dislodged.

Bile ducts are not necessarily dilated in gallstone obstruction. A history of biliary colic overrides in significance failure to detect choledocholithiasis or dilatation of the biliary system by ultrasound. Nonetheless the first and most important imaging investigation is ultrasound which reliably demonstrates dilated bile ducts but is not very accurate in showing the cause of the obstruction. Endoscopic retrograde cholangiopancreatography (ERCP) is the next step in visualizing the biliary tree and it also offers the benefit of therapeutic intervention (Clements et al 1993, Jacyna & Summerfield 1992).

Cholangitis

Presents with fever, rigors, right upper quadrant pain and tenderness, tender hepatomegaly and jaundice. If untreated, these patients rapidly develop septicemia, therefore prompt antibiotic treatment and drainage is necessary. Laboratory abnormalities show leukocytosis and elevation of alkaline phosphatase and aminotransferases.

Helminthic disease

Ascaris may migrate into the biliary system and intrahepatic ducts, although most frequently they are found in the common bile duct. They may lay their eggs and migrate. There are studies showing that they may predispose to calcium bilirubinate precipitation and calculi.

Clinically this presents as a biliary colic with nausea and vomiting and jaundice in 20% of cases. The ascaris can be visualized on a plain abdominal X-ray or with ultrasound and cholangiography. Treatment may be surgical or endoscopic removal of the worm.

Fasciola hepatica (in Europe) and *Clonorchis sinensis* (in China) are trematodes that have predilection for the biliary tract and can cause a picture of intrahepatic cholestasis with eosinophilia or recurrent cholangitis.

Primary sclerosing cholangitis

The prefix denotes the absence of any features of choledocholithiasis or previous biliary surgery to account for a fibrotic inflammatory cholangitis. Etiology and pathogenesis of primary sclerosing cholangitis (PSC) are unknown. The association with inflammatory bowel disease is seen in 70% of cases. It affects large intrahepatic and extrahepatic bile ducts leading to biliary tract obstruction. Its immunologic pathogenesis is supported by its association with extrahepatic syndromes such as vitiligo, autoimmune thyroid disease, arthralgias and also because of the presence of antineutrophil cytoplasmic antibodies (ANCA).

Diagnosis. The commonest presentation is a high alkaline phosphatase on routine testing for follow-up of patients with inflammatory bowel disease. In jaundiced patients the alkaline phosphatase and GGT are very high. ANCA antibodies may be encountered. ERCP is the procedure of choice, revealing an irregular caliber of bile ducts. In the jaundiced patient with PSC it is mandatory to administer antibiotics to prevent cholangitis as a complication of ERCP. Alternating narrowing and dilatations of bile duct caliber present a beaded appearance and coexisting saccular diverticula of the bile duct wall are virtually diagnostic.

Exclusion of cholangiocarcinoma may be difficult and any sudden deterioration (jaundice and weight loss) suggests this diagnosis, as well as dilatation of intrahepatic bile ducts on ultrasound; in these cases CT scanning or MRI may prove useful. Histologically it is characterized by portal tract inflammation, fibroobliterative lesions of medium and large size bile ducts, bile duct disappearance, heavy periportal copper accumulation and later, piecemeal necrosis and cirrhosis.

Treatment. PSC can be treated with ursodeoxycholic acid, but the disease invariably progesses to cirrhosis and then the treatment of choice is liver transplantation.

Timing of liver transplantation. In contrast to PBC, the clinical course of PSC is more variable and less predictable. The major difficulty is anticipation of complicating carcinoma which will occur in 20% of cases and should be carefully excluded clinically or by imaging. Indications for transplant are deepening jaundice, progressive, not fluctuating; intractable pruritus; weight loss and muscle wasting; and decompensated cirrhosis.

Vanishing bile duct syndrome (VBDS)

An important endpoint for numerous pathologic processes affecting the hepatobiliary tree is destruction of the biliary apparatus, thus leading to cholestatic clinical features. The syndrome of VBDS may be caused by a variety of conditions (Elias & Burra 1992, Hubscher et al 1993a). Both intra- and extrahepatic segments of the biliary tree can be involved but are not usually surgically correctable.

Cholangiocarcinoma

This can be divided into intrahepatic or extrahepatic. Intrahepatic cholangiocarcinoma is associated with primary sclerosing cholangitis and

---

Box 19.2 Vanishing bile duct syndrome – etiology

Neonatal cholestatic syndromes	Liver transplant rejection
PBC	Graft versus host disease
PSC	Histiocytosis X
Sarcoidosis	Hodgkin's disease
Mucoviscidosis	Chronic drug-induced cholestasis
Suppurative cholangitis	Infections (*Cryptosporidium* and CMV in
Caroli's disease	AIDS patients)
	Intraarterial chemotherapy (floxuridine)

chronic infestations with liver flukes. It usually presents in the sixth decade of life and the symptoms depend on the site of the tumor; if it is at the junction of the right and left hepatic ducts jaundice is typical in the absence of pain. But if it is more peripheral there will be constitutional symptoms such as nausea, anorexia, abdominal pain and jaundice. Intermittent jaundice has been described by tumor emboli from intrahepatic cholangiocarcinoma (Capizzi et al 1992).

Laboratory abnormalities do not differ from other causes of obstructive jaundice and serum α-fetoprotein is not elevated. Cholangiography may show the characteristic appearance of an intraductal tumor and combination of cholangiographically guided fine-needle aspiration and exfoliative biliary cytology may show improved diagnostic sensitivity (Dalton-Clarke et al 1986). In extrahepatic cholangiocarcinoma, CT scan, PTC and ERCP should be successful in imaging the obstructive lesion in nearly all cases.

The anticipated course of these patients is recurrent biliary tract obstruction with infectious complications with death at 6 months to 1 year despite treatment. Surgical treatment can be an option depending on the stage of the disease (Bismuth et al 1992).

Periampullary tumors

These tumors are defined as those presenting within 1 cm of the papilla of Vater. The clinical presentation is usually painless jaundice. Pain may be a prominent feature and in 15% clinical and biochemical markers of pancreatitis are present. These patients require biopsy/cytology through endoscopy and ERCP/PTC for diagnosis. ERCP has the advantage of permitting visualization and biopsy of ampullary lesions, demonstration of both biliary and pancreatic duct systems and a better therapeutic potential (Freeman & Martin 1991).

Fluctuating jaundice with anemia due to iron deficiency of blood loss is a well-recognized presentation for carcinoma of the papilla of Vater.

Carcinoma of the head of pancreas

Painless jaundice is associated with carcinoma of the pancreas when the tumor originates in the head, close to the bile duct, and carries at least a small prospect of curative surgery. Carcinoma arising elsewhere in the pancreas presenting with pain is due to perineural tumor infiltration and is virtually incurable. Nausea, anorexia and weight loss usually accompany jaundice. Pain, jaundice or both are present in over 90% of patients (Warshaw & Fernandez del Castillo 1992). A palpable enlarged liver is often found and frequently a distended gallbladder. Only 15% of patients present with an abdominal mass.

Laboratory tests are not very useful in the diagnosis. CT scan may show a mass but ERCP with visualization of bile duct and pancreatic duct is more useful since it permits cytologic assessment of pancreatic juice. Guided percutaneous needle biopsy can be performed with CT scan or ultrasound guidance.

Resectability is only possible in 20% of tumors, although surgical palliation can be obtained (Watanapa & Williamson 1992).

Miscellaneous extrahepatic cholestasis

Chronic pancreatitis may produce jaundice transiently but only rarely persists due to compression of the distal bile duct by fibrotic changes in the pancreatic head. (Singh & Reber 1990). Annular pancreas is a rare congenital abnormality that is being increasingly diagnosed by ERCP in adults and can cause extrahepatic obstructive jaundice (Baggott & Long 1991).

Chronic cholestasis

It is exceedingly rare for cholestatic hepatitis to persist for more than 6 months, yet due to some drug reactions, notably with chlorpromazine, prochlorperazine and ajmaline, cholestatic jaundice may persist for more than a year. In all cases of prolonged cholestasis it is important to obtain good quality cholangiography to exclude cholangiocarcinoma and to establish the diagnosis of primary or secondary sclerosing cholangitis.

Causes of prolonged cholestatic jaundice include:

- primary biliary cirrhosis
- primary sclerosing cholangitis
- secondary sclerosing cholangitis
- secondary biliary cirrhosis
- cholangiocarcinoma
- chlorpromazine and other drugs.

Intrahepatic cholestasis and other miscellaneous causes of jaundice

Primary biliary cirrhosis

Primary biliary cirrhosis (PBC) is a chronic inflammatory disease presumed to be due to autoimmunity and leading to an early destruction of small intrahepatic bile ducts and early cholestasis manifested by an elevation of alkaline phosphatase and the occurrence of pruritus. It has a female predominance and extrahepatic syndromes are frequently encountered, such as sicca syndrome, Raynaud's phenomenon, CREST syndrome, adult celiac disease, Sjögren's syndrome, arthralgias and thyroiditis which leads to hypothyroidism.

Early in the course of the disease liver histology shows lymphocytic infiltration of portal tracts, lymphocytic follicles and granulomatous destruction of interlobular bile ducts, but at later stages when cirrhosis ensues it may be difficult to differentiate it from other etiologies.

Etiology. The etiology of PBC is still unknown. Antimitochondrial antibodies are the most specific diagnostic markers as well as indicators of a specific defect in immunoregulation, the M2 mitochondrial antigen identified on the inner mitochondrial membrane being the most important. This antigen is the E2 subunit of the pyruvate dehydrogenase complex.

Diagnosis. The following three criteria need to be established in nearly all jaundiced patients in order to make a positive diagnosis of PBC:

1. exclusion of large duct obstruction by ERCP;
2. compatible (or diagnostic) liver biopsy;
3. positive mitochondrial antibodies.

Laboratory tests. Biochemically the disease is characterized by very high alkaline phosphatase and γ-glutamyl transferase (GGT) in nearly all patients. Serum IgM levels are elevated in 60% of patients. Mitochondrial antibodies are present in 95% of patients with PBC and in a much smaller proportion of patients with chronic active hepatitis, drug-induced jaundice and cryptogenic cirrhosis.

Treatment. Immunosuppressive therapy is not effective for PBC. Treatment is directed towards improvement of symptoms such as pruritus, mainly with cholestyramine and restitution of liposoluble vitamin supplements and calcium. Ursodeoxycholic acid (URSO) has for some time been seen to be efficient for patients with PBC, regarding their symptoms and biochemical tests (James 1990), but only recently has a controlled trial suggested that it slows the progression of the disease and reduces the need for liver transplantation (Poupon et al 1994). Many immunosuppressant drugs have been tested but largely abandoned because of their failure to prolong life, inability to improve hepatic histology or side-effects (Sherlock 1994).

Transplantation should be considered when the patient's quality of life is reduced to the point of being housebound. Uncontrollable itching and lethargy are the main symptoms that determine transplantation; other parameters are bilirubin >180 μmol/L or 10 mg/dL, diuretic-resistant ascites, spontaneous bacterial peritonitis, hepatic encephalopathy, progressive muscle wasting and recurrent variceal bleeding (Elias & Neuberger 1994). Timing for the transplant can be difficult, the rise of the serum bilirubin being the best indicator of deterioration (Neuberger 1989).

Primary biliary cirrhosis was the first disease for which it was shown that liver transplantation prolongs survival, with better results if referral is early (5-year survival rate of 69%) (Hubscher et al 1993b). Recurrence of the disease has been shown after transplantation but with very few exceptions has remained asymptomatic.

α-1-antitrypsin deficiency

Homozygous PiZZ α-1-antitrypsin (α1-AT) deficiency is an autosomal recessive disorder associated with a 85–90% reduction in serum concentration of α1-AT, premature development of emphysema and liver disease. Emphysema results from a deficient serum and lower respiratory tract α1-AT concentrations, allowing elastolytic attack on the lung, while liver disease seems more related to the hepatic accumulation of α1-AT.

Clinical factors. Ten to twenty percent of α1-AT PiZZ homozygotes will develop liver dysfunction, neonatal cholestatic jaundice being the commonest clinical manifestation. Jaundice usually appears within the first 1–4 months of life, is commoner in males than females and laboratory testing shows a cholestatic pattern.

Less commonly, α1-AT deficiency presents as liver failure in adult life in patients with no antecedent history of liver disease. The liver is characteristically very small and portal hypertension advanced with moderate splenomegaly and incipient hepatic encephalopathy. Cholestatic jaundice deepens rapidly in the preterminal phase.

Biochemical factors. Serum total α1-AT levels measured by immunodiffusion are usually very low, 10–15% of the normal serum levels of 200–400 mg/dL in homozygous PiZZ individuals and reduced to a lesser extent in heterozygotes.

Treatment. Patients are encouraged to stop smoking. Replacement therapy with synthetic or plasma-derived α1-AT decreases the presentation of emphysema and improves the quality of life (Perlmutter 1991). Liver transplantation is indicated in endstage liver disease and is associated with a change in the recipient's phenotype.

The hepatic porphyrias

Protoporphyria. Jaundice is a rare complication of this hereditary disorder, but when it does occur, it typically appears in the third or fourth decade of life (Bloomer 1988, Magnus et al 1961). The diagnosis will usually have been established many years before the onset of jaundice, during prior investigation of photosensitivity manifested as pruritus and erythema on exposure to sunlight. Complications include gallstones containing protoporphyrin.

The condition is caused by autosomal dominantly inherited deficiency of the enzyme ferrochelatase (heme synthase) which catalyzes conversion of protoporphyrin to heme (Bonkowsky et al 1975). Excess protoporphyrin is formed and excreted via the liver in bile. The diagnosis is confirmed by measurement of protoporphyrin in circulating erythrocytes or in feces. In patients with jaundice due to liver involvement, erythrocyte proto-porphyrin levels are usually >2000 µg/dL (n:<65 µg/dL) and the ratio of daily fecal protoporphyrin excretion to total red cell protoporphyrin mass is less than 0.05. Liver biopsy in the late stages reveals black tissue. Treatment with cholestyramine may induce protoporphyria excretion and reduce hepatotoxicity. Neurologic complications occur very late and in the peritransplant period (Herbert et al 1991).

Porphyria cutanea tarda (PCT). This is the commonest form of porphyria. Blistering with fragile bullae on the hands and other exposed parts are characteristic and these heal by scarring. Usually the patients have a long history of alcohol intake or estrogen ingestion. PCT may rarely be a paraneoplastic manifestation of hepatic neoplasia (Tio et al 1957) but more commonly primary liver cancer develops in elderly cirrhotic males with a mean latent period in one series of 23 years from onset of cutaneous disease (Salata et al 1985). The disease has both familial and sporadic forms.

Deficiency of the enzyme uroporphyrinogen-decarboxylase (URO-D), the fifth enzyme in the heme biosynthetic pathway, is confined to the liver in the commoner sporadic form but found in all tissues including erythrocytes in the very rare familial form (de Verneuil et al 1987). The screening test involves estimation of uroporphyrin excretion in urine which is increased more than tenfold in PCT (Elder et al 1985).

Treatment by venesection remains the first choice for management of PCT, often producing remission of cutaneous symptoms. Antimalarials have also been used with success but have potential side-effects on the retina and the liver (Bonkowsky 1991).

Hemochromatosis

Hemochromatosis can be primary (genetic-idiopathic) or secondary (acquired) due to iron-loading anemias such as thalassemia major, particularly when large amounts of blood have been transfused or, more rarely, due to dietary iron overload ('Bantu' type).

Clinical factors. The typical patient is male, 40 years or more and has hepatomegaly. Presentations at a younger age are associated with ingest-ion of supplementary iron, alcoholism and hereditary anemia. Depending on the stage of the disease, endocrine insufficiency with diabetes mellitus and testicular atrophy, bronzed pigmentation of sun-exposed parts, arthropathy and cardiomyopathy suggest this diagnosis rather than any other. The majority of patients with cirrhosis and hemochromatosis have palpable hepatomegaly and some degree of splenomegaly. Jaundice is not

Table 19.1   Diagnosis of hemochromatosis

	Hemochromatosis	Normal
Serum Fe	>220 µg/dL	<125 µg/dL
Total iron-binding capacity (TIBC)-saturation	>50%	30%
Ferritin	>1000 µg/L	Women <150 µg/L Men <200 µg/L
Hepatic iron concentration	>60 µmol/g weight	<30 µmol/g weight
Hepatic iron concentration index (hepatic iron concentration/age years)	>2.0	<2.0
HLA-A3	In 75% of hemo-chromatotic patients.	In 30% of normal patients
CT scan	Increased density	
MRI	Decreased T2 relaxation times	–
Liver biopsy	Periportal fibrosis	–
	Blue deposits	–

usually a feature of presentation. In females iron accumulation is tempered by menstruation and pregnancy with the result that clinical manifestations of the disease usually appear a decade or two later.

There is often a history of excess alcohol consumption and occasionally there may be difficulty in differentiating between alcoholic siderosis and hemochromatosis. Diabetes occurs in about two-thirds of those with hemochromatosis (Dymock et al 1972). Chondrocalcinosis may give painful knees and arthritis is common in the metacarpophalangeal joints of the index and middle finger, being the cause of much pain and disability (Bombford et al 1991).

In one study, extensive fibrosis or cirrhosis due to hemochromatosis was confined to those with hepatic iron concentrations greater than 400 µmol/g unless a second cause of liver damage, notably alcoholism, could be identified (Bassett et al 1986).

The relative density of the liver on CT scanning may also provide useful information about hepatic iron content (Howard et al 1983); later, the changes are those of cirrhosis. MRI shows marked decreases in T2 relaxation times in iron overload but as with CT scanning, is not sufficiently precise to predict iron concentration with accuracy.

In biochemical screening of siblings of probands with hemochromatosis it was shown that the predictive accuracy of increased transferrin saturation (>50%) and an elevated ferritin concentration was 94% sensitive and 86% specific for the detection of homozygous genetic hemochromatosis (Bassett et al 1984). Fasting transferrin saturation above 62% has been proposed as an initial index of hemochromatosis during screening among blood donors and has greatest sensitivity after an overnight fast (Edwards et al 1988).

Treatment is with venesection, with one unit (500 mL) of blood removed being equivalent to 250 mg of iron and in a typical patient with a 20 g iron overload, 80 weekly venesections will be required. Chelation therapy with desferrioxamine is particularly useful by subcutaneous infusion in multiply transfused individuals to slow disease progression. Follow-up of patients during treatment is with ferritin levels and follow-up of cirrhotic patients should be with α-fetoprotein to screen for the development of hepatic carcinoma. Family screening with ferritin, serum iron and total iron-binding capacity are useful.

Liver transplantation is indicated when the patient has decompensated cirrhosis or when early primary liver cancer is discovered during serial screening of serum α-fetoprotein and liver ultrasound. Contraindications include cardiomyopathy and diabetic microvascular disease or advanced atheroma.

Alcoholic liver disease

Jaundice does not occur with alcoholic fatty liver per se and its presence indicates alcoholic hepatitis and/or cirrhosis.

Clinical factors. The patient who is jaundiced due to alcoholic hepatitis is typically plethoric with multiple spider angiomata and mild to moderate ascites. There may be proximal muscle wasting, bruising of the skin, cheilosis and glossitis. Development of encephalopathy in acute alcoholic hepatitis is associated with a mortality of 50% during the same hospital admission. Fever and polymorphonuclear leukocytosis may be pronounced and prolonged, prompting a detailed search for pyogenic infections. Except in the last stages of cirrhosis, the liver is enlarged; auscultation over it may reveal an audible arterial bruit, useful confirmation of a clinical diagnosis of severe alcoholic hepatitis. This sign is also present in a proportion of patients with primary hepatocellular carcinoma.

Jaundice in patients with prolonged alcohol abuse is usually attributed to alcoholic hepatitis or cirrhosis, but occasionally alcoholic cholestasis without evidence of bile duct obstruction can be present. It is important to distinguish this from cholestasis secondary to chronic pancreatitis induced by alcohol with distal common bile duct stricture.

Laboratory tests. An oxalate specimen for blood alcohol estimation provides useful evidence when, as often occurs, the patient denies its abuse. A constellation of abnormalities with a particular pattern should suggest alcoholic liver disease. These include a very high GGT, macrocytosis, low blood urea, lipemia, hyperuricemia and hyponatremia. In addition, patients with alcoholic liver disease are prone to hypocalcemia, hypomagnesemia and hypokalemia (Finlayson 1993).

In the presence of jaundice due to alcoholic hepatitis, the serum GGT is elevated usually to 5–20 times normal and the AST to 2–10 times normal, but not to the much higher levels characteristic of acute hepatitis due to viruses, drugs and other toxins. If both AST and ALT are estimated, the AST:ALT ratio is usually more than 2.0 in contradistinction to other forms of hepatitis when it is nearly always less than 1.0 (Cohen & Kaplin 1979), though higher ratios may develop when cirrhosis supervenes in non-alcoholic disease (Williams & Hoofnagle, 1988).

Detection of a continuous deposition pattern of IgA along hepatic sinusoidal walls is also a marker with high specificity for alcoholic liver disease (Kater et al 1979) and it has been shown that serum GGT, serum IgA and sinusoidal continuous IgA deposition increase in parallel to alcohol consumption (van de Wiel et al 1987). Lipemia may reach extremely high levels in severe alcoholic hepatitis, causing a spurious hyponatremia (Na:100–130 mmol/L) due to displacement of plasma water by lipids. Association of this degree of lipemia with hemolysis in alcoholic liver disease constitutes Zieve's syndrome in which red cell morphology is characteristically bizzare.

When jaundice is caused by acute alcoholic hepatitis, the prothrombin time is almost invariably prolonged, unresponsive to vitamin K and the patient characteristically deteriorates during the first weeks of hospital admission. Macrocytosis of erythrocytes is common. Anemia may be due to deficiencies, especially of folate and pyridoxine, blood loss or hemolysis. A spur cell hemolytic anemia is generally indicative of a very poor prognosis although recovery is rarely possible. There may be pancytopenia due to folate and other vitamin deficiencies. The platelet count is often low on admission, but rises over the subsequent 1–2 weeks, even to supranormal levels, probably as a rebound phenomenon due to withdrawal of toxic levels of alcohol and vitamin repletion. In severe alcoholic hepatitis a neutrophil leukocytosis may develop and reach the extremely high levels (25 000–60 000 cells/mL) of leukemoid reactions and chronic myeloid leukemias.

Liver biopsy, provided it is not contraindicated by deficient co-agulation, establishes the diagnosis and gives further evidence of the severity of the disease. Studies evaluating the role of liver biopsy in alcoholic liver disease suggest that without histological confirmation the diagnosis will be inaccurate in 10–20% of patients (Levin et al 1979).

The most effective treatment for alcoholic liver disease is abstinence from alcohol. Corticosteroids have been shown to decrease the short-term mortality in histologically proven severe alcoholic hepatitis, although they are not useful in mild or moderate alcoholic hepatitis or in decreasing the long-term mortality (Ramond et al 1993).

The issue of liver transplantation for endstage alcoholic liver disease remains controversial mainly because of ethical issues; however, it is steadily increasing as it has been seen that patients have outcomes equal to those of other patients (Osorio et al 1993). Some factors like unstable character disorder, unremitted polydrug abuse, social isolation and extrahepatic manifestations of alcohol abuse (neurologic-cardiologic), have been observed to carry a bad prognosis as to the outcome in these patients of transplantation.

Hepatic venous outflow obstruction (Budd–Chiari syndrome)

The clinical presentation depends on the degree of obstruction and on the number of hepatic vein radicles affected. There are two major clinical forms, acute and chronic.

The acute syndrome is invariably associated with extensive blockade of the major hepatic veins, resulting in hepatocyte necrosis. In a small but significant number the inferior vena cava is also occluded and the important etiological factors are related to a hypercoagulable state. A typical presentation is with upper abdominal pain followed by rapidly accumulating ascites. Jaundice is not a marked feature unless there is massive hepatic involvement. The history may reveal risk factors including oral contraception, ingestion of pyrazolidine alkaloids in the form of herbal teas or radiotherapy and chemotherapy in conjunction with bone marrow transplantation which are known to predispose to venoocclusive disease.

In the chronic form portal hypertension is characteristically associated with abnormal vascular anatomy. The causes of the chronic form are not clear but a substantial number of cases are related to an inferior vena cava membrane (Dilawari et al 1994).

Diagnosis. Hematologic conditions which present as the Budd–Chiari syndrome include polycythemia rubra vera, paroxysmal nocturnal hemoglobinuria, deficiencies of antithrombin III, protein C and protein S, the factor V Leiden mutation or the presence of lupus anticoagulant. Biochemical derangements of conventional liver function tests may be surprisingly mild. Coagulation screens reveal marked prolongation of prothrombin time as in other causes of liver failure and may make diagnosis of the primary hematological condition most uncertain. Family studies may assist in demonstrating an inheritance pattern, such as diminished values in both parents who are obligate heterozygotes in autosomal recessive diseases (e.g. protein C deficiency).

Hepatic venography confirms the diagnosis and also facilitates the canalization of the hepatic veins by percutaneous angioplasty, the treatment of choice when possible (Vickers et al 1989).

Treatment. Therapy is directed at preventing extension by heparinization and, in early cases, attempts at lysis with fibrinolytic agents. Treatment by portal decompression is reserved for progressive cases and recently transjugular intrahepatic portosystemic shunts (TIPS) have been used in cases of normal liver function (Ochs et al 1993). Some series have shown good results with side-to-side portocaval shunts associated with balloon angioplasty for associated inferior vena cava obstruction (Kohli et al 1993). The underlying hematological condition, such as a myeloproliferate disorder, is treated accordingly with hematological advice.

Liver transplantation should be considered only when a shunt has failed or is not technically feasible. Conditions that justify consideration of liver transplantation include advanced cirrhosis on biopsy, the potential to correct a primary thrombotic disorder by liver replacement, occlusion of the retrohepatic vena cava and a failed mesocaval shunt.

Hepatocellular carcinoma

Jaundice is by no means constant in this condition and the depth of jaundice has no relation to the extent of hepatic involvement. Rarely obstructive jaundice caused by hepatoma fragments in the common hepatic duct has been described (Kiev et al 1990). It is a highly malignant tumor and worldwide the most important factors that contribute to its development are hepatitis B, hepatitis C and cirrhosis; thus early diagnosis is obtained by screening these patients with known risk factors (Colombo 1992).

Imaging modalities like ultrasound and CT scan are very useful and more recently MRI has been a good test for differentiating early hepatocellular carcinoma within regenerating nodules in cirrhosis.

Hepatic resection with or without transplantation is the primary therapeutic option but is commonly ruled out during evaluation. There is no evidence that mortality can be reduced with any of the other available treatment options, such as intraarterial chemotherapy or percutaneous alcohol injections.

Selection for liver transplantation depends on the absence of vascular invasion and hilar nodes, presence of a pseudocapsule surrounding the lesion and unicentric tumors <5 cm in size, but even so, few series report long-term tumor-free survival in more than 20–30%.

Postoperative jaundice

When jaundice presents soon after surgery it may be due to blood transfusion, extravasated blood in tissues or shock. Rarely it can present with a cholestatic picture (Schmid et al 1965).

Halothane anesthetics may be followed by a hepatitis-like picture which is most frequent 1 week after surgery. Jaundice is particularly common after cardiac surgery when hypotension and hypothermia seem to play a role. It is also important to consider infectious posttransfusion hepatitis due to hepatitis B, hepatitis C and cytomegalovirus.

Jaundice in pregnancy

Jaundice may be due to viral hepatitis or gallstone disease or can be peculiar to pregnancy, such as acute fatty liver of pregnancy, obstetric cholestasis or jaundice complicating the toxemias.

Acute fatty liver of pregnancy is of unknown origin but is associated with toxemia of pregnancy and is characterized by microvesicular fat droplets in the liver (Kaplan 1985). Its onset is between the 30th and 38th week of pregnancy, with vomiting, abdominal pain and eventually jaundice. The blood films show normoblasts and characteristically there is hyperuricemia. Maternal and fetal mortality are usually due to disseminated intravascular coagulation with massive hemolysis and have been reduced with early delivery, if necessary by caesarean section.

In *pregnancy toxemia* jaundice is infrequent and is usually hemolytic and seen in the terminal phase.

Intrahepatic cholestasis of pregnancy is characterized by pruritus and biochemical cholestasis which appears late during pregnancy, persists until delivery and disappears after parturition. The condition is usually benign for the mother, but is associated with significant fetal morbidity and mortality (Fisk & Bruce Storey 1988). Treatment with S-adenosyl-methionine and ursodeoxycholic acid may prove to be of benefit.

HEPATITIC JAUNDICE

Acute viral hepatitis

Hepatocellular inflammation can occur due to a variety of etiologies such as infections (viral being the most frequent), chemicals, drugs and various metabolic disorders. There are many varieties and distinct viruses have been identified as causes of hepatitis A, B, C, D, E (Table 19.2) and in the future the alphabet will surely increase.

Hepatitis A

Acute infection can be determined when IgM anti-HAV is positive, which can persist for 6–12 months, while the presence of only IgG anti-HAV suggests previous exposure or vaccination.

Isolation of contacts and patients is not an effective method of preventing dissemination of the disease because the virus is excreted for as long as 2 weeks before the icteric phase. Prophylaxis with immune serum globulin is effective when administered to close personal contacts of the sufferers and to those exposed to epidemics in schools, prisons, hospital and other institutions. A live attenuated vaccine has been prepared from fetal monkey cell culture and recombinant vaccine is available as well, although expensive. Vaccination is recommended for

Table 19.2 Comparative features of hepatitis A, B, C, D and E

	A	B	C	D	E
Virus	RNA, 27 nm	DNA, 42nm	RNA, 55nm	RNA, 36 nm	RNA, 33 nm
Classifi-cation	Picornavirus	Hepadnavirus	Flavivirus	Unclass.	Calicivirus
Incub. (days)	15–50	28–180	15–160	21–42	21–63
Spread	Fecal-oral	Parenteral, sexual Perinatal	Parenteral, perinatal, (?sexual)	Parenteral	Fecal-oral
Clinical onset	Acute	Insidious-acute	Insidious-acute	Insidious-acute	Acute
Fulminant	Yes	Yes	Uncommon/ No	Yes, with superinfection	Uncommon (pregnancy)
Chronicity	No	Common	Common	Common	No
Hepatoma	No	Yes	Yes	No	No
Serum diagnosis	IgM anti-HAV	IgM anti-HBc HBsAg	Anti-HCV (not in acute)	IgM anti-HDV	IgM anti-HEV
Peak ALT (u/L)	800–1000	1000–1500	300–800	1000–1500	800–1000
Active immunization	Effective	Effective	Not available	Available for HBV, not HDV	Not available
Passive Immunization	Effective	Variable	Possibly protective	Effective against coinfection, not super-infection	Not known

travelers to endemic zones. Because of relative cost, if endemic anti-HAV is low it is more cost-effective not to test prior to vaccination (also it delays vaccination). The vaccine is highly immunogenic and most young people develop adequate antibody levels following the initial injection.

There is no specific treatment for a patient with acute hepatitis A and only supportive measures should be given. No specific diet is recommended for these patients.

Hepatitis B

Hepatitis B virus (HBV) is a widely distributed pathogen which produces both acute and chronic infection in man. The virion of HBV or Dane particle consists of a surface and a core. The core contains DNA polymerase.

At least four antigen-antibody systems are observed: hepatitis B surface antigen (HBsAg) and its antibody (anti-HBs); the pre-S antigens associated with HBsAg particles and their antibodies; the particulate nucleocapsid antigen (HBcAg) and anti-HBc; and an antigen structurally related to HBcAg, namely HBeAg and its antibody (anti-HBe).

The clinical course is as follows:

1. *Exposure.* It is important to be aware of possible origin of parenteral transmission such as transfusion of blood products, needlestick injuries as well as sexual intercourse. Incubation periods vary from 60 to 180 days.
2. *Prodrome.* Anorexia, nausea, pyrexia, myalgia and aversion to smoking may suggest this viral illness until jaundice ensues. Features of serum sickness-like illness such as urticarial lesions and arthropathy may be present.
3. *Clinical jaundice.* This occurs only in some of those exposed to the virus but the depth of early jaundice tends to correlate with the severity of the hepatitis. Pyrexia and malaise frequently improve when jaundice appears. The patient lacks energy and enthusiasm. Extrahepatic manifestations are often associated with circulating immune complexes containing HBsAg and can manifest as polyarteritis, glomerulonephritis, polymyalgia rheumatica, essential mixed cryoglobulinemia or myocarditis.

Epidemiology. The disease is transmitted parenterally or by intimate, often sexual, contact. Its prevalence is 0.2% in Great Britain and the USA, 3% in Greece and Italy and as high as 10–15% in Africa and the Far East. In the high endemicity areas the transmission is in childhood and probably horizontal through kissing and shared utensils as well as vertical transmission from mother to neonate at the time of birth.

Parenterally transmitted disease includes the use of equipment for dental treatment, tattooing, acupuncture, manicures etc. as well as parenteral drug users who use unsterile, shared equipment. Blood transfusions continue to cause hepatitis B in countries where donor blood is not screened for HBsAg.

Hospital staff, particularly surgeons and dentists are at a high risk of acquiring the virus from HBsAg positive patients with a positive HBeAg.

Diagnosis. Clinical features associated with liver function tests showing hepatocellular necrosis with a high ALT, AST, bilirubin and a modestly raised alkaline phosphatase usually make the diagnosis of acute hepatitis. The specific diagnosis is sought by serological markers (Box 19.3).

Box 19.3 Serologic markers of hepatitis B	
IgM anti-HBc	Acute hepatitis B. Low level may indicate chronic hepatitis B
IgG anti-HBc	Past exposure to hepatitis B
HBsAg	Acute or chronic infection
HbeAg	Hepatitis B, high levels of infectivity
HBV DNA	Continuous infectious state, useful in monitoring treatment
Anti-HBs	Recovery and immunity to hepatitis B
Anti-HBe	Indicates resolving infection

Diagnosis of acute hepatitis is made with the clinical features and HBsAg or IgM anti-HBc or both in serum. If IgM anti-HBc is absent the patient is likely to have underlying chronic hepatitis or a HBsAg carrier state. IgM anti-HBc is especially useful for confirming the diagnosis of acute HBV infection during the 'window period' between disappearance of HBsAg and the appearance of detectable anti-HBs.

Rapidly falling concentrations of HBsAg in serum and seroconversion from HBeAg positivity to anti-HBe during the first months of acute hepatitis B anticipate a satisfactory self-limiting course. Persistence of HBeAg beyond 3 months may be a harbinger of chronicity.

Hepatitis B mutants. Variations of the hepatitis B virus have been recognized due to mutations in the various reading frames. The most common variant of HBV is one in which mutations in the pre-S and S genes have resulted in significant subtype variation. Vaccination does not produce immunity against infection with some of these agents, because there is a point mutation which alters the epitope sufficiently to render the recombinant vaccine-generated anti-HBs antibodies ineffective at neutralizing the mutant virus. It is found mainly in the Mediterranean area and Far East.

Another variant is due to a mutation in the precore region which precludes the production of HBeAg, but has high disease activity with hepatitic HBcAg and liver HBV DNA (Yoffee & Noonan 1992).

Outcome. Most attacks of acute viral hepatitis B resolve completely within 3–6 months. However, a proportion progress to fulminant hepatitis or persist to become chronic hepatitis.

Prevention. Hepatitis B immunoglobulin (HBIG) is effective for passive immunization if given prophylactically or within hours of infection and usually it is given along with vaccination, specifically in needlestick injuries involving exposure to HBsAg-positive blood products, in babies born to HBsAg-positive mothers and in contacts of acute sufferers. It is also used in HBsAg-positive liver transplant patients for an indefinite period after the transplant.

Hepatitis B vaccine. There is a plasma-derived vaccine and various recombinant vaccines; both have been proven safe and effective after three doses at 0, 1 and 6 months with an antibody response of 94%. It should be administered to high-risk groups such as promiscuous patients, hemo-dialysis patients and healthcare workers, although nowadays it is being suggested it should be given to children in the general population as a universal vaccine, but logistics and costs are difficult to face. Healthcare workers accidentally exposed to infective blood products should follow certain guidelines (Box 19.4).

Chronic hepatitis B. An acute episode of hepatitis B, icteric or anicteric, may progress directly to chronicity. Chronicity is arbitrarily defined as of more than 6 months duration and is seen in 10% of patients with hepatitis

---

Box 19.4 Postexposure to possibly infectious blood

1. Check donor blood for HBsAg and victim's blood for HBsAg and anti HBc
2. Administer 1st dose hepatitis B vaccine at once plus 0.05 mL/kg HBIG
3. If donor blood was HBsAg –ve or victim was immune HBcAb +ve, no further action.
   If donor blood HbsAg +ve, continue vaccination and give anti-HBs

---

B. This process is determined by a continuous viral replication with an inadequate immunological response of the host.

It usually affects the very young or the very old and is mostly present in men. In some patients it presents as advanced liver disease with jaundice, ascites and portal hypertension, although in other cases the patient is asymptomatic and diagnosed serologically. IgM anti-HBc is usually present and HBeAg or Ab and HBV DNA are variably detected. Liver biopsy can show chronic persistent hepatitis, active cirrhosis or hepatocellular carcinoma.

Patients with HBsAg-positive chronic hepatitis should be screened periodically for hepatocellular carcinoma with α-fetoprotein and ultra-sound.

Treatment. The objective in hepatitis B virus therapy is to suppress the histological progression of the disease and diminish infectivity. Many drugs have been used but only interferon has proven to be consistently effective at doses varying from 30 million to 35 million units per week for 6 months. The ideal candidate for treatment has a low HBV DNA level and high baseline values of aminotransferases. A satisfactory response involving loss of HBeAg and HBV DNA is generally maintained after treatment in 40% of the patients (Perillo 1994). Early results indicate that the newest nucleoside analogs with antiviral activity may be useful in treatment of hepatitis B.

Liver transplantation in hepatitis patients. Liver transplantation has had limited success in patients with HBV infection due to the high mortality rate associated with high rate of recurrent infection in the allograft. The rate of recurrence is lower in patients with fulminant hepatitis and in coinfection with hepatitis D and is most likely if there is actively replicating hepatitis B pretransplantation (Martin et al 1992).

Long-term immunoprophylaxis has shown reduced risk of recurrent HBV infection and reduced mortality although the high costs and uncertainty regarding duration of treatment are negative factors (Samuel et al 1993).

Hepatitis D

Clinical factors. Hepatitis D virus (HDV) is a defective 35–37 nm RNA virus that is dependent on the presence of the hepatitis B virus for its infectivity. Transmission of HDV occurs as for HBV. D virus hepatitis should therefore be suspected in drug addicts and their sexual partners and whenever known carriers of HBsAg develop acute exacerbations of their liver disease.

Infection with HDV may be acquired at the same time as HBV infection or may occur as a superinfection in an individual who was previously HBsAg positive. Concurrent HDV and HBV infection commonly results in a severe acute or fulminant hepatitis. HDV superinfection of chronic HBV carriers tends to exacerbate preexisting liver disease with accelerated progression to cirrhosis. Serologic diagnosis of recent infection is by the presence of IgM anti-HDV, while chronic or previous infection is demonstrated with IgG anti-HDV. Liver biopsy shows a microvesicular fat pattern, intense eosinophilic necrosis and large amounts of D antigen in the liver detected by immunohistochemical staining. Immunity against hepatitis B protects against infection with HDV.

Treatment. Treatment has been unsatisfactory. Interferon suppresses replication only transiently. In liver transplant patients who have HDV, prognosis appears to be significantly better than in those who are previously infected only with HBV (Taylor 1991).

Hepatitis C

Hepatitis C was known to exist for many years as posttransfusional non-A non-B hepatitis (NANB) until 1989, when a diagnostic test was developed to detect an antibody to the virus (anti-HCV). The hepatitis C virus (HCV) is a RNA virus with one reading frame, 50–60 nm in size, but has not been visualized yet. It is a distant relative of the flaviviruses, the family of the yellow fever virus.

Epidemiology. Its prevalence in blood donors is low: 1.2–1.4% in the USA, 0.3–0.7% in the UK. Many intravenous drug users have antibodies; 48% in Germany and 81% in the UK are HCV antibody positive. Hemophiliacs have the highest antibody prevalence, being 85% positive in the UK.

Fifty percent of HCV antibody-positive patients have no known risk factor such as transfusion of blood products, drug abuse or tattooing and their mode of transmission remains uncertain because sexual transmission remains undecided and vertical transmission is very low. Hepatitis C is much less infectious than hepatitis B, needing a much bigger load of virus for transmission.

Acute hepatitis C. The incubation varies from 4 to 12 weeks, with a group of patients being asymptomatic and only 25% of patients becoming jaundiced. This disease has not been proven to be a cause of fulminant hepatitis (Feray et al 1993, Wright et al 1991). Serum aminotransferases are elevated to 15 times normal and the disease may run an undulating course before resolution or chronicity can be confirmed.

Chronic hepatitis C. These patients are often asymptomatic or only present with fatigue, over a long course of years, with fluctuating levels of aminotransferases. Thus only when it reaches endstage liver disease does jaundice become a prominent manifestation. Rare associations with HCV infection include cryoglobulinemias and porphyria cutanea tarda. Hepatocellular carcinoma has a high association with cirrhosis due to chronic hepatitis C, especially if associated with hepatitis B which acts in a synergic way (Esteban 1993).

Patients with chronic hepatitis can be given the option of treatment with interferon, usually 3 million units subcutaneously three times a week for 6–12 months. It has the inconvenience of side-effects, high cost and only 20% of the patients will have a sustained response. Thus it is recommended for symptomatic patients or those who histologically have a severe chronic hepatitis which will lead to cirrhosis (Davis 1994).

Diagnosis. Serologic tests for HCV detect antibodies to viral antigens. The original ELISA test becomes positive 4–6 months after infection and was directed against the c100-3 antigen. Second generation tests (ELISA 2 or RIBA) include c22 and c33 antigens and appear earlier after infection (11 weeks). Detection of HCV RNA by polymerase chain reaction (PCR) is a very sensitive technique, but not widely available.

Patients with hepatitis C have a good prognosis after liver transplantation once they reach endstage liver disease; although they generally have HCV RNA positivity in their liver, recurrence is not as severe a problem as in hepatitis B patients. It is important to exclude malignancy in these patients before considering them for transplantation.

Hepatitis E

Hepatitis E is an enterically transmitted acute viral hepatitis associated with a recently characterized hepatitis E virus (HEV), which is a RNA virus of 32–34 nm (Krawcyzwiki 1993). It presents in a sporadic or epidemic form after the rainy season in developing countries in North Africa, India, Pakistan, South East Asia and Mexico. The incubation period is 6 weeks (range 2–9 weeks) and it presents as a self-limiting acute hepatitis similar to hepatitis A, primarily affecting young adults. Jaundice is usually accompanied by malaise, anorexia, abdominal discomfort and liver enlargement.

A high mortality rate (20%) is seen in infected pregnant women in their third trimester, probably related to a high incidence of disseminated intravascular coagulation. Diagnosis is by its clinical features and by IgG and IgM anti-HEV. The disease may follow a cholestatic course, but chronicity has not been seen.

Other viral hepatitis

Other well-defined viruses can cause hepatic disease, such as infectious mononucleosis, yellow fever, cytomegalovirus, herpes simplex virus and others less frequently. The analysis of these diseases goes beyond this chapter. There is also the theoretical possibility of a virus that has not been identified (hepatitis F and most recently hepatitis G).

Fulminant hepatitis

This is a syndrome resulting from massive loss of hepatocytes with loss of liver function and encephalopathy occurring within 8 weeks of the onset of jaundice. Subacute hepatic failure is defined as development of hepatic encephalopathy within 6 months but after 8 weeks from the onset of symptoms. This is sometimes referred to as late onset hepatic failure or subacute necrosis.

The most frequent causes are hepatitis A, B and non-A non-B hepatitis, but it can also be caused by other viruses such as herpes simplex, CMV, Epstein–Barr and varicella virus. Hepatotoxic drugs are the second most frequent cause, mainly acetaminophen (paracetamol) overdose, which is the most common cause in the United Kingdom, non-steroidal anti-inflammatory agents and antidepressants. Halothane and isoniazid toxicity are idiosyncratic reactions not related to the dose administered (Elliot & Strunin 1993, Lee 1993). Isoniazid toxicity has been observed most frequently in women, especially in the postpartum period (Snider & Caras 1992). Recently, however, many more cases of alcohol-acetaminophen syndrome are being described in patients who are active drinkers who use therapeutic doses or moderately excessive doses of acetaminophen for pain and develop fulminant hepatitis.

Mortality is 85% for patients reaching grade III encephalopathy or grade IV coma with unfavorable signs such as a small liver, ascites and coagulopathy with a factor V less than 15%. Those who survive do not develop cirrhosis. The diagnosis of Wilson's disease should be considered for any patient under the age of 45 years. Treatment includes management of encephalopathy with protein restriction and lactulose, control of cerebral edema with mannitol, control of hypoglycemia, renal and respiratory support and antibiotic therapy. Monitoring intracranial pressure is useful in these patients although there is concern about complications with its use (Blei et al 1993).

Hepatic transplantation should be considered in those reaching grade III or IV coma and there are criteria to establish who needs transplantation in fulminant hepatitis (O'Grady et al 1989) (Box 19.5).

Liver transplantation has clearly improved the prognosis of selected patients with fulminant hepatic failure or subacute hepatic failure

---

Box 19.5 Criteria for consideration of liver transplantation in acute liver failure

Acetaminophen
pH <7.3 (irrespective of grade of encephalopathy) more than 24 hours after overdose and pH <7.25 if treated with N-acetyl cysteine.
or
PT>100 seconds and creatinine >300 mmol/L (3.4 mg/dL) in addition to coma.

Other etiologies
PT>100 seconds (irrespective of grade of encephalopathy)
or
any three of the following:
- Age <10 or >40 years
- Non-A, non-B hepatitis, halothane hepatitis, idiosyncratic drug reactions
- Duration of jaundice >7 days before encephalopathy
- PT>50 seconds
- Bilirubin >300 μmol/L (17 mg/dL)

---

compared to historical controls; the 1 year actuarial survival rate of 50–60% is reported by most centers. (Mutimer 1994).

Drug-induced hepatitis

Hepatitic, cholestatic and hypersensitivity reactions can occur with a variety of drugs and may mimic naturally occurring liver diseases.

The response of the liver to drugs depends on an interplay between absorption, environmental factors and genetics. It is estimated that 25% of fulminant hepatic failures are drug induced; continuance of therapy once a hepatitic reaction has commenced is the commonest cause of fatal outcome. In many instances challenge is the only way of linking a drug with a hepatic reaction, although it may prove ethically unacceptable (Box 19.6).

Box 19.6 Criteria for drug-induced hepatocellular injury (from Benichou 1990)

Time
From onset of drug administration: 5–90 days
From cessation of drug administration: <15 days

Course
After cessation of treatment decrease in >50% of levels ALT within 8 days

Readministration
Will induce doubling of levels of ALT

> **Box 19.7** Laboratory screening for chronic hepatitis
>
> FBC
> PT
> LFTs: bilirubin, AST, ALT, GGT, albumin, Alk. Phos.
> Serum ceruloplasmin
> Ferritin
> α-1-antitrypsin levels
> IgA, IgG and IgM
>
> ANA
> Smooth muscle antibody
> Anti mitochondrial antibody
> LKM antibody
> HBsAg
> HBeAg
> HBeAb
> Anti-HCV

Chronic hepatitis

Chronic hepatitis is defined as persistence of an inflammatory reaction in the liver beyond 6 months. It can be produced by hepatitis B, hepatitis C, drugs, autoimmune hepatitis or in Wilson's disease. Pathologically it can be a chronic persistent hepatitis, a chronic lobular hepatitis or a chronic active hepatitis, although some authors propose to change the classification because it does not guide treatment accurately (Scheuer 1991).

Clinically the patient may be asymptomatic or present with easy bruising, amenorrhea and fatigue and by the time jaundice appears there are stigmata of chronic liver disease, including portal hypertension which would suggest a chronic rather than an acute hepatitis. Biochemical tests show a variably elevated bilirubin, aminotransferases and gammaglobulin levels (Box 19.7).

Chronic viral hepatitis has already been discussed so we will focus on autoimmune hepatitis and Wilson's disease.

Autoimmune hepatitis

Autoimmune hepatitis presents histologically as a chronic active hepatitis. It is seen mainly in women and is frequently associated with extrahepatic autoimmune syndromes. It is important to consider that there is overlap with other liver conditions of immunologic origin such as primary biliary cirrhosis (PBC), primary sclerosing cholangitis (PSC) and possibly alcoholic hepatitis (Mackay 1993).

Clinical factors. Fatigue, hepatosplenomegaly and possibly jaundice are the main features. Up to one-third of patients present initially as an episode of acute hepatitis; in women amenorrhea is typical. Various groups have been classified according to the autoantibodies encountered (Manns 1992) (Table 19.3).

Treatment. This disease is very responsive to immunosuppression with prednisolone. Treatment with prednisolone and azathioprine for its steroid-sparing effect usually results in resolution of jaundice and

Table 19.3 Serum antibodies in chronic hepatitis

	ANCA	SMA	ANA	Sol. Liver Ab	LKM-1	Anti-HCV	Anti mito-chondrial
PBC	−	−	−	−	−	−	+
PSC	+	−	−	−	−	−	−
Autoimmune type 1 (classic or 'lupoid'	−	+	+	−	−	−	−
Autoimmune type 2a (LKM-1)	−	−	−	−	+	−	−
Autoimmune type 2b (LKM-1 and anti-HCV)	−	−	−	−	+	+	−
Autoimmune type 3 (soluble liver)	−	− or +	−	+	−	−	− or +
Autoimmune type 4	−	+	−	−	−	−	+

suppression of disease activity at least to subclinical levels. Improvement of biochemical abnormalities is also seen with a reduction in serum bilirubin and aminotransferases and increases in serum albumin. Relapse is frequent and there is no reliable specific marker to predict this outcome, but when retreatment is necessary it is usually effective.

Timing of transplantation. The major indications for transplantation are when patients develop one or some of the following conditions: diuretic-resistant ascites, spontaneous bacterial peritonitis, grossly disabling lethargy, progessive jaundice, muscle wasting and a low serum albumin (<26 g/L).

Wilson's disease

This is an autosomal recessive inherited disorder first described in 1912 by Wilson as a 'progressive hepatolenticular degeneration'. Patients must be homozygous to develop the disease, although heterozygous individuals may exhibit abnormalities in copper metabolism which can result in diagnostic confusion. The gene responsible for Wilson's disease (WD) has been mapped to chromosome 13 and shows linkage with esterase D. The disease affects patients mainly between the ages of 10 and 30.

The clinical sequel results from excessive deposition of copper in various body tissues. This results primarily from a decrease in biliary copper excretion thought to result from a defect in a cationic transporter protein responsible for copper excretion into bile.

Diagnosis. Diagnosis can be confirmed with the following tests:

1. *Kayser–Fleischer rings.* Must be sought with a slit-lamp examination. They may be absent with hepatic WD but are invariably seen with neurologic manifestations.

2. *Serum ceruloplasmin (n: 20–40 mg/dL).* Values <20 mg/dL are seen in 80–90% of patients with WD. Low values are seen in 10–20% of heterozygotes and because it is an acute-phase reactant, it may be normal or elevated in patients with WD who have hepatic inflammation or neoplasm, in pregnancy or while using estrogens. Despite these limitations serum ceruloplasmin is the best screening test for WD and a level >30 mg/dL virtually excludes the condition. However, hypoceruloplasminemia alone is insufficient for a diagnosis of WD.

3. *Urinary Cu excretion (n: <70 mg/day).* In WD generally >100 mg/day are excreted. Hypercupriuria is non-specific and may be seen in primary biliary cirrhosis and chronic active hepatitis and the greatest values are seen in patients with massive hepatocellular necrosis. Administration of penicillamine at 0, 6, 12 and 18 hours during a 24-hour urine collection elevates copper excretion to >1000 mg/day in WD, but is non-specific. Great care must be taken to use copper-free instruments and containers in the collection of urine, as well as for obtaining liver specimens for copper analysis.

4. *Hepatic Cu concentration (n: 15–55 μg/g of dry weight of liver).* Values in excess of this and usually >250 μg/g of dry weight occur by the time jaundice manifests in Wilson's disease. Similar values may be encountered in cholestatic disorders which have different clinical presentation.

Treatment. Treatment is based on chelation therapy with penicillamine, which usually is a life-long therapy. In patients intolerant to penicillamine, trientine and zinc have proven useful.

Liver transplantation is curative for Wilson's disease and is indicated in patients presenting for the first time with fulminant hepatitis; also for decompensated cirrhosis. Currently neurologic manifestations unresponsive to medical treatment are not an indication for transplantation in the absence of liver failure (Schilsky et al 1994).

Screening. Once a diagnosis of WD is made, it is necessary to screen family members with history and physical examination, routine biochemical liver tests, a slit-lamp evaluation and a serum ceruloplasmin level. Liver biopsy with quantitative hepatic copper and radio copper incorporation studies should be reserved for diagnostic uncertainties.

REFERENCES

Abe H, Okuda K 1975 Biliary excretion of conjugated bromosulphtalein (BSP) in constitutional conjugated hyperbilirubinemia. Digestion 13: 272–283

Arias I M, Gartner L M, Cohen M, Ben-Ezzer J 1969 Chronic non-hemolytic unconjugated hyperbilirubinemia, with glucuronosyltransferase deficiency. Clinical, biochemical, pharmacological and genetic evidence for heterogenicity. American Journal of Medicine 47: 395–409

Baggott B B, Long W B 1991 Annular pancreas as a cause of extrahepatic biliary obstruction. American Journal of Gastroenterology 86: 224–226

Bassett M L, Halliday J W, Ferris R A, Powell L W 1984 Diagnosis of hemochromatosis in young subjects: predictive accuracy of biochemical screening tests. Gastroenterology 87: 628–633

Bassett M L, Halliday J W, Powell L W 1986 Value of hepatic iron measurements in early hemochromatosis and determination of the critical iron level associated with fibrosis. Hepatology 6: 24–29

Benichou C 1990 Criteria of drug-induced liver disorders. Journal of Hepatology 11: 272–276

Bismuth H, Nakache R, Diamond T 1992 Management strategies in resection for hilar cholangiocarcinoma. Annals of Surgery 215: 31–38

Blei A T, Olafsson S, Webster S, Levy R 1993 Complications of intracranial pressure monitoring in fulminant hepatic failure. Lancet 341: 157–158

Bloomer J R 1988 The liver in protoporphyria. Hepatology 8: 402–407

Bombford A B, Dymock I W, Hamilton E B D 1991 Genetic hemochromatosis. Gut (Suppl): S111–S115

Bonkowsky H L 1991 Iron and the liver. American Journal of Medical Sciences 301: 32–43

Bonkowsky H L, Bloomer J R, Ebert P S, Mahoney M J 1975 Heme synthetase deficiency in human protoporphyria. Demonstration of the defect in liver and cultured skin fibroblasts. Journal of Clinical Investigation 56: 1139–1148

Capizzi P J, Rosen C B, Nagorney D M 1992 Intermittent jaundice by tumor emboli from intrahepatic cholangiocarcinoma. Gastroenterology 103: 1669–1673

Clements W D B, Diamond T, McCrory D C, Rowlands B J 1993 Biliary drainage in obstructive jaundice: experimental and clinical aspects. British Journal of Surgery 80: 834–842

Cohen J A, Kaplin M M 1979 The SGOT/SGPT ratio: an indicator of alcoholic liver disease. Digestive Diseases and Sciences 24: 835–838

Cohen L, Lewis C, Arias I M 1972 Pregnancy and contraceptives in chronic familial jaundice with predominantly conjugated hyperbilirubinemia (Dubin–Johnson syndrome). Gastroenterology 62: 1182–1190

Colombo M 1992 Hepatocellular carcinoma. Journal of Hepatology 15: 225–236

Crawford J M, Hauser S C, Gollan J L 1988 Formation, hepatic metabolism and transport of bile pigments: a status report. Seminars in Liver Disease 8: 105–118

Dalton-Clarke H J, Pearse E, Krause T et al 1986 Fine needle aspiration cytology in the diagnosis of hilar cholangiocarcinoma. European Journal of Surgical Oncology 12: 143–145

Davis G L 1994 Interferon treatment for chronic hepatitis C. American Journal of Medicine 96 (suppl 1A): 41S–46S

de Verneuil H, Aitken G, Nordmann Y 1987 Familial and sporadic porphyria cutanea tarda: two different diseases. Human Genetics 44: 145–151

Dilawari J B, Bambery P, Chawla Y et al 1994 Hepatic outflow obstruction (Budd–Chiari syndrome). Experience with 177 patients and a review of the literature. Medicine 73: 21–36

Dymock I W, Cassar J, Pyke D A et al 1972 Observations on the pathogenesis, complications and treatment of diabetes in 115 cases of hemochromatosis. American Journal of Medicine 52: 202–210

Edwards C Q, Griffin L M, Goldgar D, Drummond C, Skolnick M H, Kushner J P 1988 Prevalence of hemochromatosis among 11 065 presumably healthy donors. New England Journal of Medicine 21: 1355–1362

Elder G H, Urquhart A J, de Salamanca R E et al 1985 Immunoreactive uroporphyrinogen decarboxylase in the liver in porphyria cutanea tarda. Lancet ii: 229–232

Elias E 1976 Progress report. Cholangiography in the jaundiced patient. Gut 17: 801–811

Elias E 1989 Clinical and biochemical diagnosis of jaundice. Clinical Gastroenterology 3: 357–385

Elias E, Burra P 1992 Vanishing bile duct syndrome. British Journal of Surgery 79: 604–605

Elias E, Neuberger J 1994 Specific indications, primary biliary cirrhosis. In: Neuberger J, Lucey MR (eds) Liver transplantation: practice and management. BMJ Publishing, London, pp 41–47

Elliot R H, Strunin L 1993 Hepatotoxicity of volatile anesthetics. British Journal of Anasthesia 70: 339–348

Esteban R 1993 Epidemiology of hepatitis C virus infection. Journal of Hepatology 17 (suppl 3): S67–S71

Feray C, Gigov M, Samuel D et al 1993 Hepatitis C virus RNA and hepatitis B virus DNA in serum and liver of patients with fulminant hepatitis. Gastroenterology 104: 549–555

Finlayson N D C 1993 Clinical features of alcoholic liver disease. Clinical Gastroenterology 7: 627–640

Fisk N, Bruce Storey G N 1988 Fetal outcome in obstetric cholestasis. British Journal of Obstetrics and Gynaecology 95: 1137–1143

Frank B B 1989 Clinical evaluation of jaundice. A guideline to the patient care committee of the American Gastroenterological Association. Journal of the American Medical Association 262: 3031–3034

Freeman A, Martin D 1991 Editorial. New trends with endoscopic retrograde cholangiopancreatography. Clinical Radiology 43: 223–226

Gollan J L 1983 Diagnosis of hemochromatosis. Gastroenterology 84: 418–431

Herbert A, Corbin D, Williams A et al 1991 Erythropoietic protoporphyria: unusual skin and neurologic problems after liver transplantation. Gastroenterology 100: 1753–1757

Howard J M, Ghent C N, Carey L S et al 1983 Diagnostic efficacy of hepatic computed tomography in the detection of body iron overload. Gastroenterology 84: 209–215

Hubscher S G, Lumley M A, Elias E 1993a Vanishing bile duct syndrome: a possible mechanism for intrahepatic cholestasis in Hodgkin's lymphoma. Hepatology 17: 70–77

Hubscher S G, Elias E, Buckels J A C et al 1993b Primary biliary cirrhosis – histological evidence of disease recurrence after liver transplantation. Journal of Hepatology 18: 173–184

Jacyna M R, Summerfield J A 1992 Endoscopic management of biliary tract obstruction in the 1990s. Journal of Hepatology 14: 127–132

James O F W 1990 Ursodeoxycholic acid treatment for chronic cholestatic liver disease. Journal of Hepatology 11: 5–8

Johnson C D, Fine D R, Lane R H S, Karran S J 1992 Calculous disease and cholecystitis. In: Wright's liver and biliary disease, vol. 2, 3rd edn. W B Saunders, pp 1466–1467

Kaplan M M 1985 Acute fatty liver of pregnancy. New England Journal of Medicine 313: 367–370

Kater L, Jobsis A C, de la Faule Kuyper B 1979 Alcoholic hepatic disease. American Journal of Clinical Pathology 71: 51–57

Kiev J, Dyslin D C, Vitenas P, Kerstein M D 1990 Obstructive jaundice caused by hepatoma fragments in the common hepatic duct. Journal of Clinical Gastroenterology 12: 207–213

Kohli V, Pande G K, Deu V et al 1993 Management of hepatic venous outflow obstruction. Lancet 342: 718–722

Krawczynski K 1993 Hepatitis E. Hepatology 17: 932–941

Lee W M 1993 Review: drug induced hepatotoxicity. Alimentary Pharmacologics and Therapeutics 7: 477–485

Levin D M, Baker A L, Ridell R H, Rochman H, Boyer J L 1979 Non-alcoholic liver disease. Overlooked causes of liver injury in patients with heavy alcohol consumption. American Journal Medicine 66: 429

Mackay I R 1993 Editorial: toward diagnostic criteria for autoimmune hepatitis. Hepatology 18: 1006–1008

Magnus I A, Jarett A, Prankerd T A J, Rimington C 1961 Erythropoietic protoporphyria, a new porphyria with solar urticaria due to protoporphyrinemia. Lancet ii: 448–451

Martin P, Munoz S, Friedman L 1992 Liver transplantation for viral hepatitis: current status. American Journal of Gastroenterology 87: 409–418

Mutimer D 1994 Fulminant and subacute hepatic failure. In: Neuberger J, Lucey M R (eds) Liver transplantation: practice and management. BMJ Publishing, London, pp 72–85

Neuberger J M 1989 Predicting the prognosis of primary biliary cirrhosis. Gut 30: 1519–1522

Ochs A, Sellinger M, Haag K et al 1993 Transjugular intrahepatic portosystemic stent-shunt (TIPS) in the treatment of Budd–Chiari syndrome. Journal of Hepatology 18: 217– 225

O'Grady J G, Alexander G J M, Hayllar K M et al 1989 Early indications of prognosis in fulminant hepatic failure. Gastroenterology 97: 439

Okolicsanyi L, Nassuato G, Muraca M et al 1988 Epidemiology of unconjugated hyperbilirubinemia: revisited. Seminars in Liver Disease 8: 179–182

Osorio R W, Freise C E, Ascher N L et al 1993 Orthotopic liver transplantation for end stage alcoholic liver disease. Transplantation Proceedings 25: 1133–1134

Perillo R P 1994 The management of chronic hepatitis B. American Journal of Medicine 96 (suppl 1A): 34S–40S

Perlmutter D H 1991 The cellular basis for liver injury in alpha-1-antitrypsin deficiency. Hepatology 13: 172–185

Poupon R E, Poupon R, Balkau B et al 1994 Ursodiol for the long term treatment of primary biliary cirrhosis. New England Journal of Medicine 330: 1342–1347

Ramond M J, Rueff B, Benhamou J P 1993 Medical treatment for alcoholic liver disease. Clinical Gastroenterology 7: 697–716

Salata H, Cortes J M, de Salamanca R et al 1985 Porphyria cutanea tarda and hepatocellular carcinoma: frequency of occurrence and related factors. Journal of Hepatology 1: 477–487

Samuel D, Muller R, Alexander G et al 1993 Liver transplantation in European patients with the hepatitis B surface antigen. New England Journal of Medicine 329: 1842–1847

Scheuer P J 1991 Classification of chronic viral hepatitis: a need for reassessment. Journal of Hepatology 13: 372–374

Schilsky M L, Scheinberg I H, Sterlieb I 1994 Liver transplantation for Wilson's disease: indications and outcome. Hepatology 19: 583–587

Schmid M, Hefti M L, Gattiker R et al 1965 Benign postoperative intrahepatic cholestasis. New England Journal of Medicine 272: 545–550

Sherlock S 1994 Primary biliary cirrhosis: clarifying the issues. American Journal of Medicine 96 (suppl 1A): 27S–33S

Singh S M, Reber C B 1990 The pathology of chronic pancreatitis. World Journal of Surgery 14: 2–10

Suchy F J 1993 Hepatocellular transport of bile acids. Seminars in Liver Disease 13: 235–247

Taylor J 1991 Hepatitis delta virus. Journal of Hepatology 13(Suppl 4): S114–S115

Tio T H, Leijnse B, Jarratt A, Rimington C 1957 Acquired protoporphyria from a liver tumor. Clinical Science 16: 517–525

Van de Wiel, van Hattum J, Schurman H, Kater L 1987 Immunoglobin A in the diagnosis of alcoholic liver disease. Gastroenterology 94: 457–462

Vickers C R, West R J, Hubscher S G, Elias E 1989 Hepatic vein webs and resistant ascites. Diagnosis, management and implications. Journal of Hepatology 8: 287–293

Warshaw A L, Fernandez del Castillo C 1992 Pancreatic carcinoma. New England Journal of Medicine 26: 455–465

Watanapa P, Williamson R C N 1992 Surgical palliation for pancreatic cancer: development during the past two decades. British Journal of Surgery 79: 8–20

Williams A L B, Hoofnagle J H 1988 Ratio of serum aspartate to alanine aminotransferase in chronic hepatitis. Relationship to cirrhosis. Gastroenterology 95: 734–739

Wright T L, Hsu H, Donegan E et al 1991 Hepatitis C virus not found in fulminant non-A, non-B hepatitis. Annals of Internal Medicine 115: 111–112

Yarze J C, Martin P, Munoz S, Friedman L S 1992 Wilson's disease: current status. American Journal of Medicine 92: 643–654

Yoffee B, Noonan C A 1992 Hepatitis B virus, new and evolving issues. Digestive Diseases and Sciences 37: 1–9

Index

Page numbers in **bold** type refer to illustrations.